Stress, the Brain and Depression

H. M. van Praag
Emeritus Professor of Psychiatry, University of Groningen, Utrecht, Maastricht, and the Albert Einstein College of Medicine, New York

E. R. de Kloet
Professor of Medical Pharmacology, Leiden University

J. van Os
Professor of Psychiatric Epidemiology, Maastricht University, and Visiting Professor, Institute of Psychiatry, London

D1606736

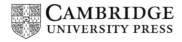

CAMBRIDGE
UNIVERSITY PRESS

CAMBRIDGE UNIVERSITY PRESS
Cambridge, New York, Melbourne, Madrid, Cape Town,
Singapore, São Paulo, Delhi, Mexico City

Cambridge University Press
The Edinburgh Building, Cambridge CB2 8RU, UK

Published in the United States of America by Cambridge University Press, New York

www.cambridge.org
Information on this title: www.cambridge.org/9781107406919

First published 2004
Reprinted 2005
First paperback edition 2012

A catalogue record for this publication is available from the British Library

Library of Congress Cataloguing in Publication Data
Praag, Herman M. van (Herman Meïr), 1929–
Stress, the brain and depression / H. M. van Praag, E. R. de Kloet, J. van Os.
    p. cm.
Includes bibliographical references and index.
ISBN 0 521 62147 X (hardback)
1. Depression, Mental – Pathogenesis.   2. Stress (Physiology) – Complications.
3. Brain – Effect of stress on.   I. Kloet, E. R. de.   II. Os, J. van (Jim van)   III. Title.
RC537.P69223   2004
616.85′27071 – dc22   2003055889

ISBN 978-0-521-62147-2 Hardback
ISBN 978-1-107-40691-9 Paperback

Contents

Preface

Can stress cause depression? This is a question of considerable importance, clinically as well as scientifically. Clinically, because an affirmative answer would elevate stress management to a prime intervention in the treatment and prevention of depression. Scientifically, because if stress constitutes a depressogenic condition, the quest for biological determinants of depression should focus primarily on the neurobiology of stress and only in the second instance on depression per se.

Traumatic life events and taxing living conditions often precede depression. In most studies it is unclear what the intensity of the emotional stress response has been. Yet, those studies generally point to a connection between adversity and depression. An associative connection; they allow no judgement on a possible causal connection. Convincing evidence of the latter would require evidence that stress may generate dysfunctions in particular brain circuitry similar to those supposedly underlying (certain components of) depression.

This, then, is the key question addressed in this book. What neurobiological changes have been ascertained in (certain types of) depression; what neurobiological changes may be induced by stress; to what extent do those changes correspond? The emphasis is laid on monoamines (MA) and stress hormones, the two systems most thoroughly studied in depression. In Chapter 7, MA ergic disturbances in depression and their possible pathophysiological significance are discussed. Chapter 8 is devoted to the CRH/HPA system, the way this system may be disturbed in depression, and the causative role these disturbances might play in the pathophysiology of depression.

In Chapter 8 the point is raised how stress affects the MA ergic and the CRH/HPA system. Human data are discussed as well as animal findings, in so far as the latter may throw light on stress effects in humans. This chapter then converges towards the question whether and to what extent the changes in the MA ergic and the stress hormone systems generated by stress and those found in (certain types of) depression overlap.

If there are reasons to assume that stress can indeed be a depressogenic factor, the question can be posited whether this applies to depression in general or to particular subtypes of depression. This is the subject matter of Chapter 9.

These key chapters are bordered by brief expositions of some related issues. First, what non-biological, clinical and epidemiological data are suggestive of a causative role of life events in depression (Chapter 4). Next the question is raised how life events are defined and assessed, including their emotional impact (Chapters 2 and 3). With regard to the biology of depression the discussion on MA ergic disturbances is complemented by a chapter on the genetics of depression (Chapter 5) and on interactional relationships between genes and environmental variables (Chapter 6). Since depression is the psychopathological construct central to this discourse, Chapter 1 was included, discussing the way depression is and could be diagnosed.

Finally, since diagnosis – i.e. the precise definition of the object of study – is the very bedrock of psychiatric research, particularly brain and behaviour research, a discussion is included on ways to refine psychiatric diagnosing, in order to make the search for biological determinants of psychopathological constructs more productive (Chapter 9).

This book, thus, is structured around three major themes: the pathophysiological role of stress in depression; the question whether a subtype of depression exists, being particularly stress-inducible; and, finally, the dilemma of diagnosing depression in a way to meet best the requirements of research into its biological underpinnings.[1]

Mrs Pauline Kruiniger deserves our special thanks for her invaluable administrative help in preparing this manuscript.

---

[1] Chapters 5 and 6 were written by van Os, Chapter 8 by de Kloet and van Praag, the remaining chapters by Van Praag.

Diagnosing depression

1.1 Diagnosing and classifying

A diagnosis is the definition of a disorder as to its nature and seat. 'Nature' refers to its phenomenology, a etiology and course; 'seat' to the underlying pathophysiology. Diagnosing is the process leading to a diagnosis. In classifying a disorder all diagnostic considerations are condensed in a single construct that receives a particular code according to the taxonomy in force.

Classification systems are by no means 'neutral', noncommittal. They influence the way disorders are being diagnosed. One is inclined to steer the diagnostic process in such a way as to arrive at a diagnosis that fits the prevailing taxonomy. The impact of classification systems on diagnosing is the more pronounced the more detailed the diagnostic criteria are spelled out. The DSM system is a typical case in point. Diagnostic criteria are stated in great detail and hence the influence of that system on psychiatric diagnosing has been enormous. Diagnoses, so to say, are made with a copy of the DSM (Diagnostic and Statistical Manual of Mental Disorders; DSM–IV: American Psychiatric Association, 1994) in one's hand, or at the least in the back of one's mind.

1.2 Diagnosing depression

Basically, there are three ways to characterize psychiatric disorders, in this case depression: the nosological or categorical, the syndromal and the dimensional/functional approaches.

1.2.1 The nosological approach

The nosological disease model conceives psychiatric disorders as discrete entities, each characterized by a particular symptomatology, course, outcome and, at least in principle, a particular pathophysiology. In principle, because so far little is known about the neurobiological underpinnings of abnormal behaviour.

This approach has dominated psychiatric diagnosing and classification since Kraepelin's days. Until 1980 nosological systems were not standardized and diagnostic criteria insufficiently spelled out. Many such systems were in circulation but none of them was internationally accepted. Moreover the various taxonomies were based on different criteria, such as aetiology, symptomatology, course and premorbid personality structure, each separately or in various combinations. The status of psychiatric diagnosing was chaotic and empirical research, based as it necessarily is on precise and standardized definition of the object of study, was thus virtually impossible.

In 1980, with the introduction of the third edition of the DSM, this situation changed dramatically. A detailed and standardized taxonomy of mental disorders was introduced in which the diagnostic criteria were carefully defined. It was solidly based on nosological principles. The system was embraced almost immediately by clinicians and researchers alike. The International Classification of Diseases (ICD) composed by the World Health Organization (WHO), a few years later, in its tenth edition, followed suit and introduced a system comparable to the one proposed in the DSM–III. Its impact on psychiatric diagnosing, however, remained modest compared with that of the DSM system.

1.2.2 Problems inherent to nosological systems

Nosological systems are by definition rigid, particularly so if disorders are characterized on a number of axes, and the defining criteria are specified in detail, as is the case in the DSM system. Patients have to meet all criteria to qualify for a particular diagnosis. Clinical realities, however, refuse to follow suit. In practice many patients are seen that do not meet all criteria required, and thus cannot be properly diagnosed and classified. This creates the need for an ever-increasing number of new diagnostic categories, at least if one wants to avoid overloading the categories 'not otherwise specified'. According to Pincus *et al.* (1992) over 150 new disorders were proposed during the DSM–IV process. The class of mood disorders is a case in point. In 1980 we started out with two main categories of depression, i.e. major depression and dysthymia. In the meanwhile a variety of new constructs have appeared, such as subsyndromal depression, atypical depression, brief recurrent depression, mixed anxiety-depression disorder, double depression and depressive personality (Angst *et al.*, 1990; Klein, 1990; Zinbarg *et al.*, 1994; Judd *et al.*, 1994, 1997; Hellerstein & Little, 1996; Herpertz *et al.*, 1998). In terms of aetiologically and phenomenology, no discontinuity has been demonstrated between those subtypes (Van Praag, 1997, 1998; Ormel *et al.*, 2001). In terms of symptomatology, course, outcome and treatment response, moreover, all those constructs show a fair degree of heterogeneity. Hence, their validity is modest at best. No doubt they show utility in clinical practice, as Kendell & Jablensky (2003) stressed, because they provide psychiatrists with a common language. For research purposes, however, they are an unsuitable starting point (Van Praag, 1997).

Particularly, the area between distress and depression has witnessed a plethora of new, so-called subthreshold entities (Sherbourne *et al.*, 1994; Olfson *et al.*, 1996). Subthreshold depressions are defined as conditions 'that do not meet the full descriptive criteria for a specific mood disorder' (e.g. having fewer than five out of the nine symptoms mentioned in the definition of major depression) but meet the 'clinical significant criterion for DSM–IV' (i.e. having clinically significant distress or impairment associated with them) (Pincus *et al.*, 1999). These conditions are distinguished from 'subclinical' conditions, in which individuals may manifest symptoms of a mental disorder, but the symptoms do not generate clinical distress or impairment (Roy-Byrne *et al.*, 1994). Taking into account that distress, used in opposition to depression, per definition generates indisposition, just as depression does, and no criteria are provided to distinguish 'clinically significant' from 'clinically nonsignificant' distress, this type of descriptive psychopathology represents diagnostic hair-splitting, or worse: diagnostic folly.

Diagnostic charting of the stretch between distress and depression has been chaotic and thus confusing. Pincus *et al.* (1999) point out that the term minor depression has been defined in nine different ways, the concept of subthreshold depression in five different ways; depressive symptoms, also called subthreshold depressive symptoms or depressive symptoms only, were defined in three different ways; mixed anxiety-depression disorder in four different ways. Two different symptom lists were used to define recurrent brief depression. The minimum number of symptoms required for a diagnosis of subthreshold mood disorder ranged from one to six. Duration has not been uniformly specified, and impairment criteria have not been standardized or are not mentioned at all.

The various subtypes of depression, moreover, show little stability; i.e. in many depressed patients diagnoses change over time, while the various subtypes often occur comorbidly (Angst *et al.*, 2000; Chen *et al.*, 2000).

The prevailing nosological classification system, meant to end all ambiguities in the diagnosis of depression, has thus set in motion a regressive movement putting us back in a chaotic situation reminiscent of that of yesteryear. The methodological concerns expressed shortly after the introduction of the DSM by Van Praag (1982a,b) are now shared by a number of investigators (Goldberg, 1996; Van Os *et al.*, 1996; Krueger *et al.*, 1998; Krueger, 1999; Vollebergh *et al.*, 2001). Judd *et al.* (1997), for instance, hypothesized a single disease hypothesis underlying the depressive spectrum and named it: unipolar depressive disease with pleiomorphic expressions. The question remains, can we and should we distinguish the various expression forms of that disease? Angst *et al.* (2000), recognizing the shortcomings of nosologically based systems, concluded that depression is better represented on a continuum, than as a category. The continuum, they propose, should be based on three dimensions, i.e. number of symptoms, duration and recurrence. Number of symptoms, however, is a crude criterion, subinformative if the nature of the symptoms is not specified.

As a consequence of the proliferation of new diagnostic constructs another problem is magnified, i.e. the comorbidity problem (Van Praag, 1996). The majority of psychiatric patients qualify for a series of (axis I and axis II) diagnoses, the group of mood disorders being a telling example. Various mood disorders often occur combined. Co-occurrence of mood disorders with anxiety disorders and with various personality disorders reaches values up to 60–80%. The greater the number of available categories, the greater the average number of diagnoses per patient will be. The comorbidity problem is thus greatly magnified and comorbidity is a true plague for psychiatric research, most particularly for biological research. By way of an example: one studies a patient with major depression and traces a biological disturbance or an effect of a particular medication. That same patient, however, qualifies for several other axis I and axis II diagnoses. What now is the behavioural correlate of the biological finding? Which of the various diagnoses responded to the medication? The depression, or one of the other diagnoses or components of those diagnoses? We do not know, and in most cases this issue is simply ignored. With avoidance behaviour, however, no problem can be properly resolved (Van Praag, 1989, 1993, 1998, 2000).

A final weakness of the nosological approach is that it forces us to draw borders; borders between discrete categories and borders between disorders and normality. The first exercise is fraught with difficulties because of substantial overlap between neighbouring entities. The latter problem is even more complicated. How can one draw the border between sadness and depression, between worrying and a pathological mood change, in a way that makes sense in terms of therapeutic measures to be taken, and in terms of predicting course and ultimate outcome of these conditions? Is it by counting the number of symptoms, by assessing their severity or duration, by measuring the degree of disability they cause, by estimating the measure in which mood state and preceding psychotraumatic experiences coincide, or in any other way? Answers are wanting; scientifically, this problem has been hardly touched. This dilemma, too, posits great problems for psychiatric research, again particularly for biological research. Suppose a test group is composed of both depressed patients and 'worriers'. The chance that one will be able to trace a biological determinant or concomitant of depression, or to provide a valid estimate of the therapeutic potential of a new antidepressant, will be considerably reduced. By way of an analogy: one would have had little chance of discovering the cause of tuberculosis if the experimental group had been composed of tuberculous patients and patients suffering from a common cold (see also Chapter 9).

In short, the nosological approach is in several major ways a diagnostic liability. True, it is handy in terms of communicability, but weak in characterizing adequately the mental disorders seen in actual practice. Convenience is obtained at the expense of diagnostic exactitude. One can even rightfully raise the question whether it will ever be possible to distinguish sorrow from depression, using discrete categories as units of classification to systematize mental pathology. So far biological research does not provide much hope. In a PET study by Mayberg *et al.* (1999), for instance, it was found that in normal sadness and depression the same changes in energy consumption occur and in the same brain regions.

1.2.3 The syndromal approach

Depressions can be diagnosed according to the prevailing syndrome. In this approach symptomatology is the only criterion used. Other relevant variables such as course, causational factors and treatment response are recorded on separate axes, independent of each other and independent of the syndrome.

This was the approach proposed by Van Praag and collaborators and used by them, from the late 1950s on, in their early biological and psychopharmacological studies of depression (Van Praag & Leijnse, 1962, 1963a,b). Three syndromes were distinguished, named vital depression, personal depression and the mixed syndromes. The symptom composition of the various syndromes was characterized as well as the impact severity has on their manifestation forms. Moreover, a standardized, structured interview was developed to assess and record those syndromes (Van Praag *et al.*, 1965).

The best fitting diagnostic analogue of vital depression in today's vocabulary, is the syndrome described under the heading of major depression, melancholic type, and that of personal depression the one subsumed under the heading dysthymia. Mixed depressions are made up of components of vital and personal depression.

The DSM system has abandoned precise syndromal differentiation. Symptomatologically, x out of a series of y symptoms suffice for a particular diagnosis, regardless of which ones. The same diagnosis, thus, covers a variety of syndromes. This approach did not refine psychiatric diagnosing. In the domain of mood disorders, for one, there is sufficient evidence that syndromal distinctions make sense, at least therapeutically (Van Praag, 1962; Heiligenstein *et al.*, 1994; Roth, 2001).

Independent scoring of the prevailing syndrome and the various non-symptomatological criteria was deemed necessary, since no clear mutual relationships had been established. Not until such relationships have been made plausible can one speak of a disease entity; or better: an entity in gestation. A true entity requires that its pathophysiology has been elucidated.

For most diagnostic constructs recognized today, mutual relationships, as referred to above, have still to be established. Yet the DSM system takes them for granted and hence the validity of the system is questionable.

1.2.4 Problems inherent to the syndromal approach

The syndromal approach to (depression) classification is also burdened with problems.

First of all, syndromes frequently appear in incomplete form or jointly with other (complete or incomplete) syndromes. This prompts clinicians and researchers alike to expand the stock of syndromes ever more. An example is the following. Quite often patients are seen with depressions showing all the symptoms of the vital depressive syndrome (in short: vital depression) save diurnal fluctuation of symptoms and in whom mood lowering is reactive, meaning that the capacity to be cheered up by positive events remains intact. We have distinguished this syndrome as 'pseudo' vital depression, from 'true' vital depression, a syndrome that fluctuates diurnally in severity and in which mood lowering is stable even if positive events happen. We realized soon that there exist many more such distinctions, and that consequently, such splitting is truly a process without an end, and thus probably fruitless.

Secondly, the severity of a syndrome is usually expressed as a sum score on a symptom rating scale. Inter-individually, and over time intra-individually, the severity of each individual symptom may vary considerably. Symptoms like anxiety, anhedonia and motor retardation as they appear in vital depression, range from being prominent to a position of minor importance. Those differences are blurred by the instruments syndromes are generally assessed with.

1.2.5 The dimensional/functional approach

A third diagnostic method is the one in which the abnormal mental state is dissected in its component parts, the psychopathological symptoms, whereupon each component is assessed as to its severity. This approach can be called dimensional.

Psychopathological symptoms, however, are actually effigies. They are the expression forms of underlying psychic dysfunctions. Psychopathological symptoms are the way those dysfunctions are experienced by the patient and observed by the investigator. Hearing voices for instance is a symptom, a particular perceptual disturbance the underlying dysfunction. Anhedonia is a symptom, the inability to couple a particular perception to the corresponding emotion the underlying dysfunction.

Symptom analysis of an abnormal mental state, therefore, should be followed by attempts to elucidate, assess and preferably measure the underlying psychic dysfunctions. This was the method Van Praag proposed when syndromal classification proved to be difficult to handle in clinical practice and research (Van Praag & Leijnse, 1965; Van Praag, 1997, 2001) The name *functional psychopathology* was coined for this approach. The advantages it yields are considerable.

Psychic dysfunctions are measurable, many of them even quantitatively; this in contrast to syndromes and disease entities. Via the functional approach psychiatric diagnosing will, at last, be elevated to a true scientific level. Moreover, this method provides the diagnostician with a map of the 'psychic apparatus', indicating which of its components function within normal limits and which of them are disrupted. This is of great importance for clinicians: it provides them with focal points to direct treatment at; biological as well as psychological treatment. It is equally important for the researcher, particularly the biological researcher, because it provides a precise delineation of the behavioural aberrations, the biological underpinnings of which one aims to elucidate.

The methods to implement functional analysis of psychopathological states do not yet lie ready. Partly they have still to be developed, partly they have to be refined. In order to accomplish this task intensive collaboration of research psychiatrists and experimental clinical psychologists is needed.

The shortcomings of the dimensional/functional method are of a practical nature. Diagnoses cannot be condensed any more into a single construct, such as major depression or dysthymia. It requires a mouthful of scores and this will hamper professional communication.

1.3 Multi-tier diagnosing

The various diagnostic strategies are by no means mutually exclusive but rather complementary. They should be combined in a comprehensive diagnostic approach consisting of the following steps.

1 Characterization of the nosological cluster the mental disorder belongs to.
2 Precise syndrome analysis.
3 Symptom analysis of the syndrome or (part of) syndromes the disorder consists of.
4 Analysis of the psychic dysfunctions underlying the psychopathological symptoms. This effort still lies largely in the experimental realm.
5 Assessment of the severity, duration, course of the syndrome and of premorbid personality features, *independent* of the syndrome and *independent* of each other.
6 The disabilities the disorder has inflicted will be charted.

This comprehensive approach is not being used in present-day psychiatry, neither in practice nor in research. The nosological approach governs and controls psychiatric diagnosing. Whatever the aim is of the research programme: the biology of depression, its response to psychotropic drugs or psychological interventions, its epidemiology or any other issue, starting point and endpoint are the discrete categories distinguished by the DSM system, or any of the new constructs not yet DSM–sanctioned. Psychiatric diagnosing is locked up in a nosological straitjacket, and thus immobilized. Syndromal precision is a thing of the past. Symptom analysis remains in abeyance. Functionalization of psychiatric diagnosis as we have advocated for many years (Van Praag & Leijnse, 1965; Van Praag *et al.*, 1987; Van Praag, 2001) is not an idea that has so far sufficiently caught on and has not received large-scale investigational attention. The shortcomings of the nosological approach are disregarded, and diagnostic business continues to be carried out as usual.

This situation is harmful for psychiatric research, and life event research is particularly sensitive. Adversity leads inevitably to mood lowering. Mood disturbances seldomly appear alone but are generally accompanied by disturbances in other psychic domains resulting for instance in anxiety, irritability, loss of appetite, sleep disturbances or diminished susceptibility for pleasurable stimuli. Those appear in various combinations and different degrees of prominence.

Consequently, the border between distress and depression is blurred, not yet established and possibly impossible to ascertain. The study of the psychological impact of life events in an all or none fashion – i.e. investigating whether case-depression does or does not appear after adversity – is a limited approach, too distanced from real-life situations. Life event research, per excellence requires dimensional/functional analysis of stress-related psychopathology whereby the type of stress phenomena, their duration and intensity, their disruptive effects on professional, family and social life, and possible predisposing personality traits are each carefully studied, assessed and recorded. These issues seem to be at least as relevant as the question whether life events have or have not contributed to the aetiology of case-depression.

Yet, life event/stress research is not (yet) carried out in this manner. Hence, most data reviewed and discussed in this monograph, from sheer necessity, have reference to the construct of depression, as defined by the DSM, with the additional restriction that most studies pertain to major depression.

1.4 Conclusions

Several methods have been employed to diagnose mental pathology, in this case depression.

The nosological approach characterizes disorders conceived as discrete and separable entities. A certain resemblance notwithstanding, most of the entities so distinguished are utterly heterogeneous and seem to consist of a variety of conditions different with regard to symptomatology, course, outcome and treatment response. A nosological diagnosis, thus, provides no more than a crude impression of the character of the mental disorder one is dealing with.

The syndromal approach characterizes the phenomenology of the disorder and recognizes a number of discrete symptom clusters. This approach, too, runs frequently up against obstinate clinical realities. Syndromes rarely appear alone and in complete form, appearing much more frequently incomplete and jointly with other (incomplete) syndromes. Syndromal diagnoses, like their nosological counterparts, fail to define individual psychiatric patients in any detailed fashion.

The dimensional-functional approach dissects the syndrome(s) the patient presents, in its component parts, i.e. the psychopathological symptoms. Those symptoms are considered to be the expression forms of underlying disturbances in psychic regulatory systems. Attempts are being made to characterize, measure and record those dysfunctioning psychic domains. The dimensional-functional approach provides a detailed, precise and truly scientific depiction of an abnormal mental state. This approach find itself still largely in the experimental realm.

All three methods should be utilized to reach a precise understanding of the psychopathological structure of abnormal mental conditions. Unfortunately this is not the direction modern psychiatry has taken. Generally a diagnosis consists of just a nosological construct. Following this trend, most attention in stress research and life event research is focused on the question as to whether case-depression can be a stress product. The psychopathological consequences of life events and stress, however, can be very diverse, and to analyse those in detail the dimensional-functional approach is indispensable. So far, researchers in this field, however, do not walk in this way and therefore we have only a limited view on the psychological damage life events and resultant stress may inflict.

REFERENCES

American Psychiatric Association (1994). *Diagnostic Criteria from the DSM–IV*. Washington, DC: APA.

Angst, J., Merikangas, K., Scheiddeger, P. & Wicki, W. (1990). Recurrent brief depression: a new subtype of affective disorder. *J. Affect. Disord.*, **19**, 87–98.

Angst, J., Sellaro, R. & Merikangas, K. R. (2000). Depressive spectrum diagnoses. *Compr. Psychiatry*, **41** (suppl. 1), 39–47.

Chen, L.-S., Eaton, W. W., Gallo, J. J., Nestadt, G. & Crum, R. M. (2000). Empirical examination of current depression categories in a population-based study: symptoms, course, and risk factors. *Am. J. Psychiatry*, **157**, 573–80.

Goldberg, D. (1996). A dimensional model for common mental disorders. *Br. J. Psychiatry*, **168**, 44–9.

Heiligenstein, J. H., Tollefson, G. D. & Faries, D. E. (1994). Response patterns of depressed outpatients with and without melancholia: a double-blind, placebo-controlled trial of fluoxetine versus placebo. *J. Affect. Disord.*, **30**, 163–73.

Hellerstein, D. J. & Little, S. A. S. (1996). Current perspectives on the diagnosis and treatment of double depression. *CNS Drugs*, **5**, 344–57.

Herpertz, S., Steinmeyer, E. M. & Sass, H. (1998). On the conceptualisation of subaffective personality disorders. *Europ. Psychiatry*, **13**, 9–17.

Judd, L. L., Rapaport, M. H., Paulus, M. P. & Brown, J. L. (1994). Subsyndromal symptomatic depression: a new mood disorder? *J. Clin. Psychiatry*, **55**, 18–28.

Judd, L. L., Akiskal, H. S. & Paulus, M. P. (1997). The role and clinical significance of subsyndromal depressive symptoms (SSD) in unipolar major depressive disorder. *J. Affect. Disord.*, **45**, 5–18.

Kendell, R. & Jablensky, A. (2003). Distinguishing between the validity and utility of psychiatric diagnoses. *Am. J. Psychiatry*, **160**, 4–12.

Klein, D. N. (1990). Depressive personality: reliability, validity and relation to dysthymia. *J. Abnorm. Psychol.*, **99**, 412–21.

Krueger, R. F. (1999). The structure of common mental disorders. *Arch. Gen. Psychiatry*, **56**, 921–6.

Krueger, R. F., Caspi, A., Moffit, T. E. & Silva, P. A. (1998). The structure and stability of common mental disorders (DSM–III–R): a longitudinal-epidemiological study. *J. Abnorm. Psychol.*, **107**, 216–27.

Mayberg, H. S., Liotti, M., Brannan, S. K. *et al.* (1999). Reciprocal limbic-cortical function and negative mood: converging PET findings in depression and normal sadness. *Am. J. Psychiatry*, **156**, 675–82.

Olfson, M., Broadhead, W. E., Weissman, M. M. *et al.* (1996). Subthreshold psychiatric conditions in a prepaid primary care group practice. *Arch. Gen. Psychiatry*, **53**, 880–6.

Ormel, J., Oldehinkel, A. J. & Brilman, E. I. (2001). The interplay and etiological continuity of neuroticism, difficulties, and life events in the etiology of major and subsyndromal, first and recurrent depressive episodes in later life. *Am. J. Psychiatry*, **158**, 885–91.

Pincus, H. A., Frances, A. F., Davis, W. W., First, M. B. & Widiger, T. A. (1992). DSM–IV and new diagnostic categories: holding the line on proliferation. *Am. J. Psychiatry*, **149**, 112–17.

Pincus, H. A., Davis, W. W. & McQueen, L. E. (1999). "Subthreshold" mental disorders. *Br. J. Psychiatry*, **174**, 288–96.

Roth, M. (2001). Unitary or binary nature of classification of depressive illness and its implications for the scope of manic depressive disorder. *J. Affect. Disord.*, **64**, 1–18.

Roy-Byrne, P., Katon, W., Broadhead, W. E. & Stein, M. B. (1994). Subsyndromal ("mixed") anxiety-depression in primary care. *J. Gen. Intern. Med.*, **9**, 507–12.

Sherbourne, C. D., Wells, K. B., Hays, R. D., Rogers, W., Burnam, M. A. & Judd, L. L. (1994). Subthreshold depression and depressive disorder: clinical characteristics of general medical and mental health specialty outpatients. *Am. J. Psychiatry*, **151**, 1777–84.

Van Os, J., Fahy, T. A., Jones, P. *et al.* (1996). Psychopathological syndromes in the functional psychoses: associations with course and outcome. *Psychol. Med.*, **26**, 161–76.

Van Praag, H. M. (1962). A critical investigation of the significance of monoamine oxidase inhibition as a therapeutic principle in the treatment of depression. Thesis, Utrecht, 1962.

(1982a). A transatlantic view of the diagnosis of depression according to the DSM III. I. Controversies and misunderstandings in depression diagnosis. *Compr. Psychiatry*, **23**, 315–29.

(1982b). A transatlantic view of the diagnosis of depression according to the DSM III. II. Did the DSM III solve the problem of depression diagnosis? *Compr. Psychiatry*, **23**, 330–7.

(1989). Diagnosing depression. Looking backward into the future. *Psychiatry Develop.*, **7**, 375–94.

(1993). Barking up the wrong tree. Towards a more effective system of psychiatric diagnosing. *Neuropsychopharmacology*, **9**, 52S–53S.

(1996). Comorbidity (psycho-) analysed. *Br. J. Psychiatry*, **168**, 129–34.

(1997). Over the mainstream: diagnostic requirements for biological psychiatric research. *Psychiatry Res.*, **72**, 201–12.

(1998). Inflationary tendencies in judging the yield of depression research. *Neuropsychobiology*, **37**, 130–41.

(2000). Nosologomania: a disorder of psychiatry. *World J. Biol. Psychiatry*, **1**, 151–8.

(2001). Anxiety/aggression-driven depression. A paradigm of functionalization and verticalization of psychiatric diagnosis. *Progress Neuro-Psychopharm. Biol. Psychiatry*, **25**, 893–924.

Van Praag, H. M. & Leijnse, B. (1962). The influence of so-called mono-amineoxydase-inhibiting hydrazines on oral loading-test with serotonin and 5-hydroxyindoleacetic acid. *Psychopharmacology*, **3**, 202–3.

(1963a). Die bedeutung der Monoamineoxydasehemmung als antidepressives Prinzip I. *Psychopharmacology*, **4**, 1–14.

(1963b). Die bedeutung der Monoamineoxydasehemmung als antidepressives Prinzip II. *Psychopharmacology*, **4**, 91–102.

(1965). Neubewertung des syndroms. Skizze einer funktionellen pathologie. *Psychiatry Neurol. Neurochir.*, **68**, 50–66.

Van Praag, H. M., Uleman, A. M. & Spitz, J. C. (1965). The vital syndrome interview. A structured standard interview for the recognition and registration of the vital depression symptom complex. *Psychiatry Neurol. Neurochir.*, **68**, 329–46.

Van Praag, H. M., Kahn, R., Asnis, G. M. *et al.* (1987). Denosologization of biological psychiatry or the specificity of 5-HT disturbances in psychiatric disorders. *J. Affect. Disord.*, **13**, 1–8.

Volleberg, W. A. M., Ledema, J., Bijl, R. V., De Graaf, R., Smit, F. & Ormel, J. (2001). The structure and stability of common mental disorders. *Arch. Gen. Psychiatry*, **58**, 597–603.

World Health Organization (1992). The International Classification of Mental and Behavioural Disorders (Tenth Revision). Geneva: WHO.

Zinbarg, R. E., Barlow, D. H., Liebowitz, M. *et al.* (1994). The DSM–IV field trial for mixed anxiety depression. *Am. J. Psychiatry*, **151**, 1153–62.

Traumatic life events: general issues

2.1 History

Cannon (1929) used the term stress to designate forces that act on the organism, disturb its homeostasis (a term he coined) and cause 'strain'. He showed that both physical stimuli such as cold, heat or fasting, and psychological stimuli, such as exposing a cat to a barking dog, could evoke similar physiological reactions, e.g. the release of substances from the adrenal medulla, later to be identified as catecholamines.

Yet Selye (1936) is considered to be the father of stress research and is certainly the one who made that field popular. He discovered that a variety of physical stimuli such as extracts of the ovary, the kidney or any other organ, and physical stimuli that provoke cold, heat or pain, led to a predictable syndrome consisting of degeneration of lymphatic structures, ulceration of the gastrointestinal tract and increased activity of the adrenal cortex. He called this the general adaptation syndrome and considered it to be a nonspecific response, an 'alarm reaction' of the body, to any noxious stimulus (a phrasing later to be replaced by 'any demand') (Selye, 1936).

The first phase of the general adaptation syndrome was called the *alarm phase* and was thought to consist of two components. Directly after exposure to the stressor, homeostatic processes are disrupted and rapid changes occur in such functions as blood pressure, heart rate, circulating glucose levels and electrolyte balance. The so-called shock responses are followed by attempts to counteract them through increased release of corticosteroids by the adrenal cortex and adrenalin by the adrenal medulla (counter-shock).

If the stressor persists, a second phase of the general adaptation syndrome develops, the so-called *resistance phase*. In this phase the organism would achieve increased adaptation to the harmful effects of the stressor, but at the same time would be more susceptible to the noxious effects of other stressors.

Upon still further exposure to the stressor a *phase of exhaustion* would be reached, with pathological changes in the immune system and gastrointestinal tract, ultimately leading to death.

Selye surmised a direct communication between the peripheral area primarily affected by the stressor and the hypothalamic-pituitary area via the so-called 'first mediator', which he was unable to elucidate.

Selye excluded psychological stressors from his research and ignored moreover the emotional arousal stressors may evoke. He was criticized for that by Mason (1971) and Mikhail (1981) who emphasized that it is the emotional response to the stressor, not the stressor itself that generates stress phenomena. Emotional turmoil provoked by a stressor constitutes the bridge between stressor and stress response. Thus the concept of a 'first mediator' is superfluous. Moreover, Mason pointed out that stress phenomena are only in part nonspecific. Some are indeed nonspecific, others are triggered to meet the specific demands provoked by the stimulus. Cold stress, for instance, will lead to conservation of heat; heat stress to attempts to get rid of excess heat. Finally, Mason and many other investigators after him (e.g. McCarty & Gold, 1996) noted that many hormonal systems respond to various stressors to variable degrees and in variable combinations. Also in this respect the stress response is much more specific, i.e. individualized, than Selye claimed.

The psychological dimension of the stress response was further elaborated by Lazarus (1966). He stated that stress occurs when (perceived) demands on the subject are taxing or seem to exceed his abilities to adjust. The heart of the matter is someone's appraisal of the threatening or frustrating situation in respect of his or her capability to withstand it. Stress phenomena appear if the appraisal has a negative outcome, and the situation is perceived to be potentially damaging and hard to cope with. Stress, thus, is not just a matter of a stimulus followed by a response, but is the outcome of a range of psychological processes in between, which Lazarus subsumed under the name appraisal.

Thus in the course of time stress research shifted from a predominantly physiologically oriented stimulus-response model to one recognizing that not only physical stimuli but also psychosocial events and situations can be a source of stress, and in which the psychological repercussions of the stressor assumed central position. Stress, in this model, became the outcome of a process. This shift in emphasis inaugurated life event research, studying the experiential, behavioural and physiological consequences of occurrences that are perceived as emotionally upsetting.

2.2 Definitions

2.2.1 The stress syndrome

A stressor can be defined as a demand on a human being. The demand can be biological or psychological in nature. The stressor is appraised by the exposed individual and rated as routine or challenging, gratifying or taxing; in the latter case as benign or harmful and in the case of negative appraisal as probably manageable or potentially overpowering and therefore threatening. Based on the outcome of the appraisal a diversity of emotions can be aroused, varying from joy to despondency, from tranquillity to anxiety, from mellowness to anger, from inward peace to guilt, from generosity to envy, from self-confidence to shame, from contentment to bitterness. They may appear in all sorts of combinations. Emotions that are aggravating and disagreeable (and to those this treatise will be restricted) evoke a state of psychic tension, of arousal that is experienced as disturbing and counterproductive. In terms of overt behaviour, stressed subjects may be irritable, tense, aggressive, distracted, disinterested, resigned, anxious or agitated. Furthermore, sleep gets disturbed; appetite often declines but may become ravenous; sexual desire generally abates. Stress, thus, is by no means a uniform syndrome, strongly influenced as it is by coping abilities and thus by personality characteristics, by living conditions and by severity, duration and number of stressors. This state of heightened arousal is usually called stress, or the psychic component of the stress syndrome. Without specification of the emotions that underlie and fuel the pressured state, and the overt behaviour it has led to, this term is just a broad and global notation with low diagnostic valence. Diagnostic specification of stress phenomena, however, is often lacking in stress research.

In addition to the psychic phenomena the stress syndrome consists of a somatic component, induced by increased production of corticotrophin releasing hormone (CRH), activation of the hypothalamic-pituitary-adrenal axis (HPA axis), and changes in the central monoaminergic (MA ergic) systems, the autonomic nervous system and the immune system (Chapters 7 and 8).

The term stress is also used when stressor is meant. This is confusing and should be avoided. Stressor refers to the igniting agent, stress to the response.

2.2.2 Coping with the stress syndrome

Coping mechanisms are brought into action to prevent, reduce or avoid stressor-induced emotional distress. The strategies used depend on the outcome of the appraisal of the situation. Thus ultimately personality variables determine the choice (Lazarus, 1966). If it seems that something can be done to remove the stressor or alleviate its consequences by direct action, so-called problem-focused coping prevails; if it seems that little can be done, emotion-focused coping predominates (Lazarus & Folkman, 1984). In the latter case only the way one attends to or interprets the stressor is changed.

The two approaches towards perceived stress described by Lazarus go back to two fundamentally different ways of coping which have been primarily distinguished in animals (Henry & Stephens, 1977; Rots et al., 1995) but also apply to humans (Vingerhoets, 1985; Petrides et al., 1997). One extreme is the active approach: 'fight or flight', the other extreme is passive in nature and characterized by conservation/withdrawal. Active coping implies goal-directed attempts to remove the stressor, to deal with the threatening situation, to find compensation for the damage inflicted or to flee from it. Seeking social support is also a powerful alleviating response. In passive coping the subject evades, submits or resigns. Intrapsychic strategies like denial, distancing and suppression are employed. The frustrations are not being fought at all, but accepted, thus avoiding defeat through resisting what might turn out to be inescapable and insurmountable. Finally, one can try to integrate the consequences of the adversity in one's life, for instance, by according it a particular meaning. Parker *et al.* (2000), pointedly, distinguished 'acting out' and 'acting in' with regard to behavioural stress responses.

Those defence patterns are not mutually exclusive but may be deployed simultaneously or in succession. The ultimate psychic effects of the stressor, thus, are far from uniform, vary inter-individually and, over time, intra-individually. Consequently and once more: they have to be diagnostically specified.

2.3 Life events and psychiatric classification

Adolph Meyer (1951, 1957) brought psychosocial stressors into aetiological prominence. He had predecessors, such as Pinel and Esquirol, but it was Meyer who put them in the centre of what he called the psychobiology of mental disorders. In that theory the interdependence of biological, psychological and social variables in the causation of mental disorders is stressed, but in point of fact psychosocial stressors were attributed an overriding aetiological significance. Mental disorders had to be considered as reactions to psychosocial adversity and as failed attempts to adapt. Diagnosis thus implied careful exploration of the circumstances having led to the mental breakdown and of the personality traits that had acted as facilitators. Treatment had to be geared towards alleviation of the psychosocial determinants (Lidz, 1966).

In the first edition of the Diagnostic and Statistical Manual of Mental Disorders published in 1952 (DSM–I), Meyer's views occupied central stage. Mental disorders were not conceived as discrete disorders, but as 'reactions of the personality to psychological, social and biological factors'.

In the third edition of the DSM (1980) this view was completely reversed. The DSM–III was fully casted in a nosological mould. Mental pathology was arranged in discrete entities and carefully defined on different axes. All criteria had to be met to qualify for a certain diagnosis. A separate axis (axis IV) was added to register psychosocial stressors, including a rating of their severity. The severity judgement had to be based 'on the clinician's assessment of the stress an 'average' person in similar circumstances and with similar sociocultural values would experience from the particular psychosocial stressor' (p. 26). Seven grades of severity were distinguished (p. 27) and adverse events grouped in 11 categories (p. 28). The decision to add axis IV signified: 'in an officially recorded fashion the realization that psychosocial factors establish a context within which disorders not only unfold but are sustained and exacerbated' (Milton, 1986).

These formulations are curious in two respects. First, severity rating of the stressor had to be based on the clinician's assessment of the stress an 'average' person would experience in similar circumstances. Generally, however, psychiatry does not deal with 'average persons', but with extraordinary people in terms of personality structure, living conditions and (presumably) of certain brain characteristics. Measuring severity of life events, while putting the individual experience in brackets, is bound to grossly under-rate life events' pathogenic power and to conceal the fact that a particular type of stressor may have very different consequences in different individuals (see Chapter 3). Actually, the difference between the assumed response of an 'average person' and the patient's response would be the true measure of a stressor's aetiological weight in a given case. The formulation objected to is a logical consequence of the prevailing tendency in present-day life event research towards de-individualization. This trend is bound to move the field away from everyday clinical realities (van Praag, 2004).

Secondly, though stressors are considered capable of contributing significantly to 'the development or exacerbation of the current disorder' (p. 26), it is not required to provide an assessment, or better an estimate of their pathogenic weight: how much did they contribute to the occurrence of the disorder in a given case.

DSM–III–R left axis IV basically unaltered. DSM–IV retained axis IV, but eliminated severity ratings, and included a checklist with only nine categories of life events to specify 'problems or stressors' judged to be relevant. Both problems that might have been involved in the initiation of the disorder as well as problems that are probably consequences of the disorder, should be listed. The DSM–IV represents, as Mazure & Drius (1998) remark, 'a continued shift away from attempts to identify aetiologically significant stressors'.

2.4 Life events and abnormal mental states

In many cases it is hard to decide whether life events and abnormal mental states coincide fortuitously, whether they are connected in a causal fashion and in the latter case: what caused what? Was the event cause or consequence of the mental state? The following conditions are considered to be suggestive of an aetiological role of the life event.

1. The event preceded the mental disorder and both are closely related in time.

    However, time of onset of a psychiatric disorder is often hard to establish with precision. Temporal closeness, moreover, is a questionable criterion.

Psychoanalytic theory presumed a tight relationship between adverse events in childhood and psychic disturbances in adulthood. This viewpoint received empirical support from recent research showing a relationship between early traumatization and increased vulnerability for mood, anxiety and certain personality disorders in adulthood (De Bellis *et al.*, 1999a,b). In posttraumatic stress disorder considerable time may pass between the event and the onset of symptoms (see Chapter 8).

Finally this criterion does not account for the fact that though the traumatic event may be short-lived, its consequences may be long lasting.

2. The severity of the event is such that it seems plausible that it has generated considerable mental turmoil.

This criterion, too, is less obvious than it seems. Severity is hard to objectify. Impact of an event is very much a function of personality structure, social connections and living conditions. A stressor relatively minor to the one, may be experienced as outright taxing by another.

3. Congruence is demonstrable between the nature of the event, personality liabilities and type or content of the ensuing mental disorder.

Such coherence may count as suggestive evidence for an event's causal significance. In mood and anxiety disorders it is not uncommon. It is rare, however, in disorders like psychogenic psychosis (brief psychotic reaction according to DSM nomenclature).

4. The mental disorder subsides when the event comes to an end.

This criterion has limited validity, because the event may be instantaneous, but its consequences may not end soon if ever.

5. Psychological interventions aimed at amelioration of the psychic consequences of the adversity initiate mental recovery.

If so, it speaks in favour of an event's aetiological significance. If not, it does not argue against it. The event might have induced brain disturbances that, once initiated, follow their own course, independent of the trigger.

All those criteria have a certain cogency, certainly if taken together. Yet definite proof of a causal relationship between stressor and mental disorder can only be derived from biology. Once it has been demonstrated that the stressor(s) disrupt neuronal circuitry involved in, for instance, mood, anxiety and aggression regulation, one has definitive proof that life events can play a causal role in mood and anxiety disorders. In case of delayed onset of the mental disorder, it has to be demonstrated that the immediate neuronal disruptions caused by the stressor endure or have returned. By and large such evidence is lacking, and thus judgements about the relationship between life events and mental disorders can be no more than probability statements. The substance of this book is a statement of that nature.

2.5 Life events and personality structure

Personality structure is a decisive factor in determining the emotional impact life events will exercise and its duration. The majority of people are able to deal adequately with adversity. They absorb the shock; disruption of professional and social life is short lasting; the painful memory is ignored, accepted as such or transmuted into an enriching experience; scars that do remain cause no disabilities. Mental breakdown due to war conditions – called 'shell shock' in World War I and 'battle fatigue' or 'war neurosis' in World War II – afflicted only a minority of soldiers. The unimaginable woes in the German extermination and concentration camps damaged some of the few survivors irreparably, while others were able to straighten themselves and live a relatively normal life. They avoided becoming prisoners of the past and managed to become future-oriented again. The self-regenerative capacity of most individuals is astonishing (van Praag, 1992).

Yet, in a segment of the population self-defence is deficient. Stressor-induced agitation is unduly severe and prolonged, and adaptation to the normal vicissitudes of life fails. This may ultimately lead to a definable mental disorder (a 'case') or to a stage of surrender, a condition nowadays referred to as being 'burned out'.

Social factors, too, constitute an important factor in determining the ultimate effect of life events. One's resilience is influenced by variables like living alone or (happily or unhappily) with a partner, being childless or having children, financial (in-)dependence, job (dis-)satisfaction, being (un-)successful in extra-professional activities, arrangements with regard to child care and housekeeping and many others. These variables, however, do not act by themselves, but via the intricacies of personality make-up. It is the person living in that situation who assesses whether a given situation has to be considered as stress-indifferent, stress-buffering or stress-promoting. It is personality make-up that, in the final instance, determines in what way social circumstances will influence someone's endurance.

Personality research, then, should be an integral part of life-event research. It is not. All too often, the design is restricted to assessing life events having occurred prior to a mental disorder, without more. Most personality studies pertain to non-clinical populations, e.g. university students (Tennant, 2002). Even if a larger range of variables is included in the design, such as situational factors and childhood experiences, a detailed exploration of personality functions is frequently lacking.

As long as biology has not provided definitive information on the interface between life events and mental disorder, congruence assessments of traumatic life event and personality frailties are essential. They are the most informative method to gain an understanding of the disrupting and hence pathogenic valence of the event.

2.6 Genetic and environmental variables influencing exposure to life events

2.6.1 Life events do not occur capriciously

The risk of being exposed to life events is influenced by genetic factors. This is particularly true for so-called dependent life events, i.e. life events that result, at least in part, from the subject's own behaviour, in this case prodromal depressive symptoms or personality features that predispose both to depression and exposure to life events (Kendler et al., 1999a,b). In other words, the exposure to life events is not entirely random, not exclusively the result of good or bad luck. Some individuals consistently experience large numbers of life events, others only few (Fergusson & Horwood, 1987; Plomin, 1994). Several lines of evidence indicate the nonrandomness of life-event exposure (Kendler & Karkowski-Shuman, 1997).

First, the number of recent life events experienced by a given individual over distinct time periods is significantly correlated. Second, specific life events, such as criminal victimization and automobile accidents seem to be repetitive in certain individuals. In other words those accidents show marked inter-individual differences. Third, the number of life events can be predicted by personal characteristics such as social class (lower social class predicts more life events), drug and alcohol intake and a series of personality factors such as self-esteem, impulsivity, frustration tolerance and risk taking. Fourth, first-degree relatives of depressed patients had significantly elevated rates both of current depression and of recent life events (Bebbington et al., 1988; McGuffin et al., 1988). Fifth, a family history of psychiatric illness predicts increased occurrence of life events (Breslau et al., 1991). Sixth, life events frequencies over the entire lifespan are significantly correlated in twins and most pronounced in monozygotic twins (Plomin et al., 1990). Curiously, one can be susceptible to adversity.

2.6.2 Genes and environment

Apparently, the risk of experiencing traumatic life events is influenced both by genetic and familial-environmental factors. Kendler et al. (1993) calculated that each group accounts for around 20% of the variance. Network events (directly affecting individuals' social network through for instance death or illness) were predominantly influenced by familial-environmental factors, while personal events, such as personal illness, financial difficulties or being robbed, were predominantly influenced by genetic factors. In an elegant study Kendler & Gardner (2001) identified some individual-specific environmental risk factors for depression that are definitely not genetic, amongst others: maternal protectiveness, conflictual parent–child relationships, divorce and financial difficulties. They reached that conclusion in a study of 72 monozygotic twin pairs discordant for lifetime history of major depression. They compared the affected and nonaffected member on a number of variables. Since these twin pairs are genetically identical and were reared in the same family through adolescence, all differences must result from differences in environmental experiences specific for the individual twin.

Genetic factors and environmental factors might act independently, rather then additionally, on the risk of being exposed to traumatic life events but two interactive models have been proposed (Kendler & Karkowski-Shuman, 1997). First, genes might render an individual vulnerable to the impact of environmental experiences. This could basically be a matter of personality (Clayton *et al.*, 1994). The depressogenic valence of (certain) life events, for instance, varies and is strongly influenced by personality traits, and many of those are partly under genetic control (Eaves *et al.*, 1989). This has been demonstrated for such traits as neuroticism, extraversion and openness to experience. This could explain why it is that the genetic influence on life-event vulnerability has been demonstrated for controllable life events, both desirable and undesirable, but not for uncontrollable life events (Saudino *et al.*, 1997).

Another possibility is that increased stressor vulnerability is caused by a direct effect of genes on the cerebral machinery, resulting, for instance, in reduced plasticity of circuits involved in mood, anxiety and aggression regulation, making them basically unstable. This will increase the risk of severe stress reactions in response to adversity. A direct effect of genes on brain development could also increase the risk of abnormal personality development, which ultimately might contribute to inabilities to process traumatic experiences adequately.

A second interactive model of genes and environment proposed by Kendler & Karkowski-Shuman (1997) and Kendler *et al.* (1999a,b) holds that genes influence the risk of exposure to life events by causing individuals to select themselves high-risk environments. In this model, too, personality factors seem to be the intermediaries (Plomin *et al.*, 1990; McGuffin *et al.*, 1991; Foley *et al.*, 1996). To a certain extent people create or choose their own 'Umwelt'. For instance, an impulsive, 'sensation-seeking', touchy individual will be at increased risk of alcohol abuse and repetitive interpersonal conflicts leading for instance to serious marital discord. 'Neurotics' tend to repeat the same type of behaviours over and over again, however counterproductive they have proven to be. They seem to be unable to learn from experience. Freud's observations in this respect were apt indeed. Of course genes, also in this scenario, do not cause life events. They contribute to rather stable personality traits that make someone the person she or he is.

In conclusion, then, the risk of being exposed to life events is partly under genetic control. Genes may act via a direct effect on the brain's plasticity or via contributions to personality make-up. Gene–environment interplay will be discussed in more detail in Chapter 6.

2.7 Conclusions

Since the ground-breaking work of Canon and Selye, stress research gradually shifted from a physiologically oriented stimulus-response model towards a model in which the psychological repercussions of the stressor assumed a central position. That shift was accompanied by an increasing interest in, and sophistication of, life-event research, where major issues have been: proper assessment; assessing the causal significance of traumatic life events; and determining the impact of genetic and environmental factors on the risk of being exposed to life events.

Life-event research has been to a large extent de-individualized. In judging the factor impact, it is not the opinion of the stricken individual that counts. Impact estimates are based on the clinician's assessment of what amount of stress an 'average' person in similar circumstances and with similar sociocultural values would have experienced from a particular stressor. As a consequence, studies on the importance of personality-bound factors on the appraisal and impact of particular events are relatively scarce. This is unfortunate. Those factors seem crucial for the ultimate psychological consequences a traumatic experience will exercise. Personality structures are pre-eminently individually shaped, and cannot be 'averaged'. That holds true even more for psychiatry, a profession that does not deal with 'average persons', but mostly with persons with extraordinary personalities. Using 'average persons' as a benchmark will lead to under-estimation of the destabilizing effect of traumatic life events.

Definitive statements on the pathogenic effects of stress have to await further advancements of biological psychiatry. Only when it has been demonstrated that the biological consequences of stress correspond with the biological underpinnings of a given psychiatric disorder, for instance a mood or anxiety disorder, will one have definitive proof that stress may indeed cause psychiatric disorders.

REFERENCES

Bebbington, P. E., Brugha, T. S., MacCarthy, B. et al. (1988) The Camberwell collaborative depression study, I: depressed probands: adversity and the form of depression. Br. J. Psychiatry, 152, 754–65.

Breslau, N., Davis, G. C., Andreski, P. & Peterson, E. (1991). Traumatic events and posttraumatic stress disorder in an urban population of young adults. Arch. Gen. Psychiatry, 48, 216–22.

Cannon, W. B. (1929). Body Changes in Pain, Hunger, Fear and Rage. New York: Appleton.

Clayton, P. J., Ernst, C. & Angst, J. (1994). Premorbid personality traits of men who develop unipolar or bipolar disorders. Eur. Arch. Psychiatry Clin. Neurosci., 243, 340–6.

De Bellis, M. D., Baum, A. S., Birmaker, B. *et al.* (1999a). Developmental traumatology, Part II: biological stress systems. *Biol. Psychiatry*, **45**, 1259–70.

De Bellis, M. D., Keshavan, M. S., Clark, D. B. *et al.* (1999b). Developmental traumatology, part II: brain development. *Biol. Psychiatry*, **45**, 1271–84.

Eaves, L. J., Eysenck, H. J., Martin, N. G. *et al.* (1989). *Genes, Culture and Personality: An Empirical Approach.* Oxford: Oxford University Press.

Fergusson, D. M. & Horwood, L. J. (1987). Vulnerability to life events exposure. *Psychol. Med.*, **17**, 739–49.

Foley, D. L., Neale, M. C. & Kendler, K. S. (1996). A longitudinal study of stressful life events assessed at interview with an epidemiological sample of adult twins: the basis of individual variation in event exposure. *Psychol. Med.*, **26**, 1239–52.

Henry, J. P. & Stephens, P. N. (1977). *Stress, Health and the Social Environment: A Sociobiological Approach to Medicine.* New York: Springer.

Kendler, K. S. & Gardner, C. O. (2001). Monozygotic twins discordant for major depression: a preliminary exploration of the role of environmental experiences in the aetiology and course of illness. *Psychol. Med.*, **31**, 411–23.

Kendler, K. S. & Karkowski-Shuman, L. (1997). Stressful life events and genetic liability to major depression: genetic control of exposure to the environment? *Psychol. Med.*, **27**, 539–47.

Kendler, K. S., Neale, M., Kessler, R., Heath, A. & Eaves, L. (1993). A twin study of recent life events and difficulties. *Arch. Gen. Psychiatry*, **50**, 789–96.

Kendler, K. S., Karkowski, L. M. & Prescott, C. A. (1999a). Causal relationship between stressful life events and the onset of major depression. *Am. J. Psychiatry*, **156**, 837–41.

  (1999b). The assessment of dependence in the study of stressful life events: validation using a twin design. *Psychol. Med.*, **29**, 1455–60.

Lazarus, R. S. (1966). *Psychological Stress and the Coping Process.* New York: McGraw-Hill.

Lazarus, R. S. & Folkman, S. (1984). *Stress, Appraisal and Coping.* New York: Springer.

Lidz, Th. (1966). Adolph Meyer and the development of American psychiatry. *Am. J. Psychiatry*, **123**, 320–32.

Mason, J. W. (1971). A re-evaluation of the concept of 'non-specificity' in stress theory. *J. Psychiat. Res.*, **8**, 323–33.

Mazure, C. M. & Drius, B. G. (1998). A historical perspective on stress and psychiatric illness. In *Does Stress Cause Psychiatric Illness?*, ed. C. M. Mazure. Washington, DC: American Psychiatric Press.

McCarty, R. & Gold, P. E. (1996). Catecholamines, stress and disease: a psychobiological perspective. *Psychosom. Med.*, **58**, 590–7.

McGuffin, P., Katz, R. & Bebbington, P. (1988). The Camberwell collaborative depression study, III: Depression and adversity in the relatives of depressed probands. *Br. J. Psychiatry*, **152**, 775–82.

McGuffin, P., Katz, R. & Rutherford, J. (1991). Nature, nurture and depression: a twin study. *Psychol. Med.*, **21**, 329–35.

Meyer, A. (1951). *The Collected Papers of Adolph Meyer.* Baltimore: Johns Hopkins.

  (1957). *Psychobiology: a Science of Man.* Illinois: Springfield, Charles C. Thomas.

Mikhail, A. (1981). Stress: a psychophysiological conception. *J. Human Stress*, **7**, 9–15.

Milton, T. (1986). On the past and future of the DSM III: personal recollections and projections. In *Contemporary Directions in Psychopathology: Towards the DSM IV*, ed. T. Milton & G. L. Klerman. New York: Guilford.

Parker, G., Roy, K., Wilhelm, K. & Mitchell, P. (2000). 'Acting out' and 'acting in' behavioural stress responses: the relevance of anxiety and personality style. *J. Affect. Disord.*, **57**, 173–7.

Petrides, J. S., Gold, P. W., Mueller, G. P. *et al.* (1997). Marked differences in functioning of the hypothalamic-pituitary adrenal axis between groups of men. *J. Appl. Physiol.*, **82**, 1979–88.

Plomin, R. (1994). *Genetics and Experience: The Developmental Interplay between Nature and Nurture*. Thousand Oaks, CA: Sage.

Plomin, R., Lichtenstein, P., Pedersen, N., McClearn, G. E. & Nesselroade, J. R. (1990). Genetic influence on life events during the last half of the life span. *Psychol. Aging*, **5**, 25–30.

Rots, N. Y., Cools, A. R., de Jong, J. & de Kloet, E. R. (1995). Corticosteroid feedback resistance in rats genetically selective for increased dopamine responsiveness. *J. Neuroendocrinol.*, **7**, 153–61.

Saudino, K. J., McClearn, G. E., Pedersen, N. L., Lichtenstein, P. & Plomin, R. (1997). Can personality explain genetic influences on life events? *J. Pers. Soc. Psychol.*, **72**, 196–206.

Selye, H. (1936). A syndrome produced by diverse nocuous agents. *Nature*, **138**, 32.

  (1956). *The Stress of Life*. New York: McGraw-Hill.

Tennant, Chr. (2002). Life events, stress and depression: a review of recent findings. *Aust. N. Z. J. Psychiatry*, **36**, 173–82.

Van Praag, H. M. (1992). *Make Believes in Psychiatry or the Perils of Progress*. New York: Brunner Mazel.

  (2004). The debit balance of present day's stress research. *World J. Biol. Psychiatry*, in press.

Vingerhoets, A. (1985). *Psychosocial Stress: an Experimental Approach. Life Events, Coping and Psychobiological Functioning*. Lisse: Swets and Zeitlinger.

Life events and depression: preliminary issues

3.1 The agenda

Can traumatic life events cause depression? Intuitively one tends to answer this question in the affirmative. After all, adverse happenings will lower one's spirit and generate feelings of sadness and frustration. One step further, so it seems, and one enters the realm of depression. Such inferences take it for granted that:

1 The border between distress and depression is well-established.
2 The term 'life event' is well delineated.
3 Life events and the emotional impact they exercise, are properly measurable.
4 It has been made clear what in this context is meant by the term causation.

We will verify whether these preconceived notions are justified.

3.2 Border issues

3.2.1 Distress versus depression

The border between depression and nondepression seems well demarcated. Brown & Harris (1989) introduced the concept of 'caseness', defining in symptomatological terms a depression that could definitely be conceived as a disorder, a pathological state. The concept was later adopted by Spitzer *et al.* (1978) in developing the Research Diagnostic Criteria and by the composers of the DSM–III and ICD–X. It has, however, not resolved the border issue (Pincus *et al.*, 1992). The problem is not so much defining a 'case', but lies in defining the non-case, and indicating where the border lies between distress and worrying on the one hand and 'case'- depression on the other. Hence, this border is still blurred, raising the question whether traumatic life events induce sadness/distress – which is self-evident – or depression proper and, secondly, whether sadness/distress is a precursor or pacemaker of depression. These are still largely moot points.

One could argue that sadness is mostly confined to the mood sphere, whereas in depression several other psychic domains are also affected, for instance anxiety and aggression regulation, motoricity, information processing and hedonic functions. This view, however, does not line up with the facts. The psychological impact of being worried, of misery, of misfortune extends far beyond the realm of mood regulation. Mourning, for instance, may and often does generate a psychic state undistinguishable from major depression (Clayton, 1982). We studied the psychological condition of students after having failed an important exam. In the week after the results were known, more than 70% mentioned persistent dysphoria and more than 40% reported at least two of the following symptoms: decreased appetite, irritability, sleep disturbances, feelings of tension and anxiety, decreased experience of pleasure and decreased libido.

It would dilute the strength of the construct depression to homoeopathic concentrations if these individuals were diagnosed as depressives and treated accordingly. Moreover there are positive arguments against a diagnosis of depression. Subjectively these subjects did not feel ill and experienced a complete congruence between mood state and the immediate cause. They continued professional life, albeit with less motivation and energy, whereas most symptoms had largely disappeared within 3–4 weeks after the trauma.

One may conclude that the *phenomenological border* between sadness/distress and depression – if a such-like zone does exist at all – is ill-defined and poorly studied.

Is *duration* of symptoms a boundary mark? In the student study mentioned above, duration of symptoms averaged 3–4 weeks. In bereaved individuals 42% still showed a range of depressive features after 4 weeks (Clayton, 1982). Grief often persists much longer than the 2 weeks the DSM stipulates as minimum duration of symptoms to qualify for a diagnosis of (major) depression. Obviously, duration of symptoms cannot serve to differentiate worrying and grief from depression.

Can *severity* be used as a cut-off point between sadness/distress and depression? The DSM defines dysthymia as less severe than major depression but of a more chronic nature. The criterion severity, however, remains unspecified. The so-called subsyndromal forms of depression are considered to be pathological mood states and in need of (pharmacological) treatment, though they do not meet all the symptomatological criteria required for the diagnoses major depression and dysthymia (Judd *et al.*, 1997). In this category, too, severity is not specified.

To be included in a study of depression a minimum score of 16 on the Hamilton Depression Scale (Hamilton, 1960) is generally required, but that cut-off score is not satisfactory. The Hamilton Scale provides a sum-score of a number of variables. Some of those are indicative of severity, such as degree of mood lowering, anhedonia, motor retardation and suicidality; other symptoms, however, are to a much lesser degree indicative of severity, for instance somatic symptoms, anxiety and anxiety equivalents and diurnal fluctuations of symptoms. Hence one can easily suffer from a serious depression with a relatively low Hamilton score and vice versa.

Decreased *social and professional functioning* might be a useful distinguishing mark, but the method has not been worked out, let alone applied to elucidate the border issue.

The border, then, between sadness/distress and depression, is blurred and psychiatry, so far, has failed to study this issue systematically. This is a serious shortcoming for life-event research and a reason why its results should be viewed with proper reserves. By way of an analogy: if one aspires to study the pathogenetic role of pneumococcus bacteria in pneumonia one should, on penalty of flawed conclusions, avoid contamination of the test group with individuals suffering from a common cold.

3.2.2 Chronic depression versus personality-related depressive traits

Another major border issue is the one between chronic mood disorders such as dysthymia and personality disorder with depressive features (Shea & Hirschfeld, 1996). A disorder is defined as a state that is time-limited or episodic and experienced by the patient as 'ich-fremd' (ego-dystonic). Depressive personality traits or depressive personality disorder, on the other hand, are conceived as enduring mood states, part of the ego structure and experienced as 'ich-nah' (ego-syntonic), as 'just the way I am'. Over the years, many depressive personalities have been conceptualized. To mention a few: Kraepelin's (1921; Kraepelin & Lange, 1927) depressive temperament; Schneider's (1958) depressive psychopathy; Kernberg's (1987) depressive masochistic personality disorder, and Akiskal's (1983; Akiskal *et al.*, 1985) character-spectrum disorder and borderline subaffective type.

The distinction between a mood disorder and depressivity as a personality trait is less clear than it seems. A substantial proportion of depressed patients show a partial treatment response; residual symptoms remain (Fava *et al.*, 2002). Dysfunctional personality features, on the other hand, may defy the stability definition. Feelings of sadness, of discomfort, of pessimism, of inadequacy, of emptiness may wax and wane, sometimes synchronous with the coming and going of (minor) events or disturbing thoughts, sometimes without obvious reason.

Uncertainty as to whether one is dealing with a chronic depression, residual symptoms of a depressive episode, with a depressive personality disorder, or with depressive personality traits, may raise serious problems in the study of the causal significance of life events in mood disorders.

3.3 Meaning of the term life event

3.3.1 Definition

A *life event* is defined as a rather sudden and short-lasting occurrence (short enough to be dated), and severe enough to provide a substantial disturbance in psychic homeostasis. Though this definition requires that the occurrence can be demarcated in time, such as in the case of rape, dismissal, sudden death of a partner, its (after-) effects may be long-lasting. Over time, the perceived intensity of a stressor may seem to abate and memories appear to have faded away, but those observations might be deceitful. In reality the getting-over time may last for months or years, if not forever. Taxing conditions of a more lasting nature, such as suffering from a chronic disease, under-appreciation at the work-place or marital problems, are called *long-term difficulties*. The border between events and difficulties, however, is blurred, since many life events act subacutely (such as impending departure of a child from home or the strenuous period preceding an important exam), whereas, as noted, the consequences of an acute event may be long-lasting.

A third category of troubling happenings are the so-called *daily hassles*, defined as bad lucks, more minor disappointments, little frustrations, that one has to deal with on a regular, sometimes daily, basis. Though as such rather insignificant, they become a nuisance if repetitive or accumulating. The distinction between hassles and difficulties, however, is often hard to make. A number of hassles together may grow into a major frustration, particularly in individuals with deficient adaptive skills. Untidiness of a housewife, for instance, may become a major burden for a somewhat rigid, obsessive spouse.

3.3.2 Heterogeneity

External events

Life events are very heterogeneous in nature. They can be forthright desirable, generating feelings of satisfaction and joy. Psychiatrists have little to do with that type of event. They might become involved if life events occur that are as such desirable and challenging but demanding to such an extent that self-confidence is negatively affected. In general, however, psychiatrists deal with individuals who have experienced negative, i.e. psychotraumatic life events. Difficulties and hassles have, by definition, a negative connotation.

Events as well as difficulties may originate in very different spheres of life, such as health, work, home, family, finances and social network (Rahe, 1995). They are likewise heterogeneous as far as context is concerned. They may, for instance, relate to losses – loss of physical abilities or material goods, of loved ones, of respectability and self-esteem, or of religious/spiritual anchorage. They may pertain to defamation or serious violation of someone's physical integrity (e.g. rape) or be related to environmental catastrophes, as in the case of fire, explosions, floods and the like.

Internal events

Psychotraumatic events and difficulties may originate primarily in the 'milieu exterieure', but likewise in the inner world, the psychic life of an individual. I am referring to what might be called 'cognitive life events', i.e. thoughts that are disquieting. Thoughts of having failed others or one's own aspirations, of being unable to arouse other people's interest, of being unloved, unappreciated, of being emotionally deprived, of having no real friends, of being sexually undesirable, of being physically unattractive, of being dominated by others and lacking defence, of being bored with life and so forth and so on. Such thoughts may be bothering someone continuously or may pop up once in a while, apparently unprovoked or precipitated by generally minor incidents or particular encounters. These thoughts may provoke feelings of grief, despair, (auto-)aggressiveness, hopelessness, helplessness and the like. Generally it concerns neurotic individuals, people with personality traits that make them vulnerable for frustrations in the relational sphere. Such individuals are numerous in the realms of psychiatry and clinical psychology, though they remain unclassified in the present-day's psychiatric classification systems.

'Internal' or 'cognitive' events and difficulties, however, are not subsumed under the heading of life events, thus not explored, not registered and not measured in life-event research. Life events are defined: 'as a change in the external environment . . . changes in mood or perception which are solely subjective . . . should not be regarded as life events' (Jenaway & Paykel, 1997). I do not share this viewpoint. As I noted before, life-event research without taking into account the (purely) subjective components of adversity, and disregarding internal events, becomes sterile and literally unreal (van Praag, 2004).

Dependent and independent life events

A crucial issue in the study of the aetiological weight of life events, finally, is the question whether a life event occurs beyond someone's control – e.g. the sudden death of one's partner or job loss due to economic malaise – or whether it happened because of a person's own behaviour. In the first case life events are called independent, in the latter case dependent. Event-facilitating behaviour can be a result of the mental condition of the individual, depression being a case in point. Another possibility is that personality traits act as facilitators of exposure to negative events, ultimately leading to a state of depression. The first possibility is more thoroughly studied than the latter.

Hammer (1991), for instance, showed that women with unipolar depression went through more dependent events, as compared with normal controls and women with a chronic medical illness. Patients with recurrent depression, moreover, experienced significantly more dependent events than first-onset depressives in the 12 months preceding the depression (Harkness *et al.*, 1999). Event-proneness, moreover, continues in states of remission (Kessler & Magee, 1993). Cui & Vaillant (1997) carried out a longitudinal prospective study in 113 men, who were followed biannually from age 26 until age 62. In comparison with a normal control group people suffering from recurrent depression reported a higher frequency of dependent negative life events after the first depressive episode. Apparently, depressive disorder promotes the occurrence of self-induced negative life events. This fact probably contributes to depressive relapses.

Which variables facilitate exposure to negative life events? First of course the *depressive condition* itself. Symptoms such as irritability, fatigue, lack of concentration, apathy and anhedonia will increase the chance of adverse encounters. Remission is quite often incomplete, and residual symptoms might have a similar effect. Depressive symptoms, moreover, may disrupt social networks and, secondarily, promote adversity and the ability to cope with it. Events associated with the depressed condition may, as said, contribute to the chronicity of the disorder. This does not imply responsibility for the first episode.

A second possibility is that event susceptibility is caused by *personality features*. Depressions – all types of depressions – are strongly intertwined with a variety of personality disorders (Hirschfeld *et al.*, 1983, 1997; Boyce *et al.*, 1991; Sato *et al.*, 2001). Personality frailties may lower the threshold for the traumatizing 'weight' of life events, and thus increase the risk of depressions, both first-onset and relapse depressions (Segal *et al.*, 1992).

There is little doubt about an association between the traumatizing sequelae of adverse events and personality structure, as well as one between depression and personality structure. Yet in life-event research, analysis of personality structure is not regarded as an indispensable link between event and psychopathology. This detracts from its validity.

Controllability

Most people strive for mastery of their own situation. Being thrown in a situation one cannot influence, and hence is being perceived as unpredictable, generates a great deal of anxiety and tension. Understandably, then, uncontrollable events, such as the sudden death of a loved one, have a greater destabilizing potential than the ones that one feels able to control or remedy, such as financial losses.

Type of event

In relation to the onset of depression, losses – e.g. loss of loved ones, money, influence, self-esteem – and 'exits', i.e. separations or threat of separations from the social field, have been studied most extensively. Most studies found an excess of loss- and exit-events prior to illness onset (Paykel *et al.*, 1969). In comparing depressed patients with members of the general population and psychiatric patients with other diagnoses, it was found that interpersonal losses become increasingly more pathogenic with increasing age (Paykel, 1982). This is particularly true for loss of important others (Paykel *et al.*, 1969; Jenaway & Paykel, 1997). Loss and separation are also common in depressed suicide attempters (Hawton & van Heeringen, 2000).

Entrance events, as opposed to exit-events, appeared not to be related to depression (Paykel *et al.*, 1969; Fava *et al.*, 1981).

Events that undermine someone's sole or main source of self-esteem were shown to be 2–3 times as depressogenic as the same events in individuals who dispose of additional resources keeping up the level of self-esteem (Ormel, 1999).

Conclusion

Without further specification, the term life event is too global to be informative. It requires specification as to the sphere of life that has been affected, the nature of the event, controllability, context in which it occurred, whether it concerned an independent or possibly dependent event, whether the event was external or rather 'internal' (cognitive) in nature, and to what extent personality traits have probably amplified its emotional effects.

Much life-event research falls short of providing complete information. This has to be taken into account in appraising this literature.

Specification of the attributes of an event is important. Indispensable, however, is information about its emotional effects and their duration. Are these variables assessable? This issue will be discussed in the next section.

3.4 How to assess life events

3.4.1 Checklists

Initially, life events were ascertained with the help of a checklist (Rahe, 1995). Patients were requested to tick from a list of possible life events those that had happened over a given period of time. The events had been rank-ordered as to severity, defined as the degree of change in psychosocial equilibrium they would have produced in an average individual. The score of each event had been determined by asking a random sample from the general population to rank-order a series of events according to severity. In that way death of a spouse received the highest score, minor violations of the law, the lowest, while the score of events like death of a close friend and change to a different line of work ended up in the middle. Yearly life change estimates were expressed as life-change units.

The initial list published by Rahe and Holmes in 1963 contained 43 life events and was called the Schedule of Recent Events. It was later extended to 74 recent life-change events and renamed Recent Life Changes Questionnaire (Rahe, 1995; Miller & Rahe, 1997).

3.4.2 Structured interviews

Checklists are easy to apply, but 'bare'. They fail to provide specifications, as mentioned in the preceding section. They omit, furthermore, to individualize the event; that is to approximate the meaning of the event and the emotional impact it has had on the exposed individual. And finally, self-administered checklists are subject to high fall-off rates, meaning that a considerable number of events are not remembered or not accurately recalled. The rate of fall-off is about 5% per month. Moreover, they do not permit careful ascertainment of illness onset.

Subsequently another method to explore life events and difficulties has been developed, i.e. the semi-structured interview. Presently two such instruments are in use: the Bedford College Life Events and Difficulties Schedule (LEDS) (Brown & Harris, 1978) and the Interview for Recent Life Events (Paykel, 1997). Major areas of the patient's existence are screened for carefully defined events that exceed a preformulated threshold of severity, and time of occurrence is determined. The LEDS includes attempts to reach an understanding about the value system, and aspirations of the stricken individual, as well as of the quality of his or her social relationships. Are the latter supportive or rather strained and unsettling? Subsequently an independent rater or preferably a panel of raters will review the data and provide an estimate of the significance of the event and its emotional impact, given the biography and current circumstances of the person 'ignoring anything the person says about his or her reaction' (Brown *et al.*, 1987). The question to be answered is *not*, what impact the life event has had on the individual in question, but the impact it would have had on an average person in the general population living under comparable conditions and with a somewhat similar outlook on life. Manuals give strict definitions of which incidents can be counted as events.

This approach to rating life events, termed 'contextual', though time consuming and labour-intensive, meant considerable sophistication of life-event research. It takes into account that the same event may mean different things to different people. The death of a partner may be an insurmountable blow for one, an unspoken relief to another. Directories provide many examples of precedents of contextual meaning.

The interview method has several advantages. Fall-off rates are much lower than with the subject-completion checklists; approximately 1% per month provided the interviewer has been adequately trained (Neilson *et al.*, 1989); disease onset is carefully scrutinized; various spheres of life are systematically screened for adversities; and context is taken into account.

3.4.3 De-subjectivation

Yet the interview method ignores, just as the checklist method does, the event-stricken individual him- or herself – the way he or she has experienced the misery (Lazarus & Folkman, 1984; Lazarus, 1993). It relies in this respect on indirect estimates. The emotional response is assessed in a de-individualized fashion. An approach in which the respondent is invited to assign a subjective weight to the events they had experienced (Sarason *et al.*, 1978) 'has been rejected as confounding measurement with emotional reaction to the event' (Kessler, 1997).

In a way this viewpoint makes sense. The mental state of the event-stricken individual may affect and distort reporting about the emotional repercussions the event preceding that mental state has had. A depressed patient, for instance, may over-emphasize its impact in order to find an explanation for his mood state, or, on the contrary, play down its effects to take the full responsibility of the mood state upon himself. Experimental induction of mood lowering has been shown to lead to a significant increase in reporting adverse events (Cohen *et al.*, 1988), possibly through overrating of in themselves insignificant occurrences. Such distortions can at least partially be corrected by interviewing life companions and re-interviewing the patient after remission.

In another way this viewpoint makes no sense. Individual, subjective experiences aroused by shocking events and possibly magnified or subdued through interference of particular personality traits, should be the core business of life-event research. Not that events as such are potentially damaging, but their psychic impact might be. The self-evident should not be sacrificed for the sake of objectivity. Psychiatry, as said, does not deal with average individuals but with extraordinary ones; extraordinary in the sense of being carriers of specific vulnerabilities. Only the subject exposed to adversity can adequately report the subjective experiences he went through. Experiences of the average person under similar conditions provide a crude image at best. Interviewers of an adversely exposed individual are bystanders. What they perceive of the emotional response is an effigy, not the real thing. Moreover they not only perceive, they pass judgements. Perceptions are filtered by the interviewer's own emotional make-up. He may find the response exaggerated, subdued, pathetic or otherwise hard to sense. His judgement, however, is irrelevant. The filtering process shapes or at least influences the judge's judgement. Subjective experiences should be judged by the subject. The subjective account of an emotional experience is the most direct, in a way the most objective evidence of what happened inwardly. To take contextual issues into account, is not enough. Suppose a researcher would assess someone's aesthetic experiences evoked by a Verdi opera by averaging the aesthetic experiences of a sample of somewhat similar individuals listening to the same piece of music. Such a strategy, I guess, would be considered odd and would procure little insight in the musical taste and aesthetic tuning of the person studied (Van Praag, 1990, 1992a).

Individual experiences are what they are: private states of mind. By desubjectivizing them they cease being just that. It is like reading notes, without hearing the music.

In our days psychiatric research aspires to an approach that is maximally objective and value-free. This is a laudable effort. One cannot, however, with impunity ignore or neglect extensive domains of psychopathology, because they are subjective in nature. Diagnostically we need both objective data and experiential data, the latter being inherently subjective (Van Praag, 1992a,b). Methods to assess the latter, moreover, are available. The experience sampling method is well suited to gauge mood states and connected cognitions (Wheeler & Reiss, 1991; De Vries, 1992; Van Eck *et al.*, 1998). Regrettably this method has so far been largely ignored in life-event research. The task of research diagnosticians will be to refine available methods to document subjective data, with maximum precision and reproducibility. This is an exercise pivotal to life-event research.

3.4.4 Conclusion

In life-event research the subjective experiences of the afflicted subject are deliberately excluded in assessment procedures. In addition, analysis of personality structure – after all a pivotal determinant of the emotional response to life events – is a rare feature. This situation is seriously handicapping this research endeavour.

3.5 What is meant by the term causation?

Causation of a (mental) disorder is a complex matter. First of all one has to distinguish pathogenesis from aetiology (Van Praag & Leijnse, 1964, 1965). The first concept refers to the complex of neuronal dysfunctions underlying a particular abnormal mental state. The factor aetiology comprises all variables that have contributed to destabilization of that circuitry. Aetiological factors can be of a biological or psychological nature. The former may be genetically determined or acquired during life, and in the latter case may have acted on the brain in the present or in the past. Often combinations of those factors have been operative.

Disruptions of neuronal circuitry are an indispensable component in the causation of mental disorders. They 'carry' such conditions. Without them behaviour and experience would not be disturbed. The pathogenic weight of an aetiological factor, on the other hand, may vary. It can be *necessary and sufficient* to generate the disorder. This does not imply that it is the only factor capable of generating the disorder. Next, an aetiological factor can be *necessary, but not sufficient* to elicit the disorder. It may play a causal role, but only in combination with other triggers will the disorder manifest.

Finally, an aetiological factor can be *neither necessary nor sufficient* in the causation of the disorder. It plays a role in that it reinforces the pathogenic weight of another variable. Such factors are of a predisposing nature, increasing the vulnerability for a certain disorder, and potentially contribute to its continuation.

Only when the pathophysiology of a particular disorder has been fully elucidated, can the causal weight of aetiological factors be definitively assessed. This is not the case for mood disorders. Only fragments of the underlying pathogenesis are known. Hence, the role of life events in the causation of depression can only be evaluated tentatively.

3.6 Conclusions

Several methodological problems will make it difficult to deduce conclusions from life-event research regarding the depressogenic significance of life events.

A major issue is the ill-defined border between distress and depression. Few will question a direct connection between adversity and distress. To demonstrate a causal relation between life events and depression, however, is a different matter.

Reliable data on the relation between life events and disease depend heavily on a clear dateable onset of the disease. This is often not the case for depression, since so frequently it is preceded by periods of distress, while the cut-off point between distress and depression is hard to establish.

'Internal' or 'cognitive' events are not included in the definition of life events, and with that a host of traumatic experiences, generally repetitive in nature, are not being studied as to their depressogenic impact.

Many people experience adversity, relatively few break down. Among the vulnerability factors, personality frailties leading to inadequate coping strategies, play – supposedly – a dominant role. Yet, personality research has only been weakly represented in life-event research.

Life-event research excludes the subjective experiences of the afflicted individual from assessment procedures. This makes it very hard to judge the destabilizing effect of life events in an individual case. De-subjectivation of psychiatric research (which, of course, is a laudable aim) should not mean shutting out the individual. It should mean developing methods to register, reproducibly and reliably, *all* psychopathological phenomena – those observable objectively as well as those that remain largely within the realm of subjective experiences.

Since we have as yet only scant insight into the biological determinants of depression, it is not yet possible to investigate whether stress leads to brain dysfunctions known to underlie depression. Definitive conclusions about the depressogenic significance of life events can only be drawn after those data become available.

REFERENCES

Akiskal, H. S. (1983). Dysthymic disorder: Psychopathology of proposed chronic depressive subtypes. *Am. J. Psychiatry*, **140**, 11–20.

Akiskal, H. S., Chen, S. E., Davis, G. C., Puzantian, V. R., Kashgarian, M. & Bolinger, J. M. (1985). Borderline: an adjective in search of a noun. *J. Clin. Psychiatry*, **46**, 41–8.

Boyce, P., Parker, B., Barnett, B., Cooney, M. & Smith, F. (1991). Personality as a vulnerability factor to depression. *Br. J. Psychiatry*, **159**, 106–14.

Brown, G. W. & Harris, T. (1978). *Social Origins of Depression*. London: Tavistock Publications. (1989). Depression. In *Life Events and Illness*, ed. T. O. Harris. London: Guilford Press.

Brown, G. W., Bifulco, A. & Harris, T. O. (1987). Life events, vulnerability and onset of depression. Some refinements. *Biol. Psychiatry*, **150**, 30–42.

Clayton, P. J. (1982). Bereavement. In *Handbook of Affective Disorders*, ed. E. S. Paykel. Edinburgh: Churchill Livingstone.

Cohen, L. N., Towbes, L. C. & Flocco, R. (1988). Effects of induced mood on self-reported life events and perceived and received social support. *J. Pers. Soc. Psychol.*, **55**, 669–74.

Cui, X. J. & Vaillant, G. E. (1997). Does depression generate negative life events? *J. Nerv. Ment. Dis.*, **185**, 145–50.

De Vries, M. (Ed.) (1992). *The Experience of Psychopathology: Investigating Mental Disorders in their Natural Setting*. Cambridge: Cambridge University Press.

Fava, G. A., Munari, F., Pavan, L. & Kellner, R. (1981). Life events and depression: a replication. *J. Affect. Disord.*, **3**, 159–65.

Fava, G. A., Fabbri, S. & Sonino, N. (2002). Residual symptoms in depression: an emerging therapeutic target. *Prog. Neuro-Psychopharmacol Biol. Psychiatry*, **26**, 1019–27.

Hamilton, M. (1960). A rating scale for depression. *J. Neurol. Neurosurg. Psychiatry*, **23**, 56–62.

Hammer, C. (1991). Generation of stress in the course of unipolar depression. *J. Abnorm. Psychol.*, **100**, 555–61.

Harkness, K. L., Monroe, S. M., Simons, A. D. & Thase, M. (1999). The generation of life events in recurrent and non recurrent depression. *Psychol. Med.*, **29**, 135–44.

Hawton, K. & van Heeringen, K. (Ed.) (2000). *The International Handbook of Suicide and Attempted Suicide*. Chichester: John Wiley & Sons.

Hirschfeld, R. M., Klerman, G. L., Clayton, P. J. & Keller, M. B. (1983). Personality and depression: empirical findings. *Arch. Gen. Psychiatry*, **40**, 993–8.

Hirschfeld, R. M., Shea, M. T. & Holzer, Ch. E. (1997). Personality dysfunction and depression. In *Depression. Neurobiological, Psychopathological and Therapeutical Advances*, ed. A. Honig & H. M. van Praag. Chichester: John Wiley & Sons.

Jenaway, A. & Paykel, E. S. (1997). Life events and depression. In *Depression. Neurobiological, Psychopathological and Therapeutical Advances*, ed. A. Honig & H. M. van Praag. Chichester: John Wiley & Sons.

Judd, L. L., Akiskal, H. S. & Paulus, M. P. (1997). The role and clinical significance of subsyndromal depressive symptoms (SSD) in unipolar major depressive disorder. *J. Affect. Dis.*, **45**, 5–18.

Kernberg, O. (1987). Clinical dimensions of masochism. In *Masochism: Current and Psychotherapeutic Contributions*, ed. R. A. Glick & D. I. Meyers. Hillsdale, NJ: Analytic Press.

Kessler, R. C. (1997). The effect of stressful life events on depression. *Ann. Rev. Psychol.*, **48**, 191–214.

Kessler, R. C. & Magee, W. J. (1993). Childhood adversity and adult depression: basic patterns of association in a U.S. National Survey. *Psychol. Med.*, **32**, 679–90.

Kraepelin, E. (1921). *Manic-depressive Insanity and Paranoia*. Edinburgh: E&S Livingstone.

Kraepelin, E. & Lange, J. (1927). *Psychiatrie* (Neunte Auflage). Leipzig: Ambrosius Barth.

Lazarus, R. S. (1993). From psychological stress to the emotions: a history of changing outlooks. *Ann. Rev. Psychol.*, **44**, 1–21.

Lazarus, R. S. & Folkman, S. (1984). *Stress, Appraisal and Coping*. New York: Springer.

Miller, M. A. & Rahe, R. H. (1997). Life changes scaling for the 1990's. *J. Psychosomatic Res.*, **43**, 279–92.

Neilson, E., Brown, G. & Marmot, M. (1989). Myocardial infarction. In *Life Events and Illness*, ed. G. Brown & T. Harris. London: Urwin Hyman.

Ormel, J. (1999). Depressie. De rol van levensgebeurtenissen, persoonlijkheid en erfelijkheid. In *Handboek stemmingsstoornissen*, ed. J. A. den Boer, J. Ormel, H. M. van Praag, H. J. M. Westenberg & H. d'Haenen. Maarssen: Elsevier/De Tijdstroom.

Paykel, E. S. (1982). Life events and early environment. In *Handbook of Affective Disorders*, ed. E. S. Paykel. Edinburgh: Churchill Livingstone.

(1997). The interview for Recent Life Events. *Psychol. Med.*, **27**, 301–10.

Paykel, E. S., Myers, J., Dienelt, M., Klerman, G., Lindenthal, J. & Pepper, M. (1969). Life events and depression: a controlled study. *Arch. Gen. Psychiatry*, **21**, 753–60.

Pincus, H. A., Frances, A. F., Davis, W. W., First, M. B. & Widiger, T. A. (1992). DSM–IV and new diagnostic categories: holding the line on proliferation. *Am. J. Psychiatry*, **149**, 112–17.

Rahe, R. H. (1995). Stress and psychiatry. In *Comprehensive Textbook of Psychiatry*, vol. 2, 6th edition, ed. Kaplan & Sadock. Baltimore: Williams and Wilkins.

Sarason, I. G., Johnson, J. H. & Siegel, J. M. (1978). Assessing the impact of life change: development of the life Experience Survey. *J. Consult. Clin. Psychol.*, **46**, 32–46.

Sato, T., Narita, T., Hirano, S., Kusunoki, K., Sakado, K. & Uehara, T. (2001). Is interpersonal sensitivity specific to non-melancholic depression? *J. Affect. Disord.*, **64**, 133–44.

Schneider, K. (1958). *Psychopathic Personalities*. Springfield, IL: Charles C. Thomas.

Segal, Z., Shaw, B., Vella, D. & Katz, R. (1992). Cognitive and life stress predictors of relapse in remitted unipolar depressed patients: test of the congruency hypothesis. *J. Abnorm. Psychol.*, **101**, 26–36.

Shea, M. T. & Hirschfeld, R. M. A. (1996). Chronic mood disorder and depressive personality. *Psychiat. Clin. North America*, **19**, 103–120.

Spitzer, R. L., Endicott, J. & Robins, E. (1978). Research diagnostic criteria: rationale and reliability. *Arch. Gen. Psychiatry*, **35**, 773–82.

Van Eck, M., Nicolson, N. A. & Berkhof, J. (1998). Effect of stressful daily events on mood states: relation to global perceived stress. *J. Pers. Soc. Psychol.*, **75**, 1572–85.

Van Praag, H. M. (1981). Socio-biological psychiatry. *Compr. Psychiatry*, **22**, 441–50.

(1990). (Re)-minding our business. *Hum. Psychopharm.*, **5**, 1–2.

(1992a). Reconquest of the subjective. Against the waning of psychiatric diagnosing. *Br. J. Psychiatry*, **160**, 266–71.

(Ed.) (1992b). *Make Believes in Psychiatry or The Perils of Progress.* New York: Brunner Mazel.

Van Praag, H. M. & Leijnse, B. (1964). Die Bedeutung der Psychopharmakologie für die klinische Psychiatrie. Systematik als notwendiger Ausgangspunkt. *Nevenarzt*, **34**, 530–7.

(1965). Neubewertung des Syndroms. Skizze einer funktionellen Pathologie. *Psychiat. Neurol. Neurochir.*, **68**, 50–66.

(2004). The debit balance of present day's stress research. *World J. Biol. Psychiatry*, in press.

Wheeler, L. & Reiss, H. T. (1991). Self-recording of everyday life events: origins, types and uses. *J. Personal. Dis.*, **59**, 339–54.

Life events and depression: is there a causal connection?

4.1 What kind of evidence is needed?

What data could be considered as tentative evidence in favour of a causal connection between traumatic life events and depression?

If,

– depressions or certain types of depression were frequently preceded by life events;
– the events would have taken place in close temporal proximity to the onset of depression, and
– would have induced a marked degree of inner turmoil (stress),
– while relief or amelioration of the event's traumatic consequences would lead to alleviation or clearing of the depression,

a causal relationship between event and depression would seem likely. Available evidence for this is discussed in this chapter.

Definitive proof of a causal relation would be the showing that the traumatic life events had led to alterations in brain circuits considered to be associated with (certain) depressive symptoms or syndromes.

Available evidence for this is discussed in Chapter 8.

4.2 Life events preceding depression

4.2.1 Acute events

The frequency of life events as well as their gravity is increased prior to major depression. This is probably also true for other depression types, but empirical data are scarce (Dolan et al., 1985; Kendler et al., 1993a,b). This was shown in community studies comparing individuals meeting criteria for depression with nondepressed individuals in the general population, and in case–control studies comparing depressives under psychiatric treatment with nondepressed controls (Brown & Moran, 1994; Dohrenwend et al., 1995). The relationship has been studied in two ways. Severe events were found to be related to the onset of depression, and the onset of depression was shown to be associated with an excess of recent life events. It generally concerns retrospective studies, focusing on major depression, over a specified recall period which is usually no longer than 1 year.

Approximately 75% of patients with major depression report negative life events prior to depression; in a control population this percentage amounted to 25 over the same period (Jenaway & Paykel, 1997). After a severe stressor, such as bereavement, the risk of major depression comes to 17–31% (Kim & Jacobs, 1995). These figures were found both in the general population and in depressed patients under psychiatric care (Brown & Harris, 1989). In the literature the relative risk of depression after exposure to negative life events varies from a factor of 3 to 10 (Ormel, 1999). The relative risk is the ratio between the incidence of a certain disorder (in this case depression) in those exposed to a particular risk factor (in this case life events) and the incidence of that same disorder in those who were not. It is, thus, a measure of the magnitude of the risk factor.

The few prospective studies available point in the same direction. Surtees (1995), for instance, showed that in the year after a fateful event 25% of the cohort studied showed depressive symptoms and 10% developed a full-blown depression. His data hint at a degree of event/outcome specificity. In women whose marital partners had recently died, depression rates increased over eight times and more than twice for anxiety disorder. In women whose husbands had recently experienced myocardial infarction the prevalence of psychiatric disorder doubled and was most pronounced for anxiety disorders.

Not surprisingly, the association with depression onset is stronger for dependent than for independent life events (Kessler, 1997; Kendler et al., 1999), while the risk of depression was higher after independent than after dependent events; in other words: independent events are better predictors of depression than dependent events (Brown & Harris, 1978). Stressful events and depression, moreover, show a dose–response relationship in that severe events show a stronger relation with depression than milder ones. The same is true for the number of events. With the number of events the depression risk increases, at least in the case of severe events (Kessler, 1997). Dose–response relationships argue in favour of a causal connection between stressor and depression. Another argument is provided by calculating the so-called 'brought-forward time'. This is a mathematical construct which makes the assumption that an episode of depression would have occurred sooner or later anyway but that the episode is brought forward by the event. In the case of severe events, Paykel (1978) calculated the brought-forward time for depression to be 2 years.

The relationship between life events and depression is particularly strong in first-onset depression. With increasing numbers of previous episodes the impact of life events decreases (Brown & Harris, 1994). A possible explanation is that repeated depression causes neuronal damage: 'scars', leading to increased vulnerability and lowering of the 'stress-threshold' (Post, 1992). Interestingly, this process seems to be 'saturable': after nine episodes, the impact of life events on depression risk remains stable (Kendler *et al.*, 2000).

Evidence exists that the enduring sequelae of an acute life event, rather than the acute event itself, account in most part for the association between life events and depression. Kessler *et al.* (1987), for instance, showed that the adverse effects of unemployment on depression are partly mediated by resultant financial troubles.

Life events, however, are by no means specifically linked to depression. Negative life events likewise frequently precede anxiety disorders and psychoses. There is some (Surtees, 1995), but scarce evidence that specific events are associated with specific psychiatric conditions.

4.2.2 Chronic difficulties

Chronic stress as a result of difficulties is a more powerful predictor of depression than acute stress (Brown & Harris, 1978; McGonagle & Kessler, 1990), and is also significantly associated with mood lowering (Pearlin, 1989; Kessler, 1997). This is in accordance with the finding in general population surveys that adults describe chronic situations more often as major sources of stress than acute events. Chronic stress, moreover, may prolong the recovery time of depression (Veroff *et al.*, 1981; Mattlin *et al.*, 1990).

The fact that chronic stressful situations have a more pronounced depressogenic effect than acute traumatic events, can, hypothetically, be explained as follows (Thoits, 1983; McGonagle & Kessler, 1990). The persistence of a problematic situation demonstrates that coping and problem-solving efforts have failed; that the situation, thus, has to be appraised as uncontrollable and generally as more threatening than the situation after acute events, that still hold the promise of resolution.

A more plausible explanation, it seems to me, is the following: chronic difficulties are frequently associated with states of chronic dysphoria, that might be classified as dysthymia or subsyndromal forms of depression (Pearlin, 1989). It is conceivable that this type of 'minor depression' predisposes for major forms of depression and increases the risk that acute events will precipitate a state of full-blown depression. Some evidence supports this view (Brown *et al.*, 1986a,b).

The relationship between chronic difficulties (chronic stress) and acute events in precipitating depression is unclear. Several authors (Brown & Harris, 1978; Van de Willige *et al.*, 1995) found the effects to be additive. Chronic difficulties together with acute events increased the depression risk ten-fold, as compared with individuals who had experienced neither (Van de Willige *et al.*, 1995). The additive effect was most pronounced if life event and chronic stress situation were 'matching', as for instance in a case of a lonely widower confronted with the death of his only friend (Brown *et al.*, 1986a,b). Life events matching the chronic stress situations were found to be three times more depressogenic than the same stressor is in individuals without a corresponding chronic strain (Ormel, 1999).

These findings correspond well with animal data indicating that rats exposed to repeated unavoidable stress lose their capacity to deal with acute stressful situations (Gambarana *et al.*, 1995).

McGonagle & Kessler (1990), on the other hand, failed to find an additive effect. On the contrary, their findings suggest that chronic stresses may *reduce* the emotional effects of acute stresses. Paradoxically, chronic stress seemed to have a stress-buffering effect. They proposed three explanations for these findings.

In the first place, chronic adversity may boost coping resources that increase resilience in times of acute adversity. Secondly, the ongoing stressful situation leads to a more rapid mobilization of coping mechanisms than would have occurred in the absence of chronic stress. Finally, acute stresses may lead to resolution of chronic difficulties; for instance, chronic marital difficulties may be resolved by the acute stressor: divorce.

Apparently, the relationship between acute and chronic stressors is a complex one and hard to establish when the assessment of individual emotional responses are not taken into account, and this is precisely what happens in current life-event research (see Chapter 3). Studies of chronic stress and its consequences are difficult to carry out, and thus not free of shortcomings. It is, for instance, difficult to decide what came first: the chronically depressed mood causing or contributing to the chronically stressed situation, or, alternatively, whether that situation precipitated the depressed state. In very few studies, moreover, are attempts being made to verify the accuracy of life-event reporting, for instance by interviewing important others or by consulting archival data. This is true for both acute events and difficulties. As mentioned, personality data are seldomly provided, and possible links between event, personality structure and chronic dysphoria are, in most cases, left out of consideration and exploration. The precise analysis and documentation of personality structure, chronic dysphoria, chronic difficulties and possible exposure to acute traumatic events, however, seem to be quintessential for life-event research.

Chronic difficulties, important as they seem to be in the aetiology of mood disorders, are in need of intensified and more sophisticated study.

4.3 Vulnerability

Frustrating life events occur frequently; only relatively few people develop depression subsequently. Paykel (1978) found that 25% of depressed patients had experienced an exit-event in the preceding 6 months, compared with 5% in a healthy control group. The relative rarity of depression following a traumatic event, he demonstrated in the following way.

Suppose 2% of 10 000 subjects in the general population become depressed during a 6-month period. Of those 200 individuals, 25% or 50 individuals will have experienced an exit-event. Five per cent of the remaining 9800 subjects, i.e. 490 subjects, will also have experienced an exit-event without becoming depressed. Thus of a total of 540 exit events only 50 or 9% were followed by the development of depression.

Obviously other factors play a role in the aetiology of depression, increasing someone's vulnerability for the destabilizing effects of life events. Brown & Harris (1978) identified a number of *social vulnerability factors* in an inner-city female population, i.e. lack of a confiding relationship; having three or more children under 14 years at home; lack of employment; low social class; and lack of social support. Loss of one's mother before age 11 was also identified as a vulnerability factor providing some evidence for Bowlby's (1988) attachment theory. Later studies confirmed that early adversity such as loss of a parent, divorce of parents or childhood neglect and abuse, increase the vulnerability for psychopathology, amongst others depression (Parker *et al.*, 1992; Parker, 1993) (see Chapter 8). The more vulnerability factors are operative, the more likely events will be followed by depression. Thus, a dose–response relationship is also found in this material (see Section 4.2.1). In a prospective study Bifulco *et al.* (1998) demonstrated that the chance of depression after serious life events is considerably increased in the presence of psychosocial vulnerability factors, such as low self-esteem, paucity of close relationships (Bifulco *et al.*, 1998) and adverse psychosocial work conditions (Paterniti *et al.*, 2002).

A second group of vulnerability factors, to be discussed in the next section, is related to *personality-structure* and functioning. Low self-esteem, for instance, was identified as such (Brown & Harris, 1986). This personality trait predisposes for depression and may likewise be a component of the depressive syndrome itself, underlining the importance of merging life-event studies with personality research and the urgent need of interactive models.

Personality traits can be linked to life-event exposure and impact in various ways. Firstly, coping skills may be poor. Secondly, certain personalities are prone to be exposed to life events or create social environments in which the likelihood of life-event exposure is increased. Thirdly, exposure to life events might, conceivably, alter personality traits, in such a way that the chance of life-event exposure increases or the effectiveness of defence mechanisms weakens. Disentangling those options is a tall order and has yet to be achieved.

Finally, *biological factors* may be involved in susceptibility to the destabilizing effect of traumatic experiences. Firstly, indirectly by interfering with personality development and thus impairing later coping abilities. Secondly, directly by damaging neuronal systems associated with the regulation of anxiety, aggression and mood, thus increasing the risk of failure in times of increasing demands. These issues are discussed in Chapter 7.

4.4 Life events, personality and depression

4.4.1 A triad?

In previous sections it was discussed that prior to depression the rate of life events is increased compared with that in a control group. In addition it was asserted that the emotional impact of life events cannot be detached from individual personality make-up. Personality characteristics, it was maintained, determine in a major way *stress-vulnerability*. Moreover, they may bring someone to engage in, or to create situations with increased likelihood of stressor exposure (*stressor-proneness*).

If indeed life events, personality structure and depression are so closely linked, one would expect:

– An increased rate of deviant personality traits and of personality disorder in mood disorders.
– An increased rate of life events in individuals with abnormal personality make up.
– Particular life events to be particularly damaging for individuals with particular personality traits.

4.4.2 Depression and personality

The construct of personality encompasses someone's way of thinking, emotional structure, attitudes and values, features that are more or less characteristic for that individual and show considerable stability over time (Costa & McCrae, 1986; Rutter, 1987). Ultimately it is personality make-up that determines to a large extent the outcome of event appraisal. Has the event to be considered as serious and threatening, or as relatively benign and manageable? Much adversity, whatever its origin – be it one's social environment, interpersonal encounters or inner psychic life – can be adequately processed, given an able-minded personality. Personality frailties make that process problematic. Since the traumatizing impact of life events is so closely related to personality features, whereas traumatizing life events so frequently precede depression, it comes as no surprise that many studies, both cross-sectional (Hirschfeld *et al.*, 1983; Trull & Sher, 1994; Sato *et al.*, 1999) and prospective (Clayton *et al.*, 1994; Krueger *et al.*, 1996), found an increased rate of personality pathology in patients suffering from depression. This relationship was much stronger in the former type of studies than in the latter. The confounding effect that depression may have on personality assessment had been avoided.

Certain personality types and personality traits have been identified as making an individual particularly depression-prone. Particularly vulnerable is the dependent personality, characterized by interpersonal dependency, noncompetitiveness, a need for close relationships which provide guidance and security, sensitivity for signs of rejection and disapproval, lack of self-esteem, submissiveness and introversion (Hirschfeld *et al.*, 1983). Another example of a vulnerable personality type is the ambitious personality with obsessive traits, characterized by a high level of aspiration, perfectionism, pronounced self-control, need to control others and by a desire for personal independence (Maciejewski *et al.*, 2000). A possible variant of the ambitious subject is the self-critical personality who tends to be negativistic, somewhat avoidant of others and often precipitating failures through obstructive behaviour (Goldberg *et al.*, 1989), but basically convinced about his own superiority.

These kinds of personalities were already identified as depression-prone in the psychoanalytic (Freud, 1917) and phenomenological (Tellenbach, 1961) literature. Only much later were these observations empirically verified. In nondepressed primiparous women, for instance, the risk of depression postnatally was increased up to ten-fold in those women who showed high interpersonal sensitivity and high neuroticism as measured with the Interpersonal Sensitivity Measure and the Eysenck Personality Inventory (Eysenck & Eysenck, 1964; Eysenck *et al.*, 1985; Boyce *et al.*, 1991). An association between interpersonal sensitivity and depression has been found by many authors (Hirschfeld *et al.*, 1983; Boyce & Parker, 1989; Sakado *et al.*, 1999, 2000). This trait is defined as 'undue and excessive awareness of and sensitivity to the behaviour and feelings of others' (Boyce & Parker, 1989). Nonmelancholic patients were found to be more interpersonally sensitive than melancholic patients and normal controls (Boyce *et al.*, 1993).

Neuroticism is another factor predicting future episodes of major depression (Angst & Clayton, 1986; Hirschfeld *et al.*, 1989; Boyce *et al.*, 1991). It is a personality construct proposed by Eysenck & Eysenck (1964) as a measure of emotionality, emotional instability and inefficient ways of coping and hence vulnerability to stress. Depression following loss, for instance, is more likely in those showing high than low neuroticism scores (Raphael & Middleton, 1990). Kendler *et al.* (1993a,b) found that one standard deviation difference in neuroticism translates in a 100% difference in the rates of first onsets of depression over 12 months.

Another personality trait proposed to be related to depression is low self-esteem (Brown & Harris, 1978; Brown *et al.*, 1986a,b; Hokanson *et al.*, 1989; McMiller *et al.*, 1989; Böker *et al.*, 2000). Negative views of oneself is one of the three cornerstones of Beck's (1974) 'depressive triad'. Neuroticism, however, was found by Roberts & Kendler (1999) to be a better predictor of major depression than low self-esteem. 'Overall emotionality or emotional reactivity to the environment', these authors conclude, 'reflects risk for depression better than does global self-concept'.

Prospective studies confirmed cross-sectional data. A longitudinal study carried out in New Zealand followed 1000 children born between 1972–1973, and found that the factor stress reactivity (related to the factor 'neuroticism') increased the risk of depression (Caspi *et al.*, 1996). Clayton *et al.* (1994) followed up a thousand Swiss conscripts and found that the traits aggression and autonomic lability (comparable with the factor 'neuroticism') were risk factors for depression. Possibly, however, neuroticism scores mainly reflect subclinical depression or residual depressive symptoms (Farmer *et al.*, 2002), and neuroticism is thus a metonym or substitution term for subdued depression.

Abundant evidence, thus, earmarks personality pathology as a risk factor for depression. Co-existence of depression and personality disorder, moreover, worsens the chance of remission after regular treatment (O'Leary & Costello, 2001).

As certain personality frailties are risk factors for depression, so is, according to some authors, depression a risk factor for personality dysfunctions or personality disorder (Fava *et al.*, 2002). Depressed, in comparison with nondepressed individuals, report less-supportive networks and more marital discord (Billings *et al.*, 1983; Gotlib & Whiffen, 1989); relationships are frequently characterized by conflict and hostility (Ruscher & Gotlib, 1988). Intimate relationships, moreover, are poorer in major depression than in several other psychiatric disorders such as anxiety disorders and nonaffective psychotic disorders (Zlotnick *et al.*, 2000). These findings support Coyne's (1976) notion that depressed individuals create a negative social environment leading to loss of social support which might contribute to exacerbation or continuance of the depression. This may also explain the fact that people with a history of depression experience more events than others even when in remission (Kessler & Magee, 1993). Some authors, however, failed to find depression-induced personality scars (Shea *et al.*, 1996).

Interpersonal discord may persist after remission (Coryell *et al.*, 1993). It is not clear whether this is a consequence of residual depressive symptoms, of enduring personality damage due to depression or of pre-existing personality traits, possibly magnified by going through a depressive condition.

4.4.3 Life events and personality

Several studies show that the factor *neuroticism* as defined by Eysenck & Eysenck (1964) is associated with high rates of life events, both in clinical studies (Fergusson & Horwood, 1987) and in general population studies (Costa & McCrae, 1986). In a study of the latter kind Ormel & Wohlfarth (1991) demonstrated that neuroticism had strong effects on producing psychological distress through life events. Neuroticism has been shown to be the best predictor of the occurrence of traumatic life events (Poulton & Andrews, 1992; Magnus *et al.*, 1993). Also, *other dysfunctional personality traits* of various kinds, such as schizoid, avoidant, dependent, passive aggressive (Leaf *et al.*, 1992) and so-called type A features (aggressiveness, ambitiousness combined with a hard drive to succeed) (Byrne, 1983) are all related to increased rates of life events. *Personality disorder symptoms*, particularly those from cluster A and B, were found to be associated with greater self-generated episodic stress, inter-personal chronic stress and relationship dissatisfaction, controlling for initial depression, measured over a 2-year period (Daley *et al.*, 1998).

Focusing on DSM defined *personality disorder*, as opposed to what the DSM calls accentuation of (normal) personality traits, similar relationships with life-event rates have been ascertained (Labonte & Paris, 1993; Daley *et al.*, 1998). In a prospective design, Sievewright (1998), for instance, studied a cohort of subjects before onset or worsening of an axis I defined mood or anxiety disorder. Sociopathic and passive dependent personality disorder was associated with increased rates of various kinds of life events.

Most investigations studied life events and personality disorder in relation to depression and therefore do not allow an answer to questions on the relationship between life events and personality structure. Yet the available data justify the conclusion that abnormal personality make-up does increase the risk of being exposed to life events.

4.4.4 Congruence

Beck (1987) used the term sociotropy for the dependent personality structure and the term autonomy for the personality striving towards control and independence and proposed that these personality traits act as 'vulnerability markers for depression by sensitizing individuals to certain types of negative life experiences'. This notion implies that the stressor threshold is not lowered across the board, but for specific events 'congruent' with the personality frailties. Sociotropy, for instance, would lead to hypersensitivity for losses interfering with one's sense of security and for events interpreted as signs of rejection. A strong need for autonomy would make a person particularly vulnerable for events that might interfere with one's sense of independence and those signifying disapproval, such as being dismissed, demoted or passed over.

The congruence hypothesis – suggesting life events to be particularly depressogenic if they wound vulnerable personality traits – seems self-evident but has been hard to substantiate unequivocally. Some authors found positive evidence (Clark *et al.*, 1992; Segal *et al.*, 1992). Congruency between the life event experienced and specific domains of concern for instance was found to increase the risk of onset of depression and relapse of depression as well as the severity of the depression (Hammen *et al.*, 1985; Zuroff & Mongrain, 1987; Segal *et al.*, 1992). In dependent individuals the magnitude of depression was greater after experiencing interpersonal stress, than after noninterpersonal stress (Hammen *et al.*, 1985; Zuroff & Mongrain, 1987). The risk of a relapse depression was increased in self-critical subjects in the case of achievement-related adversity, as compared to adversity without direct bearing on their specific domain of concern (Segal *et al.*, 1992). Parker *et al.* (1998) could demonstrate 'lock and key links' in depression, particularly in nonmelancholic, reactive depression. In other words, if 'locks' established by early adverse experiences are activated by 'keys' mirroring the earlier adverse experience there is a higher depression risk than after 'neutral' events.

On the other hand, negative results have also been reported. Mazure *et al.* (2000), for instance, failed to find congruency between what is called cognitive personality style – a term derived from Beck's vocabulary – and event-type in predicting the onset of depression.

The discrepancies in the results are not really surprising. Personality imperfections may be 'localized' in a particular domain of psychic functioning, the effects however may 'spill over' in other psychic domains. Apart from a need for protection, dependent individuals may show dysfunctional anxiety and fear to accept new challenges. Autonomy strivings do not generally go alone, but might be accompanied by the proclivity to incite authority conflicts and a leaning towards self-serving, egocentric behaviour. Hence, events perceived as harmful will touch psychic spheres other than the one(s) considered to be vulnerable. Congruence will be 'diluted' in this way.

This spill-over phenomenon, moreover, offers an explanation for two other phenomena. Firstly, the fact that categorical classifications of personality disorders, of old, show considerable overlap. Secondly, it may explain why it is that vulnerable personality traits are not specifically coupled to particular mental disorders. In the language of the Five-Factor Personality Inventory Model (Costa & McCrae, 1992), major depression was associated with increased neuroticism, decreased extraversion, increased openness to experience, and decreased conscientiousness, but the specificity of these factors for depression is low. Most of the deviant personality traits are also found in anxiety disorders, albeit less pronounced.

4.4.5 Conclusions

Personality make-up seems to be a key factor in the occurrence of depression after traumatic experiences. Certain personality traits and personality disorders predispose for life events and for depression, whereas life events and depression do strongly intercorrelate. It does not seem too bold an assumption to assert that personality make-up constitutes a major psychological link between life events and depression. Personality frailties, in their turn, can be primarily a consequence of biological factors – genetic or acquired in nature – primarily determined by the psychological impact of early adversities, or a product of both.

4.5 Early adversity, life events, personality and depression

Dysfunctional parenting, and in particular low care and overprotection, has been found to increase stressor vulnerability, the risk of depression and of recurrence of depression, both for melancholic and nonmelancholic depression (Perris *et al.*, 1986; Parker *et al.*, 1995; Carter *et al.*, 1999). Rather than being depression-specific, dysfunctional parenting seems to predispose for a variety of psychopathological conditions, such as substance abuse, alcoholism and most importantly a variety of personality disorders leading to diminished levels of social functioning (Gerlsma *et al.*, 1993; Carter *et al.*, 1999). Dysfunctional parenting has been hypothesized to disrupt two processes to normal personality development: the capacity to establish interpersonal bonds and to develop an identity of one's own, leading to self-determination (Blatt, 1990). Disturbed personality development is thought to be an important intermediary between dysfunctional parenting and depression (more general: psychopathology) (Akiskal *et al.*, 1983; Black *et al.*, 1988; Fava *et al.*, 1996).

Other childhood adversities, such as parental divorce, separation from parents, physical or sexual abuse and the like, were also found to be associated with an increased risk of depression and other forms of psychopathology in adult life. The association between life events and adult mental health is greater when childhood neuroticism was higher and childhood mental health poorer (Van Os & Jones, 1999). Childhood depression in its turn increases the risk for later personality disorder significantly, in particular dependent, antisocial, passive-aggressive and histrionic personality disorders (Kasen *et al.*, 2001).

These issues will be discussed in more detail in Chapter 8.

4.6 Genes, life events, personality and depression

Genes play an important, though by no means exclusive role in the causation of depression. This has been concluded from family, twin and adoption studies. These issues will be discussed only briefly in this chapter, and in more detail in Chapters 5 and 6.

In family studies the morbid risk of depression is determined in families of depressed patients and compared with control families or with the rate of depression in the general population. In first-degree relatives (parents, siblings and offspring) of patients with bipolar or unipolar depression the frequency of depression is considerably increased (Weissman *et al.*, 1984). The family data do not provide unequivocal evidence in favour of genetic transmission, because family aggregation may (partly) reflect a shared environment.

In twin studies the concordance rate for depression is studied in monozygotic twins (sharing identical genes) and compared with that figure in dizygotic twins (sharing only half of the genes). Consistently the concordance rate for depression in monozygotic twins (*c.* 60%) has been found to supersede that found among dizygotic twins (*c.* 20%) (Tsuang & Faraone, 1990; McGuffin *et al.*, 1991;

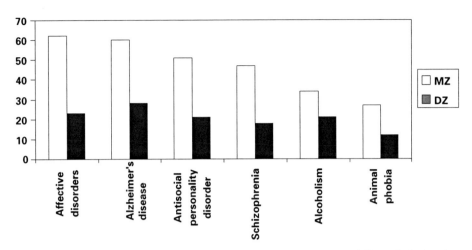

Figure 4.1. Concordance rates of some mental disorders in monozygotic (MZ) and dizygotic (DZ) twins (Ormel, 1999; Van Os & Marcelis, 1999).

Van Os & Marcelis, 1999) (Figure 4.1). The data of this approach too, though highly suggestive, still leave some reason for doubt, since intra-uterine environment is not the same for mono- and dizygotic twins: the former share the same placental circulation, the latter do not. It is conceivable, moreover, that monozygotic twins are treated differently by their parents and in their respective environments than the dizygotic twins. For this explanation, however, experimental support is lacking (McGuffin et al., 1996).

In adoption studies the fate of children born in families with depression but raised away from their parents and families is studied and, conversely, the psychiatric history of individuals from parents/families without mood disorders but raised by parents suffering from depression. In the first group the depression risk is increased, as is the case in their biological parents and relatives. In the latter group the depression risk is not increased, in spite of depression running in the foster families (Mendlewicz & Rainier, 1977; Cadoret, 1978; Wender et al., 1986). In adoption studies, too, early environmental influences – including the intra-uterine ones – cannot completely ruled out. The most convincing design would be studying monozygotic twins of which one has been raised by the biological parents and the other by a depression-free adoptive family. Such a study has not yet been carried out.

Taken together all these data strongly suggest that hereditary factors contribute to the causation of mood disorders. The hereditary component is particularly pronounced in severe depression, such as psychotic depression and major depression, melancholic type; in milder forms the genetically transmitted component does play a more modest role (McGuffin et al., 1994). On the average the contribution of nongenetic factors is estimated to be approximately 50%. The depressogenic effect of stressful life events is substantially increased in individuals at genetic risk for depression (Kendler & Karkowski-Shuman, 1997).

Genes increasing depression susceptibility may act in two ways. Firstly, *indirectly* by influencing personality structure and being (co-)responsible for the development of traits increasing emotional instability, vulnerability for the emotional impact of adversities, and the risk of being exposed to traumatic life events. These factors may result in increased susceptibility for depression. Secondly, *directly* by influencing brain development. In the latter case imperfections will occur in the development of brain circuits involved in the regulation of such psychic functions as mood, aggression and anxiety, increasing the risk of disruptions if, later in life, demands increase. In other words those subjects will be at risk for mood and anxiety disorders.

The question may be raised whether the same genes are operative in depression vulnerability, life-event risk and depressogenic personality traits. Some preliminary evidence suggests that this might be the case (Kendler & Karkowski-Shuman, 1997; Kendler *et al.*, 1999), but many more studies are still needed to make this supposition plausible.

Environmental and genetic factors, finally, do not operate independently, but interactionally. Gene–environment interactions are studied by genetic epidemiologists. Relevant data will be discussed in Chapter 6.

4.7 Life events and recovery from depression

If life events would play a significant role in the causation of depression, one would expect recovery from depression to be promoted by neutralizing events and by psychological or social interventions aimed at elimination or amelioration of the emotional consequences of the disturbing events. It has to be emphasized, however, that this reasoning is somewhat flawed in two ways. Firstly, it is conceivable that stress provokes neuronal disturbances that, once induced, follow their own course independent of the provoking variables. Secondly, the positive effects of psychotherapeutic interventions might be mere appearance, in that the depression is self-limiting and would have come to an end anyhow.

Be this as it may, several studies indicate that neutralizing the adverse effects of traumatizing events can indeed be beneficial (Tennant *et al.*, 1981; Parker *et al.*, 1986). Finding a new and satisfactory job, for instance, may ease the pain of being sacked. Conversely, continued difficulties or new blows during a depressive episode, will slow the speed of recovery from depression or may prevent it altogether. This is particularly true if new events exacerbate the adversities that triggered the depressive episode. Most of those studies were carried out in patient samples (Paykel & Tanner, 1976; Brugha *et al.*, 1990), some in community samples (Sargeant *et al.*, 1990; Mcleod *et al.*, 1992).

Several forms of psychotherapy, most notably cognitive behavioural psychotherapy and interpersonal psychotherapy have been found to be effective in the treatment of mood disorders (Paykel & Priest, 1992; Thase *et al.*, 1997; Malt *et al.*, 1999; Reynolds *et al.*, 1999). Since it is impossible to single out whether efficacy is based on reduction of the emotional impact of life events and difficulties, on strengthening of coping abilities or on direct alleviation of depressive symptoms, these data cannot count as firm evidence in favour of the hypothesis that traumatic experiences have causal significance in depression.

4.8 Conclusions

Major depression is frequently preceded by acute life events with a negative connotation, in the year prior to the onset of depression. This relationship is most pronounced in first-onset depression and decreases, up to a certain point, with increasing number of relapses. It is often difficult to exclude the possibility that the negative event was a consequence of the depression rather than an aetiological significant factor. Conversely, depressive symptoms can elicit life events or difficulties or exacerbate their effects.

The importance of personality features for appraisal of the event and in dealing with its consequences is hard to overestimate. They determine to a large extent the severity and duration of the stress phenomena subsequent to traumatic experiences, and it is these stress phenomena that destabilize neuronal circuitry and thus ultimately may lead to psychopathology. Personality should be the lynchpin of life-event and depression research. Unfortunately, this is as yet not the case.

Difficulties leading to chronic stress are often accompanied by dysphoric mood states, and the latter are probably a risk factor for major depression. The impact of chronic stress on the depressogenic power of acute traumatic events seems to be variable and probably dependent on the extent wherein the causes of chronic stress and the type of acute event 'match'. It seems likely that personality features play an important role also in this interaction but with regard to this little is known.

The aetiological 'weight' of life events is unknown. In most cases they are most probably not a sufficient cause. Paykel's studies on 'brought-forward time' suggest that frequently traumatic life events are necessary factors or accelerate the occurrence of depression at the very least. The causal impact life events exert depends on their severity and number, coping power of the subject and the presence of biological or social variables that mitigate or amplify the biological and psychological consequences of the event. It seems reasonable to assume that the aetiological significance of life events decreases with increasing strength of other risk factors for depression, such as the biological ones.

REFERENCES

Akiskal, H. S., Hirschfeld, R. M. A. & Yerevanian, B. I. (1983). The relationship of personality to affective disorders. *Arch. Gen. Psychiatry*, **40**, 801–10.

Angst, J. & Clayton, P. (1986). Premorbid personality of depressive, bipolar, and schizophrenic patients with special reference to suicidal issues. *Compr. Psychiat.*, **27**, 511–32.

Beck, A. T. (1974). The development of depression: a cognitive model. In *The Psychology of Depression: Contemporary Theory and Research*, ed. R. J. Friedman & M. M. Katz. Washington, DC: Hemisphere Publishing Corporation.

Beck, A. T. (1987). Cognitive model of depression. *J. Cogn. Psychother.*, **1**, 2–27.

Bifulco, A., Brown, G. W., Moran, P., Ball, C. & Campbell, C. (1998). Predicting depression in women: the role of past and present vulnerability. *Psychol. Med.*, **28**, 39–50.

Billings, A. G., Cronkite, R. & Moos, R. (1983). Social-environmental factors in unipolar depression: comparisons of depressed patients and nondepressed controls. *J. Abnorm. Psychol.*, **93**, 119–33.

Black, D. W., Bell, S., Hulbert, J. & Nasrallah, A. (1988). The importance of Axis II in patients with major depression: A controlled study. *J. Affect. Disord.*, **14**, 115–22.

Blatt, S. (1990). Interpersonal relatedness and self-definition: two personality configurations and their implications for psychopathology and psychotherapy. In *Depression and Dissociation: Implications for Personality, Theory, Psychopathology and Health*, ed. J. Singer. Chicago: University of Chicago Press.

Böker, H., Hell, D., Budischewski, K. *et al.* (2000). Personality and object relations in patients with affective disorders: idiographic research by means of the repertory grid technique. *J. Affect. Disord.*, **60**, 53–9.

Bowlby, J. (1988). *A Secure Base: Clinical Applications of Attachment Theory.* London: Routledge.

Boyce, P. & Parker, G. (1989). Development of a scale to measure interpersonal sensitivity. *Aust. N. Z. J. Psychiatry*, **23**, 341–51.

Boyce, P., Parker, G., Barnett, B., Cooney, M. & Smith, F. (1991). Personality as a vulnerability factor to depression. *Br. J. Psychiatry*, **159**, 106–14.

Boyce, P., Hickie, I., Parker, G., Mitchell, P., Willhelm, K. & Brodaty, H. (1993). Specificity of interpersonal sensitivity to non-melancholic depression. *J. Affect. Disord.*, **27**, 101–5.

Brown, G. W. & Harris, T. O. (1978). *Social Origins of Depression: A Study of Psychiatric Disorder in Women.* London: Tavistock/New York: Free Press.

(1986). Establishing causal links: the Beaford College studies of depression. In *Life Events and Psychiatric Disorders: Controversial Issues*, ed. H. Katschnig. Cambridge: Cambridge University Press.

(1989). *Life Events and Illness.* New York: Guilford Press.

(1994). Life events and endogenous depression: a puzzle re-examined. *Arch. Gen. Psychiatry*, **51**, 525–34.

Brown, G. W. & Moran, P. (1994). Clinical and psychosocial origins of chronic depressive episodes I. A community survey. *Br. J. Psychiatry*, **165**, 447–56.

Brown, G. W., Andrews, B., Harris, T., Adler, Z. & Bridge, L. (1986a). Social support, self-esteem and depression. *Psychol. Med.*, **16**, 813–31.

Brown, G. W., Bifulco, A., Harris, T. & Bridge, L. (1986b). Life stress, chronic subclinical symptoms and vulnerability to clinical depression. *J. Affect. Disord.*, **11**, 1–19.

Brugha, T. S., Bebbington, P. E., MacCarthy, B., Sturt, S., Wykes, T. & Potter, J. (1990). Gender, social support and recovery from depressive disorders: a prospective clinical study. *Psychol. Med.*, **20**, 147–56.

Byrne, D. (1983). Personal determinants of life event stress and myocardial infarction. *Psychosomatics*, **40**, 106–14.

Cadoret, R. (1978). Evidence of genetic inheritance of primary affective disorder. *Am. J. Psychiatry*, **133**, 463–6.

Carter, J. D., Joyce, P. R., Mulder, R. T., Luty, S. E. & Sullivan, P. F. (1999). Early deficient parenting in depressed outpatients is associated with personality dysfunction and not with depression subtypes. *J. Affect. Disord.*, **54**, 29–37.

Caspi, A., Moffitt, T. E., Newman, D. L. & Silva, P. A. (1996). Behavioral observations at age 3 years predict adult psychiatric disorder. *Arch. Gen. Psychiatry*, **53**, 1033–9.

Clark, D., Beck, A. T. & Brown, G. (1992). Sociotropy, autonomy, and life event perceptions in dysphoric and nondysphoric individuals. *Cogn. Ther. Res.*, **16**, 635–52.

Clayton, P. J., Trust, C. & Angst, J. (1994). Premorbid personality traits of men who develop unipolar or bipolar disorders. *Eur. Arch. Psychiatry Clin. Neurosci.*, **243**, 340–6.

Coryell, W., Scheftner, W., Keller, M., Endicott, J., Maser, J. & Klerman, G. L. (1993). The enduring psychosocial consequences of mania and depression. *Am. J. Psychiatry*, **150**, 720–7.

Costa, P. T. & McCrae, R. R. (1986). Crosssectional studies of personality in a national sample. *Psychol. Aging*, **1**, 140–3.

(1992). *NEO PI-R Professional Manual*. Odessa, FL: Psychological Assessment Resources.

Coyne, J. C. (1976). Toward an interactional description of depression. *Psychiatry*, **39**, 28–40.

Daley, S., Hammen, C., Davilla, J. & Burge, D. (1998). Axis II symptomatology, depression, and life stress during the transition from adolescence to adulthood. *J. Consult. Clin. Psychol.*, **66**, 595–603.

Dohrenwend, B. P., Shrout, P. E., Link, B. G., Skodol, A. E. & Stueve, A. (1995). Life events and other possible psychosocial risk factors for episodes of schizophrenia and major depression: a case-control study. In *Does Stress cause Psychiatric Illness?*, ed. C. M. Mazuri. Washington, DC: American Psychiatric Press.

Dolan, R. J., Calloway, S. P., Fonagy, P., DeSouza, F. V. A. & Wakeling, A. (1985). Life events, depression and hypothalamic-pituitary-adrenal axis function. *Br. J. Psychiatry*, **147**, 429–33.

Eysenck, S. B. G. & Eysenck, H. J. (1964). *Manual of the Eysenck Personality Inventory*. London: University Press.

Eysenck, S. B. G., Eysenck, H. J. & Barrett, P. (1985). A revised version of the psychoticism scale. *Pers. Indiv. Diff.*, **6**, 21–9.

Farmer, A., Redman, K., Harris, T. *et al.* (2002). Neuroticism, extraversion, life events and depression. *Br. J. Psychiatry*, **181**, 118–22.

Fava, M., Alpert, J. E., Borus, J. S., Nierenberg, A. A., Pava, J. A. & Rosenbaum, J. F. (1996). Patterns of personality disorder comorbidity in early-onset versus late-onset major depression. *Am. J. Psychiatry*, **153**, 1308–12.

Fava, M., Farabaugh, A. H., Sickinger, A. H. *et al.* (2002). Personality disorders and depression. *Psychol. Med.*, **32**, 1049–57.

Fergusson, D. M. & Horwood, L. J. (1987). Vulnerability to life event exposure. *Psychol. Med.*, **17**, 739–49.

Freud, S. (1917). Mourning and Melancholia. In *Collected Papers*, vol. 4. (1950). London: Hogarth Press.

Gambarana, C., Ghiglieri, O., Taddei, I., Tagliamonte, A. & Montis de, M. G. (1995). Imipramine and fluoxetine prevent the stress-induced escape deficits in rats through a distinct mechanism. *Behav. Pharmacol.*, **6**, 66–73.

Gerlsma, C., Das, J. & Emmelkamp, P. (1993). Depressed patients' parental representations: stability across changes in depressed mood and specificity. *J. Affect. Disord.*, **27**, 173–81.

Goldberg, J. O., Segal, Z., Vella, D. D. & Shaw, B. F. (1989). Depressive personality: Millon Clinical Multiaxial Inventory profiles of sociotropic and autonomous subtypes. *J. Pers. Disord.*, **3**, 193–8.

Gotlib, I. H. & Whiffen, V. E. (1989). Depression and marital functioning: an examination of specificity and gender differences. *J. Abnorm. Psychol.*, **98**, 23–30.

Hammen, C., Marks, T., Mayol, A. & deMayo, R. (1985). Depressive self-schemas, life stress, and vulnerability to depression. *J. Abnorm. Psychol.*, **94**, 308–19.

Hirschfeld, R. M., Klerman, G. L., Clayton, P. J. & Keller, M. B. (1983). Personality and Depression. Empirical findings. *Arch. Gen. Psychiatry*, **40**, 993–8.

Hirschfeld, R. M., Klerman, G. L., Lavori, P., Keller, M. B., Griffith, P. & Coryell, W. (1989). Premorbid personality assessments of first onset of major depression. *Arch. Gen. Psychiatry*, **46**, 345–50.

Hokanson, J. E., Rubert, M. P., Welker, R. A., Hollander, G. R. & Hedeen, C. (1989). Interpersonal concomitants and antecedents of depression among college students. *J. Abnorm. Psychol.*, **98**, 209–17.

Jenaway, A. & Paykel, E. S. (1997). Life events and depression. In *Depression, Neurobiological, Psychopathological and Therapeutic Advances*, ed. A. Honig & H. M. van Praag. Chicester: John Wiley & Sons.

Kasen, S., Cohen, P., Skodol, A. E., Johnson, J. G., Smailes, E. & Brook, J. S. (2001). Childhood depression and adult personality disorder. *Arch. Gen. Psychiatry*, **58**, 231–6.

Kendler, K. S. & Karkowski-Shuman, L. (1997). Stressful life events and genetic liability to major depression: genetic control of exposure to the environment. *Psychol. Med.*, **27**, 539–47.

Kendler, K. S., Neale, M. C., Kessler, R. C., Heath, A. C. & Eaves, L. J. (1993a). A longitudinal twin study of personality and major depression in women. *Arch. Gen. Psychiatry*, **50**, 853–62.

Kendler, K. S., Kessler, R. C., Neale, M. C., Heath, A. C. & Eaves, L. J. (1993b). The prediction of major depression in women: toward an integrated etiologic model. *Am. J. Psychiatry*, **150**, 1139–48.

Kendler, K. S., Karkowski, L. M. & Prescott, C. A. (1999). Causal relationship between stressful life events and the onset of major depression. *Am. J. Psychiatry*, **156**, 837–41.

Kendler, K. S., Thornton, L. M. & Gardner, Ch. O. (2000). Stressful life events and previous episodes in the etiology of major depression in women: an evaluation of the 'kindling hypothesis'. *Am. J. Psychiatry*, **157**, 1243–51.

Kessler, R. C. (1997). The effect of stressful life events on depression. *Ann. Rev. Psychol.*, **48**, 191–214.

Kessler, R. C. & Magee, W. J. (1993). Childhood adversities and adult depression: basic patterns of association in a US National Survey. *Psychol. Med.*, **23**, 679–90.

Kessler, R. C., Turner, J. B. & House, J. S. (1987). Intervening processes in the relationship between unemployment and health. *Psychol. Med.*, **17**, 949–61.

Kim, K. & Jacobs, S. (1995). Stress of bereavement and consequent psychiatric illness. In *Does Stress cause Psychiatric Illness?*, ed. C. M. Mazure. Washington, DC: American Psychiatric Press.

Krueger, R. F., Caspi, A., Moffit, T. E. *et al.* (1996). Personality traits are differentially linked to mental disorders; a multitrait–multidiagnosis study of an adolescent birth cohort. *J. Abnorm. Psychol.*, **3**, 299–312.

Labonte, E. & Paris, J. (1993). Life events in borderline personality disorder. *Canad. J. Psychiatry*, **38**, 638–40.

Leaf, R., Alington, D., Ellis, A., Digiuseppe, R. & Mass, R. (1992). Personality disorders, underlying traits, social problems, and clinical syndromes. *J. Pers. Disord.*, **6**, 134–52.

Maciejewski, P. K., Prigerson, H. G. & Mazure, C. M. (2000). Self-efficacy as a mediator between stressful life events and depressive symptoms: differences based on history of prior depression. *Br. J. Psychiatry*, **176**, 373–8.

Magnus, K., Diener, E., Fujeta, F. & Pavot, W. (1993). Extraversion and neuroticism as predictors of objective life events: a longitudinal analysis. *J. Pers. Soc. Psychol.*, **65**, 1046–53.

Malt, U. F., Robak, O. H., Madsbu, H.-P., Bakke, O. & Loeb, M. (1999). The Norwegian naturalistic treatment study of depression in general practice (NORDEP) – I: randomised double blind study. *Br. J. Med.*, **318**, 1180–4.

Mattlin, J. A., Wethington, E. & Kessler, R. C. (1990). Situational determinants of coping and coping effectiveness. *J. Health Soc. Behav.*, **31**, 103–22.

Mazure, C. M., Bruce, M. L., Maciejewski, P. K. & Jacobs, S. C. (2000). Adverse life events and cognitive-personality characteristics in the prediction of major depression and antidepressant response. *Am. J. Psychiatry*, **157**, 896–903.

McGonagle, K. A. & Kessler, R. C. (1990). Chronic stress, acute stress and depressive symptoms. *Am. J. Comm. Psychol.*, **18**, 681–706.

McGuffin, P., Katz, R. & Rutherford, J. (1991). Nature, nurture and depression: a twin study. *Psychiatr. Med.*, **21**, 329–35.

McGuffin, P., Owen, M. J., O'Donovan, M. C. *et al.* (1994). *Seminars in Psychiatric Genetics*. London: The Royal College of Psychiatrists.

McGuffin, P., Katz, R., Watkins, J. & Rutherford, J. (1996). A hospital-based twin register of the heritability of DSM IV unipolar depression. *Arch. Gen. Psychiatry*, **53**, 126–9.

Mcleod, J. D., Kessler, R. C. & Landis, K. R. (1992). Speed of recovery from major depressive episodes in a community sample of married men and women. *J. Abnorm. Psychol.*, **101**, 277–86.

McMiller P., Kreitman, N. B., Ingham, J. G. & Sashideran, S. P. (1989). Self-esteem, life stress and psychiatric disorder. *J. Affect. Disord.*, **17**, 65–75.

Mendlewicz, J. & Rainier, J. (1977). Adoption study supporting genetic transmission in manic-depressive illness. *Nature*, **268**, 326–9.

O'Leary, D. & Costello, F. (2001). Personality and outcome in depression: an 18-month prospective follow-up study. *J. Affect. Disord.*, **63**, 67–78.

Ormel, J. (1999). Depressie. De rol van levensgebeurtenissen, persoonlijkheid en erfelijkheid. In *Handboek stemmingsstoornissen*, eds. J. A. den Boer, J. Ormel, H. M. van Praag, H. G. M. Westenberg & H. d' Haenen. Maarssen: Elsevier/De Tijdstroom.

Ormel, J. & Wohlfarth, T. D. (1991). How neuroticism, long term difficulties, and changes in quality of life affect psychological distress. A longitudinal approach. *J. Pers. Soc. Psychol.*, **60**, 744–55.

Parker, G. (1993). Parental rearing style: examining for links with personality vulnerability factors for depression. *Soc. Psychiatry*, **28**, 97–100.

Parker, G., Holmes, S. & Manicavasagar, V. (1986). Depression in general practice attenders. 'Caseness', natural history and predictors of outcome. *J. Affect. Disord.*, **10**, 27–35.

Parker, G., Barrett, E. & Hickie, I. (1992). From nurture to network: examining links between perceptions of parenting received in childhood and social bonds in adulthood. *Am. J. Psychiatry*, **149**, 877–85.

Parker, G., Hadzi-Pavlovic, D., Greenwald, S. & Weissman, M. (1995). Low parental care as a risk factor to lifetime depression in a community sample. *J. Affect. Disord.*, **33**, 173–80.

Parker, G., Gladstone, G., Roussos, J. *et al.* (1998). Qualitative and quantitative analyses of a 'lock and key' hypothesis of depression. *Psychol. Med.*, **28**, 1263–73.

Paterniti, S., Niedhammer, I., Lang, T. & Consoli, S. M. (2002). Psychosocial factors at work, personality traits and depressive symptoms. *Br. J. Psychiatry*, **181**, 111–17.

Paykel, E. S. (1978). Contribution of life events to causation of psychiatric illness. *Psychol. Med.*, **8**, 245–53.

Paykel, E. S. & Tanner, J. (1976). Life events, depressive relapse and maintenance treatment. *Psychol. Med.*, **6**, 481–5.

Paykel, E. S. & Priest, R. G. (1992). Recognition and management of depression in general practice: consensus statement. *Br. Med. J.*, **305**, 1198–202.

Pearlin, L. T. (1989). The sociological study of stress. *J. Health Soc. Behav.*, **30**, 241–56.

Perris, C., Arrindell, W., Perris, H. & Eisemann, M. (1986). Perceived depriving parental rearing and depression. *Br. J. Psychiatry*, **148**, 170–5.

Post, R. M. (1992). Transduction of psychosocial stress into the neurobiology of recurrent affective disorders. *Am. J. Psychiatry*, **149**, 999–1010.

Poulton, R. & Andrews, G. (1992). Personality as a cause of adverse life events. *Acta Psychiatr. Scand.*, **85**, 35–8.

Raphael, B. & Middleton, W. (1990). What is pathological grief? *Psychiatr. Ann.*, **20**, 304–7.

Reynolds, C. F., Frank, E., Perel, J. M. *et al.* (1999). Nortriptyline and interpersonal psychotherapy as maintenance therapies for recurrent major depression. *J. Am. Med. Assoc.*, **281**, 39–45.

Roberts, S. B. & Kendler, K. S. (1999). Neuroticism and self-esteem as indices of the vulnerability to major depression in women. *Psychol. Med.*, **29**, 1101–9.

Ruscher, S. M. & Gotlib, I. H. (1988). Marital interaction patterns of couples with and without a depressed partner. *Behav. Ther.*, **19**, 455–70.

Rutter, M. (1987). Temperament, personality and personality disorder. *Br. J. Psychiatry*, **150**, 443–58.

Sakado, K., Sato, T., Uehara, T., Sakado, M., Kuwabara, H. & Someya, T. (1999). The association between the high interpersonal sensitivity type of personality and a lifetime history of depression in a sample of employed Japanese adults. *Psychol. Med.*, **29**, 1243–8.

Sakado, K., Kuwabara, H., Sato, T., Kehara, T., Sakado, M. & Someya, T. (2000). The relationship between personality, dysfunctioning parenting in childhood, and life time depression in a sample of Japanese adults. *J. Affect. Disord.*, **60**, 47–51.

Sargeant, J. K., Bruce, M. L., Florio, L. P. & Weissman, M. M. (1990). Factors associated with 1-year outcome of major depression in the community. *Arch. Gen. Psychiatry*, **47**, 519–26.

Sato, T., Sakado, K., Uehara, T., Narita, T. & Hirano, S. (1999). Personality disorder comorbidity in early-onset versus late-onset major depression in Japan. *J. Nerv. Ment. Disord.*, **187**, 237–42.

Segal, Z. V., Vella, D. D., Shaw, B. F. & Katz, R. (1992). Cognitive and life stress predictors of relapse in remitted unipolar depressed patients: test of the congruency hypothesis. *J. Abnorm. Psychol.*, **101**, 26–36.

Shea, M. T., Leon, A. C., Mueller, T. I., Solomon, D. A., Warshaw, M. G. & Keller, M. (1996). Does major depression result in lasting personality change? *Am. J. Psychiatry*, **153**, 1404–10.

Sievewright, N. (1998). *Personality Disorder and the Occurrence of Adverse Life Events.* Thesis, University of Nottingham.

Surtees, P. J. (1995). In the shadow of adversity: the evolution and resolution of anxiety and depressive disorder. *Br. J. Psychiatry*, **166**, 583–94.

Tellenbach, H. (1961). *Melancholy: History of the Problem, Endogeneity, Typology, Pathogenesis, Clinical Considerations.* Pittsburgh: Duquesne University Press.

Tennant, C., Bebbington, P. & Hurry, J. (1981). The short-term outcome of neurotic disorders in the community: the relation of remission to clinical factors and to 'neutralizing' life events. *Br. J. Psychiatry*, **139**, 213–20.

Thase, M. E., Greenhouse, J. B., Frank, E. *et al.* (1997). Treatment of major depression with psychotherapy or psychotherapy–pharmacotherapy combinations. *Arch. Gen. Psychiatry*, **54**, 1009–15.

Thoits, P. A. (1983). Dimensions of life events that influence psychological distress: an evaluation and synthesis of the literature. In *Psychological Stress: Trends in Theory and Research*, ed. H. B. Kaplan. New York: Academic Press.

(1986). Multiple identities: Examining gender and marital status differences in distress. *Am. Soc. Rev.*, **51**, 259–72.

Trull, T. J. & Sher, K. J. (1994). Relationship between the five factor model of personality and Axis I disorders in a nonclinical sample. *J. Abnorm. Psychol.*, **103**, 350–60.

Tsuang, M. T. & Faraone, S. V. (1990). *The Genetics of Mood Disorders*. Baltimore: Johns Hopkins University Press.

Van den Willige, G., Ormel, J. & Giel, R. (1995). Etiologische betekenis van ingrijpende gebeurtenissen en langdurige moeilijkheden voor het ontstaan van depressie en angststoornissen. Een nadere uitwerking. *T. Psychiat.*, **37**, 689–703.

Van Os, J. & Jones, P. B. (1999). Early risk factors and adult person-environment relationships in affective disorder. *Psychol. Med.*, **29**, 1055–67.

Van Os, J. & Marcelis, M. (1999). Nature and nurture in de psychiatrie: genetische epidemiologie. In *Handboek psychiatrische epidemiologie*, ed. A. de Jong, J. Ormel, W. van de Brink & D. Wiersma. Maarssen: Elsevier/De Tijdstroom.

Veroff, J., Douvan, E. & Kulka, R. A. (1981). *The Inner-American: A Self-portrait from 1957 to 1976*. New York: Basic Books.

Weissman, M. M., Gershon, E. S., Kidd, K. K. *et al.* (1984). Psychiatric disorders in the relatives of probands with affective disorders: the Yale University National Institute of Mental Health Collaborative Study. *Arch. Gen. Psychiatry*, **41**, 13–21.

Wender, P. H., Ketz, S. S., Rosenthal, D., Schulsinger, F., Ortman, J. & Lunde, I. (1986). Psychiatric disorders in the biological and adoptive families of adopted individuals with affective disorders. *Arch. Gen. Psychiatry*, **43**, 923–9.

Zlotnick, C., Kohn, R., Keitner, G. & Grotta della, S. A. (2000). The relationship between quality of interpersonal relationships and major depressive disorder: findings from the National Comorbidity Survey. *J. Affect. Disord.*, **59**, 205–15.

Zuroff, D. C. & Mongrain, M. (1987). Dependency and self-criticism: vulnerability factors for depressive affective states. *J. Abnorm. Psychol.*, **96**, 14–22.

Genetics of depression

5.1 Introduction

In the previous chapters, the role of genetic and nongenetic factors (e.g. life events, personality traits and chronic difficulties) in relation to the onset of depression was discussed. This leads to the question, which was already touched upon earlier: to what degree do genetic and nongenetic factors interact, that is, to what degree do they influence each other? In the two following chapters this question will be dealt with in more detail. First, the genetics of depression will be discussed. In the next chapter, we will specifically deal with the gene–environment interactions that are thought to underlie depressive illness.

5.2 Genetics of depression

5.2.1 Genetic epidemiology of depression

Mental health practitioners are used to thinking in terms of 'visible' environmental risks in relation to onset and persistence of psychiatric disorders. Stressful life events, chronic difficulties and dysfunctional parental interactions are but a few examples. Traditional psychiatric epidemiology was concerned mainly with such environmental risks. Conversely, clinical genetics was until recently almost exclusively concerned with Mendelian syndromes, for which single-gene defects could be mapped by positional cloning. Over the past decades, however, there has been increasing awareness that, for common psychiatric disorders, 'hidden' genetic factors can have a substantial influence on the effect of environmental exposures or even pose as risk factors. As genes can be considered as a conventional epidemiological risk factor in association studies (Sham, 1996), and epidemiological theory can be readily applied to genetically sensitive data sets (Susser & Susser, 1989; Ottman, 1990), epidemiologists and human geneticists have been gradually integrating their respective fields of research into a new discipline called genetic epidemiology (Khoury *et al.*, 1993). Within genetic epidemiology, the term *ecogenetics* refers to the study of specific gene–environment relationships such as gene–environment interaction and gene–environment correlation that will be described in the next chapter (Motulsky, 1977).

The unique feature of genetic epidemiology is that the genetic risk factors can be studied without direct measurement, by examining familial clustering of associated traits. These can be physically observable traits on the one hand (exophenotypes or simply phenotypes), such as motor retardation or low mood, or measurable biological traits (endophenotypes) on the other, such as plasma cortisol, nonsuppression on the dexamethasone suppression test or other traits described by Gottesman as 'data not available to the naked eye that are intermediate to the phenotype and the genotype . . .' (Gottesman, 1994). Thus, familial clustering of a disease phenotype can be demonstrated by studying the rate of disorder in the first-degree relatives of individuals with the disease (the probands), and comparing this with the rate of disease in first-degree relatives of controls. Twin studies, adoption studies and special types of family studies can subsequently be used to disentangle the respective roles of genes and environment in the causation of familial aggregation (Table 5.1). The principle of these studies involves comparisons in which either genetic similarity is varied randomly while environmental similarity is held constant, or vice versa. This can be accomplished through knowledge that certain family relationships are not as similar genetically or environmentally as others. For example, genetic effects can be traced by examining the degree of resemblance of reared-apart genetically identical twins (who share the same genes but not the environment), whereas familial environmental effects can be traced by examining the degree of resemblance of nongenetically related adoptive relatives (who share the same environment but no genes). The strength of this approach is that statements can be made on the relative contributions of genes and environments through inference, without the need of direct measurement. This is not to say, of course, that direct measurement of genes and environments is not desirable.

5.2.2 Molecular genetics of depression

With the advent of molecular genetic techniques, it has now also become possible to examine genetic variation at the molecular level, and to relate these to particular phenotypic outcomes. Molecular genetic studies are based on the principle that disease occurrence can be linked to a genetic marker of some sort. An *allele* is one of the alternative versions of a gene (such as the different alleles of the gene determining the colour of the flowers of Mendel's pea plants). If a gene has two or more alleles with a frequency of at least 1% in the population, it is customary to speak of a *polymorphism*. The *locus* is the position of the gene on the chromosome, which may thus be occupied by different alleles in different individuals.

Knowledge about the relative frequencies of the different alleles of such a polymorphism in diseased and nondiseased individuals in the same family can yield information about the location of genes that influence the risk of disease. For

Table 5.1. Most common types of studies in epidemiological and molecular genetics.

	Aims	Remarks
Family studies	Identification of familial aggregation of diseases Study of familial syndromal overlap Identification of biological markers of genetic transmission (endophenotypes) Study of interaction of familial with other biological/ social factors	Main advantage of family studies is the possibility of selection of epidemiological, representative samples yielding generalizable results. Main disadvantage is difficulty to separate genetic from environmental influences.
Twin studies		
Twins traditional	1 MZ vs. DZ similarity as a test of genetic aetiology 2 Quantification of contribution of genes and environment to phenotypic variance	MZ pairs may be treated more alike by their parents than DZ twins, which may contribute to the greater degree of phenotypic resemblance of MZ twins, and may inflate the associated heritability estimates.
Twins reared apart	Direct estimate of the magnitude of heritable effects	Furthermore, there is evidence that MZ twins are more similar than DZ twins with regard to important
Twins reared apart vs. twins reared together	Direct estimate of the magnitude of common rearing environment	risk factors for psychiatric disorders such as complications of birth and pregnancy, which may
Discordant MZ twins	1 Identification of nongenetic contributors to disease 2 Identification of correlates of disorder	also lead to spuriously high heritability estimates. Traditional twin methodology does not take into account assortative mating (which would tend to lower heritability estimates), and nonadditive gene effects and genotype–environment interactions
Offspring discordant twins	Confirmation of unexpressed genotypes	(which would tend to inflate heritability estimates). The generalizability of results obtained from twin studies to the general population is uncertain.

(*cont.*)

Table 5.1. (*cont.*)

	Aims	Remarks
Adoption studies		
Adoptee study	Resemblance between biological affected parents and adopted-away offspring indicates shared heredity	Adoptive parents are in the main a biased sample, having been screened by adoption organizations for elevated social stability and absence of mental disorder.
Adoptee rearing environment study	Variation of expression of disease in high-risk adoptees as a function of adoptive rearing environment indicates genotype–environment interaction	Biological parents of adoptees are a similarly biased sample, because of high rates of mental disorder and low level of social stability.
Adoptee's family study	Resemblance between affected adoptees and biological parents indicates shared heredity	Selective placement by adoption organizations according to ethnic, religious, socioeconomic status and other characteristics may introduce bias.
Cross-fostering study	Resemblance between affected adoptees with normal biological parents and affected adoptive parents indicates effect of rearing environment	
Molecular genetic studies		
Linkage studies	Making a statement about the likelihood of close physical proximity of disease and marker alleles by comparing the frequency of variants of a marker polymorphism in affected and unaffected members in groups of closely related individuals	Linkage studies are heavily dependent on unknown parameters such as gene frequencies and penetrance. Newer linkage methods using sib-pairs partly avoid such problems.
Association studies	Making a statement about the likelihood of close physical proximity of disease and marker alleles on the basis of a comparison of the frequencies of variants of a marker polymorphism in groups of cases and controls.	Linkage studies are suitable for detecting genes of major effect, whereas it is likely that psychiatric disorders in most families involve multiple genes of small effect. Association studies are simpler to carry out than linkage studies but are 'near sighted': they can detect genes of small effect, but only those that are very close to the marker. They are also prone to confounding but newer methods avoid this by using within-family control groups for allelic association analyses.

example, if in a large family with a high rate of disease X over several successive generations most of the diseased individuals have allele A of marker gene Y, whereas most of the nondiseased have allele B, it can be inferred that the locus of the disease gene is apparently so tightly linked (i.e. is very close) to the locus of the marker gene Y that their alleles (allele A and B for gene Y and the disease and nondisease alleles for the disease gene) are transmitted together (or co-segregate) most of the time in this family. Had this tight linkage not existed, then the alleles of marker gene Y and the disease gene would have been subject to the normal process of *recombination*, whereby new combinations of paternal and maternal alleles would have been created, and individuals with the disease would have displayed allele A as frequently as allele B. If linkage has been established and the site of gene Y is known, it can be inferred that the disease gene must be in close proximity to the locus of gene Y on its particular chromosome. This chromosomal region can then be characterized further with molecular genetic techniques to identify the genetic variation. Linkage thus refers to a relationship between loci on a chromosome, and can be examined by studying patterns of transmission within pedigrees of a few generations of multiply affected families.

The related term *association* refers to a relationship between alleles, which can be identified by comparing a group of affected individuals with a group of controls. The assumption here is that all cases come from the same ancestral family many generations ago, i.e. that they will share tiny segments of chromosomes that have 'survived' recombination. If, on these tiny segments, the disease allele lies near a marker allele, the cases will, in the case–control association analysis, have a statistically more than random chance of having this marker allele than the controls. In this case, allelic association has been established.

The discovery of polymorphic DNA markers throughout the genome and the development of efficient methods of genotyping have enabled the application of linkage and association analysis to the mapping of disease loci. This approach is called positional cloning because it is based on the estimation of genetic distances from the co-transmissions or co-occurrences of alleles, and not on knowledge of gene function. Positional cloning has been successful in mapping the genes responsible for hundreds of simple Mendelian diseases. However, application of this approach to complex disorders such as depression has so far been less successful; most initial reports of linkage have been weak and subsequently replicated in only a proportion of studies.

5.3 Genes and environment

Environmental and genetic influences on the phenotype can be divided into familial and nonfamilial components. Since the genes of an individual are always derived from the parents, nobody's DNA in a family is unique (i.e. genetic factors are

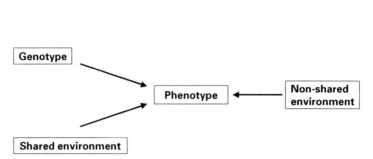

Figure 5.1. Factors influencing the phenotype.

always familial). However, environmental factors may be either shared with other relatives, or may be unique to the individual. For example, all the children in a family living together may share the same crowded housing conditions; these same children, however, may all go to different schools whose environments they do not share with their siblings. These familial and nonfamilial environmental and genetic influences on the phenotype are summarized in Figure 5.1.

Genetic and environmental influences predict both differences and similarities between relatives. Consider full siblings living in the same family. Such siblings who share on average 50% of their genes should resemble each other more on genetically influenced traits than individuals picked at random from the general population, who do not share the same genetic material. However, they should also *differ* from each other more than genetically identical twins, because full siblings also differ in 50% of their genes whereas identical twins share 100% of their genetic material. Similarly, genetic epidemiology predicts that individuals in the same family should resemble each other because they share a multitude of environmental influences (shared familial environment), such as parental social class, housing, parental illness and parental rearing practices. However, environmental influences on phenotypic variance also operate to make siblings *different* from each other, to the extent that the environmental factors are *not* shared with the sibling (nonshared environment). These include, for example, differential parental treatment, experiences at school, peer influences and personal illness or accidents.

5.4 The depression exophenotype

As explained above, phenotypes such as depression are the result of the influence of genotype and environment. However, phenotypes may be discrete (e.g. affected or not affected with hypertension) or continuous (e.g. blood pressure). In the case of a continuous phenotype, genetic and environmental influences are expressed as the degree to which phenotypic deviations from the mean (phenotypic variance) for some character in a population are a function of these environmental and genetic influences. In the case of discrete phenotypes, an underlying continuously distributed disease *liability* is assumed to exist, representing a quantitative measure of underlying vulnerability. The variance of this underlying liability can also be modelled as a function of environmental and genetic influences.

5.4.1 Depression as a discrete and a continuous trait

The depression phenotype can be characterized in a variety of different ways, which may have consequences for the outcome of genetic investigations. For example, the traditional view is to conceive of depression as a categorically defined qualitative (discrete) phenotype, that can be reliably assessed using DSM (American Psychiatric Association, 1994) or ICD (World Health Organization, 1992) criteria. However, depression can alternatively be conceived of as a quantitative (continuous) phenotype, i.e. as a characteristic that can occur along a continuum of severity in the general population with no clear qualitative distinction between cases and non-cases (Lewis & Wessely, 1990; Anderson *et al.*, 1993; Goldberg, 1996; Whittington & Huppert, 1996; Kessler *et al.*, 1997; Judd *et al.*, 1998; Kendler & Gardner, 1998; Angst & Merikangas, 2001; Preisig *et al.*, 2001).

5.4.2 Genetics of the qualitative phenotype

The estimated point prevalence of the qualitative phenotype varies between around 5–7% in studies using ICD criteria and 2–3% in studies using DSM criteria. The lifetime prevalence is, depending on the site and instrument used, between 5–12%, but may be higher than 15% according to more recent studies using sensitive instruments such as the most recent versions of the Composite International Diagnostic Interview (CIDI) (Kessler *et al.*, 1994; Bijl *et al.*, 1997). The prevalence is highest in women (about twice the risk of men after adolescence) and in the age group 25–45 years. Part of the age effect may be due to the fact that depression is getting more prevalent in each successive birth cohort after World War II, and therefore more prevalent in cohorts of younger people than in cohorts of older people (Burke *et al.*, 1991). This is referred to as the cohort effect in depression. The exact cause of the cohort effect is not known, but it is thought to represent changes in the prevalence of some underlying nongenetic risk factor for depression.

Family studies

Family studies are a powerful tool to demonstrate transmission of disease from one generation to the other, and the factors influencing that transmission. Depression tends to cluster in families (Slater & Cowie, 1971). Many studies have consistently shown that the lifetime risk of depression in the first-degree relatives of patients with depressive disorder (the familial morbid risk) is around 2–4 times higher than the general population risk (Rice *et al.*, 1987; McGuffin *et al.*, 1988; Sullivan *et al.*, 2000), and only a small part of this elevated risk can be explained by the fact that relatives of patients tend to seek help at an earlier stage because they have been 'sensitized' to the use of therapy (Kendler *et al.*, 1995a). An earlier age of onset in the patient (usually referred to as 'probands' in family studies) is associated with greater familial morbid risk (Weissman *et al.*, 1984, 1988; Bland *et al.*, 1986), although probands with onset in childhood do not appear to have higher familial rates of depression (Harrington *et al.*, 1997), and not all studies controlled for year of birth (i.e. excluded the cohort effect described above). A clinical feature of depression that is consistently associated with increased familial morbid risk is tendency to recurrence (Gershon *et al.*, 1986; McGuffin *et al.*, 1987, 1996). Relatives of probands with bipolar disorder also have a three- to four-fold higher lifetime risk of unipolar depression (Rice *et al.*, 1987), but relatives of probands with unipolar depression do not have a higher risk of bipolar disorder (Rice *et al.*, 1987), with the possible exception of relatives of postpubertal adolescent probands (Harrington *et al.*, 1997).

Twin studies

Family studies can only rarely be used to distinguish between, let alone quantify, genetic and cultural transmission. Twin studies and adoption studies are the main approaches towards separating and quantifying genetic and cultural transmission. The value of the three adoption studies of major depression is limited in view of their numerous methodological limitations to do with, for example, confounding by adoption and typically very small numbers (von Knorring *et al.*, 1983; Cadoret *et al.*, 1985; Wender *et al.*, 1986). However, a range of methodologically sound twin studies have been carried out in the last decade (Kendler *et al.*, 1995b, 2000; McGuffin *et al.*, 1996; Lyons *et al.*, 1998; Bierut *et al.*, 1999). Some of these studies were population-based (representative samples), whilst others were clinically based (more selected samples). Whilst results were similar for both types of studies, indicating substantial genetic effects on the liability to depression (Box 5.1), the results must be viewed with caution for a number of reasons (Box 5.2) (Goodman, 1991; Malhi *et al.*, 2000; Kendler, 2001; Rutter *et al.*, 2001). One critical argument is that there are very few twin studies that attempt to incorporate interactions between genes and environment, even though these interactions are believed to form the core of the aetiology of depression. If interactions between genes and environment are not included, estimations of the contributions of genes and environment to the liability of depression may be imprecise. In other words, any heritability estimate is highly dependent on the particular mix of underlying and largely unmeasured gene–environment relationships in that particular population (Van Os & Sham, 2002). This issue will be discussed in more detail in the next chapter.

Box 5.1. Summary findings of twin studies of depression.

1. Around 40% of the variance in liability to depression is due to the effect of genes, and may be as high as 70%.
2. Environmental influences that are aetiologically important are those that are specific to the individual (nonshared environment).
3. Environmental influences that are common to family members (shared environment) do not appear to contribute to the liability of depression: familial clustering is due to shared genes rather than shared environment. However, the shared family environment may contribute indirectly by influencing interpersonal relations, social support, and substance use/misuse.
4. Although the heritability in men and women appears to be of similar magnitude, the genes involved may be partly different.
5. The genes that influence depression may also, in part, influence the liability for other behavioural phenotypes such as anorexia, neuroticism, smoking, alcoholism and anxiety disorders.

Box 5.2. Possible criticisms on results of twin studies.

1. Twin models rarely include separate contributions of interactions between genes and environment, yet these interactions are at the base of most aetiological models of depression.
2. The absence of shared environmental effects is conceptually rather meaningless: all aspects of the shared environment can contribute to the aetiology of depression in as much as they will be interpreted uniquely (i.e. become nonshared environmental effects) by the person.
3. The absence of shared environmental effects is unlikely to apply to extremely adverse environments that are shared between siblings, such as a climate of abuse and neglect during development.
4. Twin studies have low statistical power to detect moderate to small contributions of the shared family environment on top of a large genetic contribution.
5. Identical, monozygotic twins may be more concordant for depression not because they share more of their genes than nonidentical, dizygotic twins, but because they are more likely to share environmental aetiological factors.
6. In comparison with singletons, twins are in many respects unique, and depression in twins may not be comparable to depression in singletons.

5.4.3 Genetics of the quantitative phenotype

Instruments exist from which a depression 'score' can be derived, consisting, for example, of the total number of depressive symptoms, with weightings for duration and severity (Lindelow *et al.*, 1997). A consistent finding is that when the

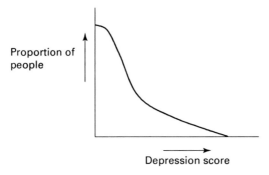

Figure 5.2.   Distribution of depression scores in the population. The half-normal distribution indicates that while the majority of people have none or minimal complaints, there is a continuous spread of more severe depressive states in the population.

distribution of such scores in the general population samples is plotted, the shape of the curve typically is half-normal (Figure 5.2). The half-normal distribution indicates that although the majority of people have none or only minimal depressive complaints, beyond this 'healthy' group there is a continuous increase in the number of depressive complaints over a significant segment of the population.

Although virtually all twin, family and adoption studies in depression have focused on the qualitative phenotype, epidemiological and genetic studies suggest that the quantitative phenotype may be the more valid one (i.e. closer to how the depression really exists in nature). In a recent study using a genetically sensitive design (a design in which it is possible to separate environmental and genetic effects), for example, it was shown that the milder, 'subsyndromal' forms of depression (i.e. not fulfilling formal DSM criteria) were continuous with the more severe syndromes fulfilling DSM criteria. A point of rarity separating subsyndromal and 'full' syndromes was not detectable, leading the authors to conclude that major depression, as articulated by DSM–IV, may be merely a diagnostic convention imposed on a continuum of depressive symptoms of varying severity and duration (Kendler & Gardner, 1998).

There have been few genetically sensitive studies of the quantitative phenotype. One study investigated the source of individual differences in self-reported depressive symptoms across two large twin samples and their families. The estimated heritability of depressive symptoms was 30–37%, i.e. in the same order as that reported for depressive disorder (Kendler et al., 1994). A twin study of depressive symptoms in childhood found evidence of substantial heritability, which increased with age (Thapar & McGuffin, 1994). However, these data do not shed light on the question whether the genes that contribute to the variation in depressive symptoms are the same as those that contribute to the liability of the dichotomously defined

DSM–IV depressive disorder. One twin study compared the contributions of genes and environment to the quantitative and the qualitative phenotype of depression. This study found that 70% of the variance in genetic risk factors and 24% of the variance in environmental risk factors was shared by a diagnosis of lifetime major depression and total depression symptom score on a self-report depression scale (Foley *et al.*, 2001). This study therefore suggests that much, but not all of the genetic influence to the quantitative and the qualitative phenotype is shared, whereas only a small proportion of the environmental variance is shared.

5.4.4 Genetics of the comorbid phenotype

The same genetic influence may impact on more than one phenotype (pleiotropy). There is evidence from various twin studies that the genes that contribute to the liability to depression also contribute, in varying degrees, to other behavioural phenotypes such as anorexia, smoking, alcohol dependence and, in particular, generalized anxiety disorder (Kendler *et al.*, 1993b; Kendler, 1996; Prescott *et al.*, 2000; Wade *et al.*, 2000). The results of a large multivariate twin analysis, in which the lifetime history of phobia, generalized anxiety disorder, panic disorder, bulimia nervosa, major depression and alcoholism was assessed and analysed simultaneously, suggested that the genetic influences on these six disorders were neither highly specific nor highly nonspecific. Neither a model that contained a discrete set of genetic factors for each disorder nor a model in which all six disorders result from a single set of genes was well supported (Kendler *et al.*, 1995c).

5.5 The depression endophenotype

As mentioned earlier, a promising approach in elucidating the aetiology of depression lies in the identification of associated biological traits, or endophenotypes, that are transmitted together with the depression exophenotype. For example, the well-known mood-lowering effect of tryptophan depletion can be used in the first-degree relatives of patients with depressive disorder in order to examine whether these individuals at high genetic risk have a similar, greater or lower response to tryptophan depletion. Several studies have suggested that individuals at enhanced genetic risk for depression have a greater reduction in mood after tryptophan depletion than controls (Benkelfat *et al.*, 1994; Klaassen *et al.*, 1999). Another, related line of work is that of pharmacogenetics (Steimer *et al.*, 2001). For example, there is work that suggests that the therapeutic response to certain antidepressant drugs tends to cluster in families in the same way as the depressive disorder itself (Tsuang & Faraone, 1990). Knowledge has been obtained in recent decades about the genetic basis of pharmacokinetic variability. Genetic tests suitable for the routine laboratory are now available for some important metabolizing enzymes, that aid in the identification of individuals who are slow or fast metabolizers of certain drugs. In comparison with the genetics of pharmacokinetics, the genetic basis of pharmaco-dynamic variability is less well studied. There have been reports, without consistent results, on serotonin transporter gene polymorphisms and their influence on the response to antidepressive therapy with SSRIs as a possible diagnostic tool in assessing the chances of response to the most popular group of antidepressants at present (Kim *et al.*, 2000; Weizman & Weizman, 2000; Serretti *et al.*, 2001).

5.6 The genetics of personality and depression

The personality trait neuroticism (N), representing stress-sensitivity or trait-anxiety, is a robust risk factor for depression (Parker, 1980; Fergusson *et al.*, 1989; Andrews *et al.*, 1990; Boyce *et al.*, 1991). Twin studies suggest that a large part of this association is due to the fact that a substantial part of the genetic liability to depression is shared with neuroticism (Eaves *et al.*, 1989; Kendler *et al.*, 1993a; Lauer *et al.*, 1997). This suggests that N reflects the familial liability for depressive disorder. Longitudinal cohort studies indicate that children who have high levels of N are more likely to develop depression as adults (Rodgers, 1990; Van Os & Jones, 1999). These data therefore suggest that it may be feasible to collect large samples of individuals at genetic risk for depression on the basis of their level of N, thus facilitating the search for the genes that contribute to depressive symptoms in the general population.

5.7 Development and genes

Support for a developmental hypothesis of depression (postulating that depression is the result of a cascade of developmental events) can be derived from the observation that the occurrence of depression is strongly age-dependent. Population studies examining the entire age range have shown that the rate of depression is much higher in the youngest age groups. For example, in the US National Comorbidity Survey, the 12-month prevalence of affective disorder in the age group 15–24 years was 67% higher, and the 12-month prevalence in the 25–44 year olds around 30% higher than in the age group 45–54 years. Such a dose–response relationship in the association between age and affective disorder in the general population suggests that the occurrence of affective symptoms continues to be related to underlying developmental processes. Although the mechanisms driving age-related variation in depression remain ill understood, there is some evidence that part of the association between age and depression may be related to age-dependent expression of risk genes. Thus, the genes that contribute to depression or to the risk factors of depression may not be 'switched' on until a certain age is reached. A recent twin study by Silberg and colleagues showed that the occurrence of life events, a well-established risk factor for depression, was partly under genetic control. In addition, however, their data suggested that the influence of genes on the occurrence of life events was not stable, but instead showed a developmentally related increase from pre-puberty to puberty (Silberg *et al.*, 1999). Thus, in as much as the risk factor life events is under genetic control, its impact may increase with age, resulting in higher rates of depression.

5.8 Molecular genetic findings

The combined evidence of family, adoption and twin studies suggests that a substantial part of the differences in vulnerability for depression in a given population are due to genetic differences. The relatively small number of molecular genetic studies conducted so far have not yielded consistent results, but work in a number of carefully selected samples using the continuous phenotype approach may yield results in the coming years (Boomsma *et al.*, 2000; Kirk *et al.*, 2000; Sham *et al.*, 2000).

5.9 Do environmental factors create enduring liabilities to depression?

In a review of psychosocial adversity in relation to psychopathology, Rutter makes the point that there is a need to shift attention to the role of psychosocial risk factors in the persistence and recurrence of disorders rather than the traditional study of life-event related precipitation of disease (Rutter, 1999). An interesting study from the developmental point of view is a 30-year longitudinal follow-up of 1824 adults who were recruited in the study as foetuses and on whom detailed information was available on pre- and perinatal events. Individuals who as children had lived in lower-income households had higher risks of reporting an emotional or nervous condition as adults, independent of income level as adults. In addition, there was evidence that the effect of birth problems, such as low birth weight, small for gestational age and pre-term delivery, on adult mental health was modified by the childhood social environment, in that the effect of birth problems on adult mental health was higher in those who were brought up in low-income households (Fan & Eaton, 2001).

Another possible developmental mechanism whereby social factors may create enduring liabilities is the effect of the wider social environment, such as the neighbourhood environment, on child and adolescent development (Leventhal & Brooks-Gunn, 2000). Thus, Kalff and colleagues studied child problem behaviour in 36 neighbourhoods of a medium-size city in the Netherlands. Children living in more deprived neighbourhoods had higher rates of problem behaviour, independent of individual-level measures of socio-economic status and other individual-level risk factors (Kalff *et al.*, 2000). Another study, conducted in the

US, similarly showed that lower neighbourhood incomes were associated with greater child psychological distress (Shumow et al., 1998). These studies therefore suggest that the wider social environment contributes to the onset of child problem behaviour. Such evidence may carry great significance for a developmental hypothesis of depression, because the onset of child problem behaviour in itself creates enduring developmental liabilities over time that contribute to adult illness onset and persistence. For example, Champion and colleagues showed in a 20-year follow-up of a sample of inner London school children that emotional or behavioural disturbance in childhood predicted a strong increase in the rate of severely negative events and difficulties some two decades later, independent of adult psychiatric disorder (Champion et al., 1995). Similarly, children with established psychiatric disorders were shown to have higher rates of behaviour-dependent severe events and major adversities than either a sample of community controls or a sample of patients with chronic physical illness (Sandberg et al., 1998).

5.10 Conclusion

Family, twin and to a lesser extent adoption studies all point towards a genetic influence on depressive disorder. However, this influence appears to be rather moderate and to date no replicable molecular genetic findings have been produced. Early onset and higher recurrence rate is associated with a greater risk in the relatives of patients. There is uncertainty as to what actually constitutes the depression phenotype. All studies also point to important environmental influences that may be accumulated over the developmental period to produce enduring liabilities in adulthood.

Given this state of affairs, the question now becomes to what degree depression is the result of the interplay of genes and environment rather than the effects of either factor alone. It is highly unlikely that genes are not sensitive to the effects of the environment and vice versa. In the next chapter, therefore, we will focus on the interplay of nature (genes) and nurture (environment) in the causation of depression.

REFERENCES

American Psychiatric Association (1994). Diagnostic Criteria from the DSM–IV. Washington, DC: APA.

Anderson, J., Huppert, F. & Rose, G. (1993). Normality, deviance and minor psychiatric morbidity in the community. Psych. Med., 23, 475–85.

Andrews, G., Stewart, G., Morris Yates, A., Holt, P. & Henderson, S. (1990). Evidence for a general neurotic syndrome. Br. J. Psychiatry, 157, 6–12.

Angst, J. & Merikangas, K. R. (2001). Multi-dimensional criteria for the diagnosis of depression. *J. Affect. Disord.*, **62**, 7–15.

Benkelfat, C., Ellenbogen, M. A., Dean, P., Palmour, R. M. & Young, S. N. (1994). Mood-lowering effect of tryptophan depletion. Enhanced susceptibility in young men at genetic risk for major affective disorders. *Arch. Gen. Psychiatry*, **51**, 687–97.

Bierut, L. J., Heath, A. C., Bucholz, K. K. *et al.* (1999). Major depressive disorder in a community-based twin sample: are there different genetic and environmental contributions for men and women? *Arch. Gen. Psychiatry*, **56**, 557–63.

Bijl, R. V., van Zessen, G. & Ravelli, A. (1997). [Psychiatric morbidity among adults in The Netherlands: the NEMESIS- Study. II. Prevalence of psychiatric disorders. Netherlands Mental Health Survey and Incidence Study]. *Ned. Tijdschr. Geneeskd.*, **141**, 2453–60.

Bland, R. C., Newman, S. C. & Orn, H. (1986). Recurrent and nonrecurrent depression. A family study. *Arch. Gen. Psychiatry*, **43**, 1085–9.

Boomsma, D. I., Beem, A. L., van den Berg, M. *et al.* (2000). Netherlands twin family study of anxious depression (NETSAD). *Twin Res.*, **3**, 323–34.

Boyce, P., Parker, G., Barnett, B., Cooney, M. & F. S. (1991). Personality as a vulnerability factor to depression. *Br. J. Psychiatry*, **159**, 106–14.

Burke, K. C., Burke, J. D., Jr., Rae, D. S. & Regier, D. A. (1991). Comparing age at onset of major depression and other psychiatric disorders by birth cohorts in five US community populations. *Arch. Gen. Psychiatry*, **48**, 789–95.

Cadoret, R. J., O'Gorman, T. W., Heywood, E. & Troughton, E. (1985). Genetic and environmental factors in major depression. *J. Affect. Disord.*, **9**, 155–64.

Champion, L. A., Goodall, G. & Rutter, M. (1995). Behaviour problems in childhood and stressors in early adult life. I. A 20 year follow-up of London school children. *Psychol. Med.*, **25**, 231–46.

Eaves, L. J., Eysenck, H. J. & Martin, N. G. (1989). *Genes, Culture and Personality*. New York: Academic Press.

Fan, A. P. & Eaton, W. W. (2001). Longitudinal study assessing the joint effects of socio-economic status and birth risks on adult emotional and nervous conditions. *Br. J. Psychiatry Suppl*, **40**, 578–83.

Fergusson, D. M., Horwood, L. J. & Lawton, J. M. (1989). The relationships between neuroticism and depressive symptoms. *Soc. Psychiatr. Epidemiol.*, **24**, 275–81.

Foley, D. L., Neale, M. C. & Kendler, K. S. (2001). Genetic and environmental risk factors for depression assessed by subject-rated symptom check list versus structured clinical interview. *Psychol. Med.*, **31**, 1413–23.

Gershon, E. S., Weissman, M. M., Guroff, J. J., Prusoff, B. A. & Leckman, J. F. (1986). Validation of criteria for major depression through controlled family study. *J. Affect. Disord.*, **11**, 125–31.

Goldberg, D. P. (1996). A dimensional model for common mental disorders. *Br. J. Psychiatry*, **168**, 44–9.

Goodman, R. (1991). Growing together and growing apart: the non-genetic forces of children in the same family. In *The New Genetics of Mental Illness*, ed. P. McGuffin & R. Murray. London: Butterworth-Heinemann.

Gottesman, I. I. (1994). Schizophrenia epigenesis: past, present, and future. *Acta Psychiatr. Scand. Suppl*, **384**, 26–33.

Harrington, R., Rutter, M., Weissman, M. *et al.* (1997). Psychiatric disorders in the relatives of depressed probands. I. Comparison of prepubertal, adolescent and early adult onset cases. *J. Affect. Disord.*, **42**, 9–22.

Judd, L. L., Akiskal, H. S., Maser, J. D. *et al.* (1998). A prospective 12-year study of subsyndromal and syndromal depressive symptoms in unipolar major depressive disorders. *Arch. Gen. Psychiatry*, **55**, 694–700.

Kalff, A. C., Kroes, M., Vles, J. S. H. *et al.* (2000). Neighbourhood-level and individual-level effects on child problem behaviour: a multilevel analysis. *J. Epidemiol. Community Health*, in press.

Kendler, K. S. (1996). Major depression and generalised anxiety disorder. Same genes, (partly) different environments – revisited. *Br. J. Psychiatry, Suppl*, 68–75.

Kendler, K. S. (2001). Twin studies of psychiatric illness: an update. *Arch. Gen. Psychiatry*, **58**, 1005–14.

Kendler, K. S. & Gardner, C. O. (1998). Boundaries of major depression: an evaluation of DSM–IV criteria. *Am. J. Psychiatry*, **155**, 172–7.

Kendler, K. S., Neale, M. C., Kessler, R. C., Heath, A. C. & Eaves, L. J. (1993a). A longitudinal twin study of personality and major depression in women. *Arch. Gen. Psychiatry*, **50**, 853–62.

(1993b). Major depression and phobias: the genetic and environmental sources of comorbidity. *Psychol. Med.*, **23**, 361–71.

Kendler, K. S., Walters, E. E., Truett, K. R. *et al.* (1994). Sources of individual differences in depressive symptoms: analysis of two samples of twins and their families. *Am. J. Psychiatry*, **151**, 1605–14.

Kendler, K. S., Kessler, R., Walters, E. *et al.* (1995a). Stressful life events, genetic liability, and onset of an episode of major depression in women. *Am. J. Psychiatry*, **152**, 833–42.

Kendler, K. S., Pedersen, N. L., Neale, M. C. & Mathe, A. A. (1995b). A pilot Swedish twin study of affective illness including hospital- and population-ascertained subsamples: results of model fitting. *Behav. Genet.*, **25**, 217–32.

Kendler, K. S., Walters, E. E., Neale, M. C., Kessler, R. C., Heath, A. C. & Eaves, L. J. (1995c). The structure of the genetic and environmental risk factors for six major psychiatric disorders in women. Phobia, generalized anxiety disorder, panic disorder, bulimia, major depression, and alcoholism. *Arch. Gen. Psychiatry*, **52**, 374–83.

Kendler, K. S., Myers, J. M. & Neale, M. C. (2000). A multidimensional twin study of mental health in women. *Am. J. Psychiatry*, **157**, 506–13.

Kessler, R. C., McGonagle, K. A., Zhao, S. *et al.* (1994). Lifetime and 12-month prevalence of DSM-III-R psychiatric disorders in the United States. Results from the National Comorbidity Survey. *Arch. Gen. Psychiatry*, **51**, 8–19.

Kessler, R. C., Zhao, S., Blazer, D. G. & Swartz, M. (1997). Prevalence, correlates, and course of minor depression and major depression in the National Comorbidity Survey. *J. Affect. Disord.*, **45**, 19–30.

Khoury, M. J., Beaty, T. H. & Cohen, B. H. (1993). *Genetic Epidemiology*. Oxford: Oxford University Press.

Kim, D. K., Lim, S. W., Lee, S. *et al.* (2000). Serotonin transporter gene polymorphism and antidepressant response. *Neuroreport*, **11**, 215–19.

Kirk, K. M., Birley, A. J., Statham, D. J. *et al.* (2000). Anxiety and depression in twin and sib pairs extremely discordant and concordant for neuroticism: prodromus to a linkage study. *Twin Res.*, 3, 299–309.

Klaassen, T., Riedel, W. J., van Someren, A., Deutz, N. E., Honig, A. & van Praag, H. M. (1999). Mood effects of 24-hour tryptophan depletion in healthy first-degree relatives of patients with affective disorders. *Biol. Psychiatry*, 46, 489–97.

Lauer, C. J., Bronisch, T., Kainz, M., Schreiber, W., Holsboer, F. & Krieg, J. C. (1997). Pre-morbid psychometric profile of subjects at high familial risk for affective disorder. *Psychol. Med.*, 27, 355–62.

Leventhal, T. & Brooks-Gunn, J. (2000). The neighborhoods they live in: the effects of neighborhood residence on child and adolescent outcomes. *Psychol. Bull.*, 126, 309–37.

Lewis, G. & Wessely, S. (1990). Comparison of the General Health Questionnaire and the Hospital Anxiety and Depression Scale. *Br. J. Psychiatry*, 157, 860–4.

Lindelow, M., Hardy, R. & Rodgers, B. (1997). Development of a scale to measure symptoms of anxiety and depression in the general UK population: the psychiatric symptom frequency scale. *J. Epidemiol. Community Health*, 51, 549–57.

Lyons, M. J., Eisen, S. A., Goldberg, J. *et al.* (1998). A registry-based twin study of depression in men. *Arch. Gen. Psychiatry*, 55, 468–72.

Malhi, G. S., Moore, J. & McGuffin, P. (2000). The genetics of major depressive disorder. *Curr. Psychiatr. Rep.*, 2, 165–9.

McGuffin, P., Katz, R. & Bebbington, P. (1987). Hazard, heredity and depression. A family study. *J. Psychiatr. Res.*, 21, 365–75.

McGuffin, P., Katz, R., Aldrich, J. & Bebbington, P. (1988). The Camberwell Collaborative Depression Study. II. Investigation of family members. *Br. J. Psychiatry*, 152, 766–74.

McGuffin, P., Katz, R., Watkins, S. & Rutherford, J. (1996). A hospital-based twin register of the heritability of DSM–IV unipolar depression. *Arch. Gen. Psychiatry*, 53, 129–36.

Motulsky, A. G. (1977). Ecogenetics: genetic variation in susceptibility to environmental agents. In *Human Genetics*, ed. S. Armendares & R. Lisker. Amsterdam: Excerpta Medica.

Ottman, R. (1990). An epidemiologic approach to gene–environment interaction. *Genet. Epidemiol.*, 7, 177–85.

Parker, G. (1980). Vulnerability factors to normal depression. *J. Psychosom. Res.*, 24, 67–74.

Preisig, M., Merikangas, K. R. & Angst, J. (2001). Clinical significance and comorbidity of subthreshold depression and anxiety in the community. *Acta Psychiatr. Scand.*, 104, 96–103.

Prescott, C. A., Aggen, S. H. & Kendler, K. S. (2000). Sex-specific genetic influences on the comorbidity of alcoholism and major depression in a population-based sample of US twins. *Arch. Gen. Psychiatry*, 57, 803–11.

Rice, J., Reich, T., Andreasen, N. C., Endicott, J., Van Eerdewegh, M., Fishman, R., Hirschfeld, R. M. & Klerman, G. L. (1987). The familial transmission of bipolar illness. *Arch. Gen. Psychiatry*, 44, 441–7.

Rodgers, B. (1990). Behaviour and personality in childhood as predictors of adult psychiatric disorder. *J. Child Psychol. Psychiatry*, 3, 393–414.

Rutter, M. L. (1999). Psychosocial adversity and child psychopathology. *Br. J. Psychiatry*, 174, 480–93.

Rutter, M., Pickles, A., Murray, R. & Eaves, L. (2001). Testing hypotheses on specific environmental causal effects on behavior. *Psychol. Bull.*, **127**, 291–324.

Sandberg, S., McGuinness, D., Hillary, C. & Rutter, M. (1998). Independence of childhood life events and chronic adversities: a comparison of two patient groups and controls. *J. Am. Acad. Child Adolescent Psychiatry*, **37**, 728–35.

Serretti, A., Zanardi, R., Rossini, D., Cusin, C., Lilli, R. & Smeraldi, E. (2001). Influence of tryptophan hydroxylase and serotonin transporter genes on fluvoxamine antidepressant activity. *Mol. Psychiatry*, **6**, 586–92.

Sham, P. (1996). Genetic epidemiology. *Br. Med. Bull.*, **52**, 408–33.

Sham, P. C., Sterne, A., Purcell, S. *et al.* (2000). GENESiS: creating a composite index of the vulnerability to anxiety and depression in a community-based sample of siblings. *Twin Res.*, **3**, 316–22.

Shumow, L., Vandell, D. L. & Posner, J. (1998). Perceptions of danger: a psychological mediator of neighborhood demographic characteristics. *Am. J. Orthopsychiatry*, **68**, 468–78.

Silberg, J., Pickles, A., Rutter, M. *et al.* (1999). The influence of genetic factors and life stress on depression among adolescent girls. *Arch. Gen. Psychiatry*, **56**, 225–32.

Slater, E. & Cowie, V. (1971). *The Genetics of Mental Disorder.* London: Oxford University Press.

Steimer, W., Muller, B., Leucht, S. & Kissling, W. (2001). Pharmacogenetics: a new diagnostic tool in the management of antidepressive drug therapy. *Clin. Chim. Acta*, **308**, 33–41.

Sullivan, P. F., Neale, M. C. & Kendler, K. S. (2000). Genetic epidemiology of major depression: review and meta-analysis. *Am. J. Psychiatry*, **157**, 1552–62.

Susser, E. & Susser, M. (1989). Familial aggregation studies. A note on their epidemiologic properties. *Am. J. Epidemiol.*, **129**, 23–30.

Thapar, A. & McGuffin, P. (1994). A twin study of depressive symptoms in childhood. *Br. J. Psychiatry*, **165**, 259–65.

Tsuang, M. & Faraone, S. D. (1990). *The Genetics of Mood Disorders.* Baltimore: Johns Hopkins University Press.

Van Os, J. & Jones, P. B. (1999). Early risk factors and adult person–environment relationships in affective disorder. *Psychol. Med.*, **29**, 1055–67.

Van Os, J. & Sham, P. (2002). Gene–environment interactions. In *The Epidemiology of Schizophrenia*, ed. R. M. Murray, P. B. Jones, E. Susser, J. Van Os & M. Cannon. Cambridge: Cambridge University Press.

von Knorring, A. L., Cloninger, C. R., Bohman, M. & Sigvardsson, S. (1983). An adoption study of depressive disorders and substance abuse. *Arch. Gen. Psychiatry*, **40**, 943–50.

Wade, T. D., Bulik, C. M., Neale, M. & Kendler, K. S. (2000). Anorexia nervosa and major depression: shared genetic and environmental risk factors. *Am. J. Psychiatry*, **157**, 469–71.

Weissman, M. M., Wickramaratne, P., Merikangas, K. R. *et al.* (1984). Onset of major depression in early adulthood. Increased familial loading and specificity. *Arch. Gen. Psychiatry*, **41**, 1136–43.

Weissman, M. M., Warner, V., Wickramaratne, P. & Prusoff, B. A. (1988). Early-onset major depression in parents and their children. *J. Affect. Disord.*, **15**, 269–77.

Weizman, A. & Weizman, R. (2000). Serotonin transporter polymorphism and response to SSRIs in major depression and relevance to anxiety disorders and substance abuse. *Pharmacogenomics*, **1**, 335–41.

Wender, P. H., Kety, S. S., Rosenthal, D., Schulsinger, F., Ortmann, J. & Lunde, I. (1986). Psychiatric disorders in the biological and adoptive families of adopted individuals with affective disorders. *Arch. Gen. Psychiatry*, **43**, 923–9.

Whittington, J. E. & Huppert, F. A. (1996). Changes in the prevalence of psychiatric disorder in a community are related to changes in the mean level of psychiatric symptoms. *Psychol. Med.*, **26**, 1253–60.

World Health Organization (1992). *The International Classification of Mental and Behavioural Disorders* (Tenth Revision). Geneva: WHO.

Gene–environment correlation and interaction in depression

6.1 Gene–environment relationships

As mentioned in the previous chapter, the term *ecogenetics* refers to the study of the interplay of genes and environment (Motulsky, 1977), the application of which to depression is relevant though still in the initial stages (Van Os & Marcelis, 1998; Malaspina *et al.*, 1999).

The models of gene–environment relationships presented below all assume that genetic and environmental factors increase the risk for depression, rather than reducing it. However, in the case of protective effects the underlying principles are the same, although some extensions of the models and their mathematical representations are sometimes necessary. Interaction between genes and environment means more than simply stating that both are involved in disease aetiology. There are several biological plausible mechanisms by which genes and environment can co-influence disease outcome (Plomin *et al.*, 1977; Kendler & Eaves, 1986; Khoury *et al.*, 1993; Ottman, 1996; Van Os & Marcelis, 1998).

6.1.1 Correlation: genes influence environmental exposure

A gene may increase the likelihood that a person becomes exposed to an environmental risk factor, which in turn increases the risk for depression. For example, liability to experience life events is influenced by genetic factors, especially controllable or dependent life events, that are within the influence of the person (Thapar & McGuffin, 1996; Kendler & Karkowski-Shuman, 1997; Saudino *et al.*, 1997). Thus, as far as life events are a risk factor for depression, part of the apparently environmental risk may be of genetic origin, and only part of it may be causal (Kendler *et al.*, 1999). Conversely, it can be envisaged that an environmental factor influences what genotype a person is going to have by influencing the rate of genetic mutations. This occurs, for example, when an environmental factor affects the rate of germline or somatic mutations in a population. These first two mechanisms are examples of what is called genotype–environment correlation. The term *correlation*

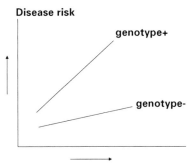

Figure 6.1.   Genotype–environment interaction: genetic control of sensitivity to the environment. In gene–environment interaction, the impact of the environmental exposure on disease risk depends on the co-presence of a certain genotype. In the example above, the effect of the environmental exposure on disease risk is much greater if the genotype is present than if the genotype is absent.

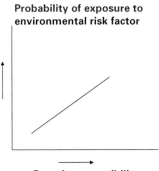

Figure 6.2.   Genotype–environment correlation: genetic control of exposure to the environment. In gene–environment correlation, the likelihood that a person becomes exposed to a certain environmental risk factor depends on the co-presence of the genetic risk factor. In the example above, the likelihood that a person becomes exposed to a certain environmental risk factor becomes greater with the degree of genetic susceptibility.

is used because if in the population the occurrence of E (the environmental risk factor) depends on the occurrence of G (the genetic risk factor) or vice versa, their prevalences will be correlated (Figure 6.1).

6.1.2 Synergism: genes and environment co-participate in the same cause

In genotype–environment *synergism*, the biological effects of G and E are dependent on each other in such a way that exposure to neither or either one alone does not result in disease, whereas exposure to both does. For example, a gene could influence the *sensitivity* to an environmental risk factor (Figure 6.2), or, conversely,

Table 6.1. Effects, measured on the additive scale, of the four exposure states occasioned by a genetic (G) and an environmental (E) risk factor for depression. For explanation see text.

Risk factor	G−	G+
E−	R	$R(G) - R$
E+	$R(E) - R$	$R(GE) - R$

an environmental factor could influence the effect of a genetic risk factor by controlling the degree of gene expression, or affecting epigenetic mechanisms such as DNA methylation (Petronis *et al.*, 1999). For example, it has been suggested that enduring changes in hypothalamic-pituitary-adrenal axis function, including corticotrophin releasing factor gene expression, may be implicated in the effect of early parental loss on human vulnerability to psychopathology, via alterations in responsiveness to stress (Agid *et al.*, 1999) (see Chapter 8). It is also possible that other nongenetic, stochastic (random) events during development affect gene expression (McGuffin *et al.*, 1994; Woolf, 1997). For example, exposure to high maternal cortisol levels during early development may influence expression of genes that modify later risk of depression.

Models describing gene–environment synergism

Describing a theory of synergism between genes and environment in nature is one thing, devising a statistical model which will aid us in quantifying such mechanisms in collected data is another. Let us assume that there are two risk factors for depression, one an environmental risk factor E, and one a single-gene risk factor G in the population. *Risk* is the proportion of individuals who get depression. If there are two risk factors G and E, there are four possible exposure states according to whether each factor is present or absent, and each of these four exposure states carry a specific risk. Thus, the risk for depression in the population exposed to E only is R(E) and the risk in the population exposed to G only is R(G). The risk of depression in the population exposed to neither E or G is R, whereas the risk in the population exposed to both G and E is R(GE). On the additive scale, the *effect* of a risk factor is expressed as a *risk difference*. For example, if R(G) is 0.25 and R is 0.10, the effect of G is $0.25 - 0.10 = 0.15$. We can thus express the effect of G as $R(G) - R$, the effect associated with E as $R(E) - R$, and the effect associated with the GE-exposure as $R(GE) - R$. Table 6.1 shows the effects associated with the four different exposure states.

As the combined effect of G and E is $R(GE) - R$, the excess of this over the sum of the solitary effects of G and E is:

$$[R(GE) - R] - [R(G) - R] - [R(E) - R] = [R(GE) - R(G) - R(E) + R]$$

If $[R(GE) - R(G) - R(E) + R] > 0$, G and E are said to interact on the additive scale. We will hereafter refer to $[R(GE) - R(G) - R(E) + R]$ as the *statistical additive interaction*.

How can we quantify the extent to which G and E act synergistically, that is in some way depend on each other, or co-participate, in disease causation? Let us consider the proportion of individuals in the population who developed depression after exposure to both G and E, or R(GE). It is possible that some of these individuals would also have contracted the disorder after exposure to either G or E alone. The degree to which some individuals would have also contracted the disorder after exposure to either G or E alone is referred to as the degree of *parallelism* (Darroch, 1997). If there is parallelism, G and E 'compete' to cause depression, and the more they compete, the smaller the proportion of individuals that contracted the disease because of the *co-participation* of G and E. Thus, parallelism can be thought of as the opposite of synergism. For example, in the extreme case of 100% parallelism where all individuals exposed to G and E had developed the disease because of the causal action of either G or E alone, no individual could have contracted depression because of the co-participation of G and E. In this case, the amount of synergism would be zero. In practice, it is impossible to assess the amount of parallelism and the amount of synergy in individuals exposed to both G and E. However, it can be shown that the amount by which synergism exceeds parallelism equals the excess of R(GE) over the sum of the solitary effects of G and E (i.e. the statistical additive interaction as shown above) (Darroch, 1997). In other words:

$$|synergism| - |parallelism| = [R(GE) - R(G) - R(E) + R]$$

Previous models of synergy tended to ignore parallelism and assumed that synergy was equal to the additive interaction (Rothman, 1986). However, assuming that parallelism does not exist may underestimate synergism. In practice therefore, the amount of synergy has to be approximated using the following equation (Darroch, 1997):

$$\frac{|synergism|}{R(GE) - R(E)} \quad \frac{|x2|}{|parallelism|} \quad \frac{R(GE) - R(G)}{R(G) - R}$$
$$\frac{|x1|}{} \quad \frac{}{R(E) - R}$$

The variables x1 and x2 are two unknowns that sum with synergism and parallelism to $[R(GE) - R(E)]$ and $[R(E) - R]$ respectively. For example, in the Virginia Twin Study, G was measured by diagnosis of depression in the co-twin (highest genetic risk: monozygotic twin, co-twin affected, lowest genetic risk: monozygotic twin, co-twin unaffected), E by the exposure to stressful life events, and the outcome variable consisted of monthly rate of onset of major depression (Kendler *et al.*, 1995). The risks associated with the depression outcome were respectively 0.5% and 1.1% for the group exposed to neither G nor E, and the group exposed to G only. R(E) was 6.2%, and R(GE) was 14.6%. Filling in these risks in the equation above results in the following estimates:

	synergism			x2		0.135
	x1			parallelism		0.006
0.084	0.057	0.141

It can be seen that |x2| must be between 0 and 0.057. Therefore |synergism| must be between 0.078 and 0.135. In other words, between 53% (0.078/0.146) and 93% (0.135/0.146) of depression cases exposed to both life events and genetic risk were attributable to the synergistic action of these two factors.

It is useful to estimate the fraction of cases attributable to the synergistic action of G and E. If the greatest proportion of depression cases exposed to G and E is due to the synergistic, co-dependent action of G and E, the incidence of depression could be reduced by targeting either G or E. However, if in the population exposed to both G and E the degree of synergism is small and parallelism is dominant, depression incidence could be reduced most effectively by targeting both G and E.

6.1.3 Genes and environment add to each other's effect

Some models of disease causation imply that there is no synergism. For example, an individual may get depression only if in possession of a certain type of vulnerability conferred by either genetic or environmental factors. An environmental factor could disrupt early brain development in the same fashion as a genetic mutation. If synergism is zero, the effect of genes and environment is said to be *additive*. As we have seen that

$$|synergism| - |parallelism| = \text{statistical additive interaction},$$

it follows that if synergism is zero, the statistical additive interaction equals − |parallelism| and is less than or equal to zero. Thus, if genetic and environmental risk factors act additively to cause disease, their joint effect equals the sum of their individual risks, after taking into account the negative effect of parallelism. It follows that if the data show that the statistical additive interaction is positive, G and E cannot act additively to cause depression, and some other model of disease causation involving synergism must apply. However, if the statistical additive interaction is zero, there may still be synergism if parallelism is not zero.

6.1.4 Genes and environment multiply each other's effects

Other disease models imply that there is no parallelism. For example, depression may be caused by genes and environment in multiple stages. The term stages in this context indicates that a disease, for example a certain type of cancer, always progresses from a precancerous stage, in which there are tissue changes that are clearly distinct from normality but also from the cancerous end stage, to the cancerous disease. If certain factors are necessary causes for the transition from normality to the precancerous stages and other factors are necessary for the transition from the precancerous stage to the cancerous end stage, the cancer in question is a disease that is caused in two stages. Under a two-stage model, the clinical manifestation of depression is the result of a second stage of disease, which can only be reached via a first stage. Genetic factors may influence risk for the first stage of disease, and the first stage only, whereas an environmental factor may influence risk for the second stage of disease, and the second stage only. Transition from stage one to depression can only take place after passing first from stage one to stage two, and stage two will only result in depression if it was first preceded by stage one. Under this model, G and E cannot 'compete' to cause disease, and therefore parallelism will be zero. If parallelism is zero, the additive statistical interaction will equal |synergism| and will therefore always be non-negative. In other words, if the additive interaction is negative, the multistage model cannot hold.

The multistage model is associated with a multiplicative model of disease causation. On the multiplicative scale, the effect of a risk factor is expressed as a *risk ratio*. Thus, the effect of G would be expressed as $R(G)/R$. For example, if $R(G)$ is 0.25 and R is 0.10, the effect of G is $0.25/0.10 = 2.5$. Under the hypothesis of a multistage model, it can be shown that the magnitude of the combined effect of G and E will be equal to the *product* of their individual effects. Thus, if the effect of G on depression is 10, and the effect of E is 2, the effect of their combined exposure will be 20. The importance of the multiplicative interaction lies not only in the possible underlying validity of the model of disease causation, but also in the fact that many of our standard statistical procedures (such as logistic regression analysis) are carried out on the multiplicative scale. Researchers presenting their results in terms of multiplicative risks should be aware of the underlying assumptions of disease causation and, for example in the case of the multistage model, their (bold) assumption that there is no parallelism.

6.2 Research findings on gene–environment interaction and correlation

6.2.1 Gene–environment correlation

There is evidence that many of the factors thought to represent environmental risks for depression are partly under the control of genetic factors. These include, apart from the life events mentioned above, substance use (Kendler & Prescott, 1998), exposure to certain pregnancy complications (Marcelis *et al.*, 1998) and head injury resulting from trauma and accidents (Lyons *et al.*, 1993; Matheny *et al.*, 1997). In the above-cited study of obstetric complications (Marcelis *et al.*, 1998), it was found that familial clustering for affective disorder increased the risk for exposure to an obstetric complication at birth. This would be a mechanism whereby the risk for environmental exposure leading to mental disorder in the offspring may be influenced by the affective disorder genotype in the parent. As environmental factors cannot be directly influenced by DNA, genetic control of exposure to such factors must be mediated by some characteristic of the person (Plomin, 1994). For example, the genetic influence on exposure to life events was shown to be mediated by personality traits such as neuroticism, extraversion and openness to experience (Saudino *et al.*, 1997), genetic control of exposure to obstetric complications could be mediated by liability to depression (Marcelis *et al.*, 1998), and accident-proneness may be associated with genetic factors through the personality trait sensation-seeking (Koopmans *et al.*, 1995; Jonah, 1997). As discussed in Chapter 4, it has been shown that part of the genetic liability to depression is expressed in the form of personality vulnerability traits, such as a high level of neuroticism (Fergusson *et al.*, 1989; Rodgers, 1990; Kendler *et al.*, 1993b). A high level of neuroticism has been shown to be associated with higher rates of controllable or dependent life event (Fergusson & Horwood, 1987; Kendler *et al.*, 1993a; Van Os & Jones, 1999; Van Os *et al.*, 2001), which in turn could facilitate the development of depressive symptoms. Thus, it can easily be envisaged that genotype–environment correlations play a significant role in the cascade of events leading to the development of depression. Indeed, a twin study showed that in women, genetic risk factors for major depression increase the probability of experiencing life events in the interpersonal and occupational/financial domains (Kendler & Karkowski-Shuman, 1997). Another example is that of head injury, which has been shown to be partly under genetic control (Lyons *et al.*, 1993; Matheny *et al.*, 1997) and also raises the risk of depression, even decades after the event (Holsinger *et al.*, 2002).

6.2.2 Gene–environment interaction

In humans, gene–environment interaction research has focused mostly on how genes may influence sensitivity to environmental risk factors (Figure 6.2). How the environment affects gene expression has been studied extensively in animals (for example see Kaufer *et al.*, 1998; Serova *et al.*, 1998), and is described in Chapter 8.

As no genes that increase the risk for depression have been unequivocally identified, gene–environment interaction studies necessarily have to do with proxy variables (i.e. variables that serve as an indirect indicator, for example family history as an indirect indicator of genetic risk) of not only genetic risk, but often also of the environmental risk factor, each of which has its particular problems (Table 6.2). Another problem common to studies of gene–environment interaction is that it is difficult to assess gene–environment interaction in the simultaneous presence of gene–environment correlation and that studies rarely are able to address this issue. This is because the assumption in mathematical models of gene–environment

Table 6.2. Studies of gene–environment interaction in depression.

Proxy genetic variable	Proxy environmental variable	Findings	Remarks
Positive family history (FH)	Experimental tryptophan depletion	Subjects with a FH more often had a lowering of mood following tryptophan depletion than subjects without a FH (Benkelfat *et al.*, 1994), suggesting genetic sensitivity to central serotonin depletion in depression	Not fully informative unless both environmental exposure status and clinical status is measured in both cases *and* all first degree relatives and analyses are adjusted for age, sex and number of relatives
	Stressful life events	Risk of major depression in relatives was 50% lower when the onset of depression in the patient was preceded by a severe life event (Pollit, 1972), suggesting existence of 'genetic' and 'environmental' subtypes of depression. Perris and colleagues were not able to replicate, however, and McGuffin and colleagues reported that the relatives of patients whose onset of depression followed life events or chronic difficulties had slightly higher lifetime rates of depression (Perris *et al.*, 1982; McGuffin *et al.*, 1988). Individuals with positive FH of depression were more sensitive to depression-inducing effects of stressful life events than those without, suggesting *synergism* between G and E (Phelan *et al.*, 1991).	Even then, however, the level of misclassification is likely to be high because many unaffected relatives may carry the high–risk genotype. Also not informative because *absence* of an association between positive FH and environmental exposure does *not* rule out gene–environment interaction, and *presence* of an association does not rule out *lack* of gene–environment interaction (Marcelis *et al.*, 1998). Experimental studies (e.g. tryptophan depletion) suffer to a lesser degree from these limitations than studies with observational environmental exposures (e.g. life events)

(*cont.*)

Table 6.2. (*cont.*)

Proxy genetic variable	Proxy environmental variable	Findings	Remarks
Having a parent with emotional disorder	Independent negative life event that did not show gene–environment correlation	There was no effect of independent life events on adolescents' depression in the absence of parental emotional disorder, but a significant effect in its presence, suggesting synergism between genes and life events	Findings suggest synergism between genes and life events. However, study used classification of genetic risk that was subject to considerable misclassification
Having an MZ (high risk) or a DZ (low risk) twin with depression	Stressful life events	In the group at lowest genetic risk, the probability of onset of major depression per month was 0.5% and 6.2%, respectively, for those unexposed and exposed to a severe life event. In those at highest genetic risk, these probabilities were 1.1% and 14.6%, respectively (Kendler *et al.*, 1995)	
MZ twin pairs are more concordant for depression than DZ twin pairs	Marital status	Having a marriage-like relationship acts as a protective factor in reducing the impact of genetic liability to symptoms of depression in the general population (Heath *et al.*, 1998)	The status of marriage-like relationship as an environmental factor is uncertain, but results are nevertheless encouraging Measures were obtained by questionnaire
Biological parent with alcoholism	Exposure to dysfunctional adoptive family environment	Major depression in females was predicted by an alcoholic diathesis only when combined with exposure to disturbed adoptive parent or sibling, suggesting the existence of a genetic factor is present for which alcoholism is at least a marker, and which exerts its effect in women as a gene–environment interaction leading to major depression (Cadoret *et al.*, 1996)	Children destined to develop depression may have contributed to dysfunctional family environment rather than the other way round Numbers were too small to show statistically significant effect of G × E

interaction is that there is no gene–environment correlation and vice versa in models of gene–environment correlation the assumption is that there is no gene–environment interaction. While some studies suggest the possibility of gene–environment interaction, it is clear that more new research and more replication research is needed. Unfortunately, the studies that have yielded the most convincing evidence so far cannot be replicated easily, with the possible exception of tryptophan depletion studies in first-degree relatives of patients (Benkelfat *et al.*, 1994). Once genes that increase the risk for depression have been identified, it will be possible to directly investigate interaction between genotype and environmental risk factors.

Recently, the first study showing gene–environment interaction using a direct measure of the genotype was presented. A functional polymorphism in the promoter region of the serotonin transporter (5-HT T) gene was found to moderate the influence of stressful life events on depression. Individuals with one or two copies of the short allele of the 5-HT T promoter polymorphism exhibited more depressive symptoms, diagnosable depression and suicidality in relation to stressful life events than individuals homozygous for the long allele (Caspi *et al.*, 2003 – see also p. 106). If replicated, this work would represent a major advance in elucidating the aetiology of depression.

6.3 Conclusion

Although research findings on gene–environment interactions and correlations remain scarce, the examples described in this chapter suggest that they are nevertheless common and of large effect. This in itself is a very important finding. As epidemiological studies are rarely, if ever, able to model specific gene–environment relationships, the question arises of how such underlying mechanisms distort our estimates of epidemiological parameters such as relative risk (RR) and the amounts of synergism and parallelism in individuals exposed to both G and E. At present, therefore, it is extremely difficult to interpret relative risk estimates from studies. For example, the effect size of recent life events on subsequent risk for depression may vary widely as a function of the underlying degree of gene–life event interactions.

Similarly, the consequences of GE interaction of family and twin studies have been examined recently by Guo (2000a,b,c). It was concluded that commonly used measures of genetic effects such as recurrence risk ratios for relative pairs, concordance rates for twins and heritability coefficients are functions not only of genetic effects and gene frequency, but also of environmental effects and the distribution of environmental factors, in the presence of GE interaction.

As discussed in the previous chapter, the discovery of polymorphic DNA markers throughout the genome and the development of efficient methods of genotyping have enabled the application of linkage and association analysis to the mapping of disease loci. The usual explanation for the lack of strong and consistent linkage findings is the limited power of linkage analysis to detect genes of small or modest effect. Although it is possible that gene effect is uniformly low in all populations, it is more likely that there are variations in gene effect according to the environment. In the presence of gene–environment interaction, the average effect of a gene may be small, but the actual effect may be quite high under certain environmental conditions. Thus, the existence of gene–environment interactions and correlations are one of the likely, yet largely ignored, reasons for the disappointing results of molecular genetic studies.

The more fundamental problem, as described in Chapter 1, is that commonly depression is modelled as a categorical disease, whereas the scientific evidence suggests that underlying dimensions of personality and depressive symptoms may be more suitable representations of the depression phenotype. As described in Chapter 9, underlying functional variation in the regulation of anxiety, aggression and mood may ultimately represent the valid phenotypic targets for the study of the co-actions of genes and environment.

More intensive use of research designs that can elucidate these interactions will enhance our understanding of the pathways of risk leading to onset and persistence of psychiatric illness in the general population. Without this knowledge, our understanding of what drives the variation of depression in the general population must remain incomplete.

REFERENCES

Agid, O., Shapira, B., Zislin, J. et al. (1999). Environment and vulnerability to major psychiatric illness: a case control study of early parental loss in major depression, bipolar disorder and schizophrenia. Mol. Psychiatry, 4, 163–72.

Benkelfat, C., Ellenbogen, M. A., Dean, P. et al. (1994). Mood-lowering effect of tryptophan depletion: enhanced susceptibility in young men at genetic risk for major affective disorders. Arch. Gen. Psychiatry, 51, 687–97.

Cadoret, R. J., Winokur, G., Langbehn, D., Troughton, E., Yates, W. R. & Stewart, M. A. (1996). Depression spectrum disease, I: The role of gene–environment interaction. Am. J. Psychiatry, 153, 892–9.

Caspi, A., Sugden, K., Moffitt, T. E. et al. (2003). Influence of life stress on depression: moderation by a polymorphism in the 5-HTT gene. Science, 301, 386–9.

Darroch, J. (1997). Biologic synergism and parallelism. Am. J. Epidemiol., 145, 661–8.

Fergusson, D. M. & Horwood, L. J. (1987). Vulnerability to life events exposure. Psychol. Med., 17, 739–49.

Fergusson, D. M., Horwood, L. J. & Lawton, J. M. (1989). The relationships between neuroticism and depressive symptoms. Soc. Psychiatry Epidemiol., 24, 275–81.

Guo, S. W. (2000a). Familial aggregation of environmental risk factors and familial aggregation of disease. *Am. J. Epidemiol.*, **151**, 1121–31.

(2000b). Gene–environment interaction and the mapping of complex traits: some statistical models and their implications. *Hum. Hered.*, **50**, 286–303.

(2000c). Gene–environment interactions and the affected-sib-pair designs. *Hum. Hered.*, **50**, 271–85.

Heath, A. C., Eaves, L. J. & Martin, N. G. (1998). Interaction of marital status and genetic risk for symptoms of depression. *Twin Res.*, **1**, 119–22.

Holsinger, T., Steffens, D. C., Phillips, C. *et al.* (2002). Head injury in early adulthood and the lifetime risk of depression. *Arch. Gen. Psychiatry*, **59**, 17–22.

Jonah, B. A. (1997). Sensation seeking and risky driving: a review and synthesis of the literature. *Accid. Analysis Prev.*, **29**, 651–65.

Kaufer, D., Friedman, A., Seidman, S. & Soreq, H. (1998). Acute stress facilitates long-lasting changes in cholinergic gene expression. *Nature*, **393**, 373–7.

Kendler, K. S. & Eaves, L. J. (1986). Models for the joint effect of genotype and environment on liability to psychiatric illness. *Am. J. Psychiatry*, **143**, 279–89.

Kendler, K. S. & Karkowski-Shuman, L. (1997). Stressful life events and genetic liability to major depression: genetic control of exposure to the environment? *Psychol. Med.*, **27**, 539–47.

Kendler, K. S. & Prescott, C. A. (1998). Cannabis use, abuse, and dependence in a population-based sample of female twins. *Am. J. Psychiatry*, **155**, 1016–22.

Kendler, K. S., Neale, M., Kessler, R., Heath, A. & Eaves, L. (1993a). A twin study of recent life events and difficulties. *Arch. Gen. Psychiatry*, **50**, 789–96.

(1993b). A longitudinal twin study of personality and major depression in women. *Arch. Gen. Psychiatry*, **50**, 853–62.

Kendler, K. S., Kessler, R. C., Walters, E. E. *et al.* (1995). Stressful life events, genetic liability, and onset of an episode of major depression in women. *Am. J. Psychiatry*, **152**, 833–42.

Kendler, K. S., Karkowski, L. M. & Prescott, C. A. (1999). Causal relationship between stressful life events and the onset of major depression. *Am. J. Psychiatry*, **156**, 837–41.

Khoury, M. J., Beaty, T. H. & Cohen, B. H. (1993). *Genetic Epidemiology.* Oxford: Oxford University Press.

Koopmans, J. R., Boomsma, D. I., Heath, A. C. & van Doornen, L. J. (1995). A multivariate genetic analysis of sensation seeking. *Behav. Genet.*, **25**, 349–56.

Lyons, M. J., Goldberg, J., Eisen, S. A. *et al.* (1993). Do genes influence exposure to trauma? A twin study of combat. *Am. J. Med. Genet.*, **48**, 22–7.

Malaspina, D., Sohler, N. & Susser, E. S. (1999). Interaction of genes and prenatal exposures in schizophrenia. In *Prenatal Exposures in Schizophrenia*, ed. E. S. Susser, A. S. Brown & J. M. Gorman. Washington, DC: American Psychiatric Press.

Marcelis, M., van Os, J., Sham P. *et al.* (1998). Obstetric complications and familial morbid risk of psychiatric disorders. *Am. J. Med. Genet.*, **81**, 29–36.

Matheny, A. P., Jr., Brown, A. M. & Wilson, R. S. (1997). Behavioral antecedents of accidental injuries in early childhood: a study of twins. 1971. *Injury Prev.*, **3**, 144–5.

McGuffin, P., Katz, R. & Bebbington, P. E. (1988). The Camberwell Collaborative Depression Study: III. Depression and adversity in the relatives of depressed probands. *Br. J. Psychiatry*, **152**, 775–82.

McGuffin, P., Asherson, P., Owen, M. & Farmer, A. (1994). The strength of the genetic effect. Is there room for an environmental influence in the aetiology of schizophrenia? *Br. J. Psychiatry*, **164**, 593–9.

Motulsky, A. G. (1977). Ecogenetics: genetic variation in susceptibility to environmental agents. *Human Genetics*, ed. S. Armendares & R. Lisker. Amsterdam: Excerpta Medica.

Ottman, R. (1996). Gene–environment interaction: definitions and study designs. *Prev. Med.*, **25**, 764–70.

Perris, H., von Knorring, L. & Perris, C. (1982). Genetic vulnerability for depression and life events. *Neuropsychobiology*, **8**, 241–7.

Petronis, A., Paterson, A. D. & Kennedy, J. L. (1999). Schizophrenia: an epigenetic puzzle? *Schizophr. Bull.*, **25**, 639–55.

Phelan, J., Schwartz, J. E., Bromet, E. J. *et al.* (1991). Work stress, family stress and depression in professional and managerial employees. *Psychol. Med.*, **21**, 999–1012.

Plomin, R. (1994). *Genetics and Experience.* London: Sage.

Plomin, R., DeFries, J. C. & Loehlin, J. C. (1977). Genotype–environment interaction and correlation in the analysis of human behavior. *Psychol. Bull.*, **84**, 309–22.

Pollitt, J. (1972). The relationship between genetic and precipitating factors in depressive illness. *Br. J. Psychiatry*, **121**, 67–70.

Rodgers, B. (1990). Behaviour and personality in childhood as predictors of adult psychiatric disorder. *J. Child Psychol. Psychiatry*, **3**, 393–414.

Rothman, K. J. (1986). *Modern Epidemiology.* Boston, MA: Little, Brown and Company.

Saudino, K. J., McClearn, G. E., Pedersen, N. L., Lichtenstein, P. & Plomin, R. (1997). Can personality explain genetic influences on life events? *J. Pers. Soc. Psychol.*, **72**, 196–206.

Serova, L., Sabban, E. L., Zangen, A., Overstreet, D. H. & Yadid, G. (1998). Altered gene expression for catecholamine biosynthetic enzymes and stress response in rat genetic model of depression. *Brain Res. Mol. Brain Res.*, **63**, 133–8.

Thapar, A. & McGuffin, P. (1996). Genetic influences on life events in childhood. *Psychol. Med.*, **26**, 813–20.

Van Os, J. & Jones, P. B. (1999). Early risk factors and adult person–environment relationships in affective disorder. *Psychol. Med.*, **29**, 1055–67.

Van Os, J. & Marcelis, M. (1998). The ecogenetics of schizophrenia: a review. *Schizophr. Res.*, **32**, 127–35.

Van Os, J., Park, S. B. & Jones, P. B. (2001). Neuroticism, life events and mental health: evidence for person–environment correlation. *Br. J. Psychiatry Suppl*, **40**, s72–7.

Woolf, C. M. (1997). Does the genotype for schizophrenia often remain unexpressed because of canalization and stochastic events during development? *Psychol. Med.*, **27**, 659–68.

Monoamines and depression

7.1 The beginnings

Systematic research into the biological determinants of depression started in the late 1950s with the introduction of the antidepressants (Van Praag, 1977). From their introduction in 1958 on, it was clear that the monoamine oxidase inhibitors (MAO I) were interfering with the degradation of monoamines (MA) – such as serotonin (5-hydroxytryptamine, 5-HT), noradrenaline (NA) and dopamine (DA) – and thus in all likelihood exerted an influence on the functioning of MA ergic systems in the brain. The second group of antidepressants, the tricyclic antidepressants (TCAs), was introduced about the same time as the MAO I. A few years afterwards, it was discovered that these compounds, too, exercise a pronounced influence on the MA ergic system, by inhibiting the reuptake of 5-HT and NA in the presynaptic nerve terminals. Both mechanisms – inhibition of MA degradation and of MA reuptake – will facilitate MA ergic transmission. Other groups of antidepressants, developed subsequently, all appeared to exert effects leading to the same final common path: activation of MA ergic transmission.

Based on these findings, the question arose whether MA ergic dysfunction in the brain might play a role in the pathophysiology of depression, particularly in those mood disorders that respond favourably to this type of treatment. These considerations set in motion an abundance of MA research in depression, an endeavour starting in the late 1950s and continuing to this day (Honig & van Praag, 1997).

A second domain of intense biological depression research concerns the hypothalamic–pituitary–adrenal (HPA) axis (Holsboer, 2000). Systematic study of diurnal cortisol secretion revealed increased plasma level of cortisol and increased urinary cortisol excretion in a subgroup of depression (Sachar *et al.*, 1973). In addition, suppression of cortisol secretion by the synthetic glucocorticosteroid dexamethasone can be defective (Carroll *et al.*, 1976). Both hypercortisolaemia and dexamethasone nonsuppression pointed to an overactive HPA axis. This conclusion was confirmed by the finding of increased production of corticotrophin releasing hormone (CRH) in the hypothalamus. These findings marked the beginning of an intensive search for the role of CRH and corticosteroids in the pathogenesis of depression (see Chapter 8).

The CRH/HPA and the MA ergic systems have been the main foci of biological depression research over the past four decades. The forthcoming chapters will be restricted to these two lines of research. Only the main findings will be discussed: in this chapter those related to the MA ergic systems, in Chapter 8 the CRH/cortisol data. The issues to be raised are the following:

– Can MA-ergic systems be disturbed in depression?
– How does stress influence the CRH and HPA systems?
– Does stress/CRH overdrive/cortisol overproduction lead to MA ergic disturbances in the brain, and if so are those similar to the ones that may be found in depression?

If the latter would be the case, this would strongly support the notion that stress might indeed *cause* depression.

7.2 Serotonin and depression

In a subgroup of patients with mood disorders disturbances in the MA ergic systems have been ascertained. They relate to the *metabolism* of MA and to the functioning of MA *receptors*.

7.2.1 Localization of serotonergic circuits

The cell bodies of 5-HT ergic neurons are located in a restricted area, i.e. the raphe nuclei located in the midbrain and the upper part of the medulla oblongata. The latter nuclei (n. raphe pallidus and obscurus) give rise to axonal projections innervating the medulla oblongata and spinal cord. The nuclei located in the mesencephalon (n. raphe dorsalis; n. raphe medianus and n. centralis superior), send their axons upward to almost all parts of the cortex cerebri and upper brain stem. Projections from both sets of nuclei, however, broadly overlap. The almost ubiquitous presence of 5-HT ergic terminals makes it understandable why it is that this system is involved in the regulation of so many psychological and physiological functions.

7.2.2 Serotonin metabolism

The major degradation product of 5-HT, 5-hydroxyindoleacetic acid (5-HIAA), is found in the cerebrospinal fluid (CSF) as well as in the brain itself. 5-HIAA in lumbar CSF originates partly in the brain, partly in the spinal cord. However, both animal studies (Mignot *et al.*, 1985) and human (postmortem) studies (Stanley *et al.*, 1985) have revealed a close correlation between brain and CSF 5-HIAA.

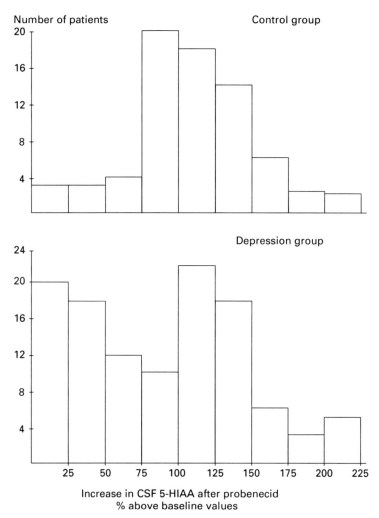

Figure 7.1. Increase of CSF 5-HIAA concentration after probenecid in patients suffering from major depression, melancholic type (bottom) and in a nondepressed control group (top). The columns indicate the number of patients showing the increase in concentration given at the bottom of the column. The distribution in the depression group is bimodal. There is a significant increase in individuals with low CSF 5-HIAA (Van Praag, 1982).

Furthermore the 5-HIAA concentration in the brain is to a large extent a function of 5-HT metabolism. Therefore CSF 5-HIAA can be considered as an indicator (albeit a crude indicator) of 5-HT metabolism in (certain parts of) the brain.

Several studies reported that in (a subgroup of) depression the CSF concentration of 5-HIAA is lower than in a nondepressed control group (Figure 7.1). This applied both to baseline and to post-probenecid concentrations (Van Praag et al., 1970;

Table 7.1. Data indicative of disturbed 5-HT metabolism in (a subgroup of) depression.

Low CSF 5-HIAA

Many antidepressants and electroconvulsive treatment increase the efficiency of 5-HT ergic
transmission

Tryptophan depletion may lead to mood lowering

Treatment with 5-hydroxytryptophan (5-HTP) may have antidepressant effects

Reduced plasma levels of tryptophan

Decreased uptake of 5-HTP into the CNS

Decreased trapping of alpha-$[^{11}C]$ methyl-l-tryptophan into the synthesis of 5-HT

Van Praag & Korf, 1971a,b; Åsberg *et al.*, 1976). Probenecid is a blocker of 5-HIAA
transport from the CSF to the bloodstream. The rise of 5-HIAA concentration in
CSF after probenecid is (again, a crude) indicator of the production rate of 5-HIAA
in the brain (Korf & Van Praag, 1971).

Low baseline and post-probenecid CSF 5-HIAA suggest a diminution of 5-HT
metabolism in the central nervous system (CNS). Subsequently this tentative conclusion was supported by several lines of evidence (Table 7.1). First, the abundant
data that the various classes of antidepressants, as well as electroconvulsive treatment, improve the efficiency of 5-HT ergic transmission, particularly of 5-HT$_{1A}$
receptor-mediated transmission. This happens either by sensitization of postsynaptic receptors or by desensitization of presynaptic receptors that normally reduce the
release of 5-HT in the synaptic cleft or inhibit the firing rate of the 5-HT nerve cell
(Blier & de Montigny, 1994).

A second group of data is derived from the so-called tryptophan-depletion strategy (Young *et al.*, 1985). Tryptophan is an essential amino acid and the precursor of
5-HT. A shortage of tryptophan will lead to a deficiency of 5-HT. Such a shortage
can be generated by ingesting a mixture of amino acids, devoid of tryptophan and
rich in competing amino acids, i.e. amino acids competing with tryptophan for
the same transport mechanism from the bloodstream into the CNS. This leads to a
rapid decrease of tryptophan in the bloodstream (Delgado *et al.*, 1990), lowering of
5-HIAA in the CSF (Williams *et al.*, 1999) and, in animals, to substantial lowering
of brain 5-HT (Moja *et al.*, 1989).

Applied to normal volunteers this procedure leads to the occurrence of mood
lowering (Young *et al.*, 1985), in particular in those individuals with a family history
of depression (but without having gone through depressive episodes themselves)
(Benkelfat *et al.*, 1994; Klaassen *et al.*, 1999a,b) (Figure 7.2). Patients in remission
from an episode of major depression, who responded to tryptophan depletion with
mood lowering, showed an increased relapse risk in the next 12 months (Moreno
et al., 2000). Depletion of 5-HT but not of NA induces a relapse in depressed

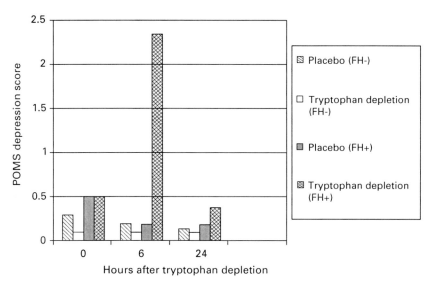

Figure 7.2.   Effect of tryptophan depletion on mood, in normal individuals with or without positive family history for depression. Tryptophan depletion generates pronounced mood lowering for a brief period (Klaassen et al., 1999a,b). FH = family history.

patients in remission after treatment with 5-HT specific antidepressants (Delgado & Moreno, 2000). Conversely, treatment with the 5-HT precursor 5-HTP, in combination with a peripheral decarboxylase inhibitor, led to amelioration of depression, in particular in patients with low CSF 5-HIAA (Van Praag & de Haan, 1980a,b) (Table 7.2).

Furthermore (some) depressed patients exhibit reduced tryptophan availability in plasma (Maes et al., 1990), reduced increase in plasma 5-HTP after an oral load with l-tryptophan (Deakin et al., 1990) and decreased uptake of 5-HTP across the blood–brain barrier (Agren et al., 1991; Agren & Reibring, 1994). These data, too, suggest a defect in the synthesis of 5-HT.

Direct measurement of 5-HT synthetic capacity is presently possible by positron emission tomography (PET), measuring the trapping of the tracer α-$[^{11}C]$methyl-l-tryptophan (α-MTrp) into the synthesis of 5-HT. α-MTrp is a synthetic analog of l-tryptophan. Its methyl group prevents incorporation of the tracer in protein metabolism (Diksic et al., 1990), but does not interfere with its incorporation in the synthesis of 5-HT. The rate of trapping of α-MTrp is considered to be an index of 5-HT synthetic capacity (Chugani & Muzig, 2000). Low 5-HT synthesis capacity has been found in impulsive subjects with borderline personality disorder (Leyton et al., 2001), a disorder often complicated by depressive symptoms, as well as in depression in particular in those patients with high impulsivity (Benkelfat et al., 2002).

Table 7.2. Number of patients who relapsed, and number of relapses, during placebo and 5-hydroxytryptophan (5-HTP) periods (van Praag & de Haan 1980a,b).

The difference in relapse rate is statistically significant both in group A ($P < 0.005$, sign test; $P < 0.05$, McNemar test) and in group B ($P < 0.005$, sign test; $P < 0.005$, McNemar test).

		No. of patients who relapsed		No. of relapses	
		Placebo period	5-HTP period	Placebo period	5-HTP period
Group A[a]	($n = 10$)	9	3	14	3
Group B[b]	($n = 10$)	8	3	10	4

[a] 1 year of 5-HTP medication, followed by 1 year of placebo medication.
[b] 1 year of placebo medication, followed by 1 year of 5-HTP medication.

Interestingly, lowering of CSF 5-HIAA in a subgroup of depression appears to be a trait-related phenomenon: it does not disappear after remission of the depression (Van Praag 1977a,b, 1992; Träskman-Bendz et al., 1984) (Figure 7.3). Marginal 5-HT production possibly represents a vulnerability factor, increasing the risk of depression in times of mounting stress (Van Praag, 1988). This hypothesis is supported by the finding that treatment with l-5-HTP, a 5-HT precursor the brain readily transforms into 5-HT, has therapeutic and prophylactic efficacy in depression, in particular in those with signs of deficient 5-HT metabolism (Van Praag & de Haan, 1980a,b) (Table 7.2).

7.2.3 In vivo receptor studies
5-HT receptors and depression

The 5-HT system operates via a great number, at least 15, probably function-specific receptors. They are subdivided in 7 subtypes, named 5-HT$_1$, 5-HT$_2$ . . . . . 5-HT$_7$ receptors. The 5-HT$_1$ receptor family is subdivided into 4 subgroups: 5-HT$_{1A}$ up to 5-HT$_{1D}$, the 5-HT$_2$ family counts 3 subtypes: 5-HT$_{2A}$ up to 5-HT$_{2C}$ receptors.

5-HT$_{1A}$ receptors are located both pre- and postsynaptically. The presynaptic 5-HT$_{1A}$ receptor is located on the cell bodies and involved in negative feedback regulation of the 5-HT neuron. Its activation leads to reduction of its firing rate. The 5-HT$_{1D}$ receptor (analogous with the 5-HT$_{1B}$ receptor in rodents) is also found pre- and postsynaptically. The presynaptic receptor is located on the presynaptic membrane and functions likewise as a '5-HT brake': its activation leads to diminution of 5-HT release. Finally α_2 adrenergic autoreceptors are present not only on NA ergic nerve terminals, but on 5-HT ergic varicosities as well. In both cases their activation leads to diminished transmitter output.

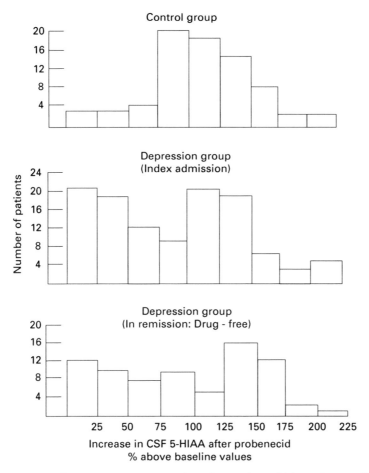

Figure 7.3.   Increase of CSF 5-HIAA concentration after probenecid in patients suffering from major depression, melancholic type (endogenous depression; vital depression) and in a non-depressed control group. The columns indicate the number of subjects. The increase in concentration is shown at the bottom of the column.

As compared with the control group, there is a significant increase in individuals with low CSF 5-HIAA in the depression group at the time of the index admission. After remission this value is still significantly increased (Van Praag, 1988).

In humans, 5-HT receptors have been predominantly studied with challenge tests. To the extent that selective ligands have become available, PET and single-photon emission computed tomography (SPECT) studies recently have assumed an ever-more important role (Table 7.3).

In challenge tests an agonist or antagonist (but generally the former) of the receptor to be studied is administered, whereupon a function mediated by that receptor system is analysed, for instance the secretion of a hormone by the pituitary gland or a physiological function, such as temperature regulation.

Table 7.3. Data indicative of reduced functioning of 5-HT(1A) receptors in (a subgroup of) depression.

Reduced hormonal response to indirect 5-HT agonists
Reduced hormonal response to relative selective (partial) 5-HT$_{1A}$ receptor agonists (azapirones)
Reduced numbers of 5-HT$_{1A}$ receptors both pre- and postsynaptically
Deletion of 5-HT$_{1A}$ receptors in the forebrain of animals induces anxiety-like behaviour
Azapirone type of partial 5-HT$_{1A}$ receptor agonists may exert antidepressant effects
Highly selective postsynaptic 5-HT$_{1A}$ receptor agonists have antidepressant effects in animal models of
    depression and exert anti-aggressive and anxiolytic effects
Presynaptic 5-HT$_{1A}$ antagonists may augment the therapeutic effects of antidepressants

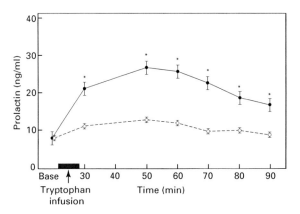

Figure 7.4.   The effect of an intravenous l-tryptophan load on plasma prolactin in patients with major depression (o) and normal controls (•). In the depressed group the response is significantly blunted: * P < 0.01 (Heninger *et al.*, 1984).

In most 5-HT receptor studies *indirect* 5-HT agonists have been used such as the 5-HT precursors tryptophan and 5-HTP as well as fenfluramine, a 5-HT releaser and inhibitor of its reuptake (Newman *et al.*, 1998). The secretion of prolactin and ACTH by the pituitary gland and of cortisol by the adrenal cortex have been mostly used as serotonergically mediated variables.

Most of those studies reported blunting of the hormonal responses to indirect 5-HT agonists in a subgroup of depression (Ansseau, 1997), indicating down-regulation of 5-HT receptors (Figure 7.4). The data from Strickland *et al.* (2002) represent a notable exception. In a group of mildly depressed women residing in the community the prolactin response to fenfluramine was found to be elevated. A hypothetical explanation for these discrepant findings is the following. The prolactin response to fenfluramine is, at least in part, mediated via 5-HT$_{1A}$ receptors. Assuming 5-HT synthesis indeed to be reduced in subtypes of depression, one could expect compensatory upregulation of 5-HT receptors and intensification of the fenfluramine/prolactin response. Sustained hypercortisolaemia, however, as may occur in depression, will reduce expression of the 5-HT$_{1A}$ receptor gene, resulting in decline of the fenfluramine/prolactin response. According to this line of reasoning the outcome of this test depends on type of depression and point of time it is carried out. This hypothesis has not yet been put to the test.

The prolactin responses to fenfluramine and to the SSRIs citalopram and clomipramine remain blunted in recovered patients (Florey *et al.*, 1998; Bhagwagar *et al.*, 2002; Golden *et al.*, 2002). The cortisol response to citalopram on the other hand does normalize. These findings suggest that some aspects of impaired 5-HT ergic transmission are trait-markers, just as low CSF 5-HIAA is.

Indirect 5-HT agonists act presynaptically and hence increase 5-HT availability throughout the entire 5-HT system. They do not provide information on which of the some 15 different subtypes of 5-HT receptors are actually downregulated. To this end one needs selective and direct agonists (or antagonists) of each of the receptor subtypes. Only a few of those are available for use in humans.

5-HT$_{1A}$ receptors

Highly selective, full, pre- or postsynaptic 5-HT$_{1A}$ agonists or antagonists have not yet been studied in humans. Data are available regarding a few azapirone derivatives, i.e. ipsapirone, giperone and buspirone. Those compounds are partial agonists of the 5-HT$_{1A}$ receptor and not very selective ones: their main metabolite 1–phenyl-piperazine, for instance, is also an α_2-adrenergic antagonist (De Vrij, 1995). Blocking of this presynaptically located adrenergic receptor, present on both 5-HT ergic and NA ergic neurons, could lead to increased 5-HT and NA release and thus contribute to antidepressant effects (Heiser & Wilcox, 1998). In addition these drugs activate the D$_2$ receptor, particularly buspirone.

Several studies reported blunted hormonal responses after an ipsapirone challenge in (a subgroup of) depression as well as attenuation of buspirone-induced hypothermia, suggesting abnormal functioning of the 5-HT$_{1A}$ receptor (Lesch *et al.*, 1990; Cowen *et al.*, 1994) (Figure 7.5) (Table 7.3). As mentioned, this receptor is located both post- and presynaptically. The presynaptic 5-HT$_{1A}$ receptors are located on the cell bodies and dendritic branches of 5-HT ergic neurons. They play an important role in feedback inhibition of the 5-HT ergic neuron. Stimulation of a 5-HT ergic nerve cell leads to release of 5-HT not only in the synaptic cleft but also in the region of the soma (cell body). The somatodendritic 5-HT$_{1A}$ receptor is thus activated which leads to inhibition of the firing rate of the 5-HT ergic neuron. Blunted hormonal responses to ipsapirone could thus mean: hyporesponsivity of the postsynaptic 5-HT$_{1A}$ receptor or hyper-responsivity of its presynaptic equivalent. Since, normally, after administration of ipsapirone, the release of hormones like prolactin and cortisol increases, activation of the postsynaptic receptor

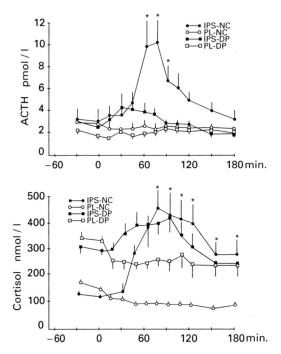

Figure 7.5. Mean plasma ACTH and cortisol responses ($\pm$ SE) as a function of time after 0.3 mg/kg ipsapirone (IPS) or placebo (PL) administered orally under double blind, random-assignment conditions to patients with unipolar depression (DP) and matched controls (NC). *P < 0.05 (Lesch *et al.*, 1990).

evidently supersedes that of the presynaptic receptor and hence blunting of the ipsapirone response can be regarded as an indication of downregulation of the postsynaptic 5-HT$_{1A}$ receptor.

PET studies provided direct evidence for 5-HT$_{1A}$ receptor pathology in depression. A widespread reduction in 5-HT$_{1A}$ receptor binding was reported in patients with major depression, both presynaptically in the raphe nuclei and postsynaptically, i.e. in several cortical regions (Drevets *et al.*, 1999; Sargent *et al.*, 2000) (Figure 7.6). After remission an increase failed to occur, another indication that 5-HT receptor disturbances in depression carry trait-character, possibly representing risk factors for depression.

If 5-HT$_{1A}$ receptor pathology is indeed involved in the pathophysiology of depression, one would expect selective, full, postsynaptic 5-HT$_{1A}$ agonists and presynaptic 5-HT$_{1A}$ antagonists with the same qualifications, to exert antidepressant effects, at least in patients with signs of 5-HT$_{1A}$ receptor pathology (Van Praag, 1996). A (small) number of studies do report antidepressant activity of the azapirone type of partial 5-HT$_{1A}$ agonists (Deakin, 1993; Pecknold, 1994). The same type of drugs

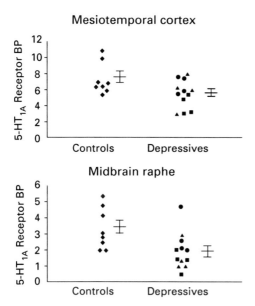

Figure 7.6.   Scatter histograms of the 5-HT$_{1A}$ receptor binding potential (BP) values for depressed patients and a control group. Within the depressed sample, circles indicate unipolar depressives with only major depressive disorder relatives, triangles indicate unipolar depressives with bipolar depressive (BD) relatives, and squares designate BD depressives with BD relatives. Mean and standard error bars appear to the right of each data set (Drevets *et al.*, 1999).

exert anxiolytic effects. This dual efficacy is explained by their partial agonistic properties (Olivier *et al.*, 1999). In anxiety states, presumed to be associated with over-stimulation of 5-HT receptors, the azapirones displace 5-HT from the post-synaptic 5-HT$_{1A}$ receptor and thus act as antagonists. In depression, supposedly associated with 5-HT deficiency, the azapirones do not have to compete with 5-HT and act as agonists. The azapirones, however, are not very selective drugs. Highly selective, postsynaptic 5-HT$_{1A}$ agonists have not yet been studied in humans.

The nonselective presynaptic 5-HT$_{1A}$ receptor antagonist pindolol (being also a β-adrenergic blocker) has been shown by some (Blier & Bergeron, 1998), but not all (Berman *et al.*, 1997) authors to speed up and augment the therapeutic effect of SSRIs and some other antidepressants. The variable results are possibly caused by suboptimal dosages (Rabiner *et al.*, 2001). There is no indication of its therapeutic activity given as monotherapy.

In animal models of depression (particularly the forced swimming test and the learned helplessness test), highly selective 5-HT$_{1A}$ receptor agonists possess anti-depressant properties (Borsini *et al.*, 1999; Muñoz & Papp, 1999; Mayorga *et al.*, 2001). In addition they exert anti-aggressive and anxiolytic effects (Borsini *et al.*, 1999; De Boer *et al.*, 1999). Mice lacking the 5-HT$_{1A}$ receptor show increased anxiety

(Parks *et al.*, 1998). Several lines of evidence indicate that these are postsynaptic effects. This was most elegantly demonstrated by Gross *et al.* (2002). They developed a method to knock out and restore the 5-HT$_{1A}$ receptor at will and demonstrated that anxiety-like behaviour was only produced if 5-HT$_{1A}$ receptors in the forebrain were deleted, not if their presynaptic counterpart in the raphe nuclei were knocked out.

Present-day antidepressants, particularly the SSRIs, increase 5-HT availability across the board via reuptake inhibition and upregulation of tryptophan hydroxylase (TPH) gene expression (Kim *et al.*, 2002). TPH being the enzyme catalysing the first and rate-limiting step of 5-HT synthesis: the transformation of 5-HT into 5-HTP. Yet, their antidepressant effects are thought to be associated with sensitization of the postsynaptic 5-HT$_{1A}$ receptor and/or desensitization of its presynaptic counterpart (Blier & de Montigny, 1994). Lithium augmentation of antidepressant effects is supposedly produced by tonic activation of (postsynaptic) forebrain 5-HT$_{1A}$ receptors (Haddjeri *et al.*, 2000). One has to keep in mind, however, that activation of postsynaptic 5-HT$_{1A}$ receptors leads to an increase of the extra-cellular NA level in the hippocampus, an effect that might contribute to antidepressant effects (Suwabe *et al.*, 2000).

All in all, much evidence points to the 5-HT$_{1A}$ receptor as an important pathophysiological factor in (some types of) depression.

5-HT$_{1B (D)}$ receptors

The 5-HT$_{1B}$ receptor (equivalent to the 5 HT$_{1D}$ receptor in humans) is located both pre- and postsynaptically. The presynaptic receptor is located on nerve endings and its activation shuts down 5-HT release. Activation of the postsynaptic receptor has strong aggression-reducing effects (Abe *et al.*, 1998). Knocking out the 5-HT$_{1B}$ receptor in mice leads to enhancement of aggressive behaviour (Sandou *et al.*, 1994).

Some animal data suggest that the 5-HT$_{1B}$ receptor is involved in antidepressant drug action in animal models of depression (Redrobe *et al.*, 1996).

In humans there is some evidence that the postsynaptic 5-HT$_{1D}$ is hyporesponsive. Challenge tests with zolmitripan, a 5-HT$_{1D}$ receptor agonist that penetrates the brain fairly well, leads to increased release of growth hormone, supposedly via activation of postsynaptic 5-HT$_{1D}$ receptors. In depression, particularly melancholic depression, the growth hormone response to zolmitripan was found to be blunted (Whale *et al.*, 2001). Human data indicating antidepressant activity of postsynaptic 5-HT$_{1D}$ receptors agonists, however, are lacking.

5-HT$_2$ receptors

The status of the 5-HT$_2$ receptor in depression is uncertain. It has been studied with challenge tests, using the relatively selective 5-HT$_{2C}$ agonist, m-chlorophenylpiperazine (mCPP). It is an anxiogenic substance and may provoke panic attacks in patients with panic disorder, while, in addition, the hormonal responses to mCPP are above average, indicating supersensitivity of this receptor. Patients suffering from generalized anxiety disorder or panic disorder, also showed increased hostility rating after mCPP administration. Normal subjects did not (Kahn *et al.*, 1988; Germine *et al.*, 1992). In depression, the sensitivity of the 5-HT$_{2C}$ receptor has been found to be both unchanged (Kahn *et al.*, 1990) and increased (Klaassen *et al.*, 2002). Anxiety may be a major component of depressive syndromes. It can be a precursor or possibly even a pacemaker of certain depressive syndromes (see Chapter 9). It is thus conceivable that, in this way, 5-HT$_2$ receptor pathology might contribute to depressive psychopathology in some depressive syndromes.

Brain-imaging studies, however, show mixed results. In a single SPECT study D'Haenen *et al.* (1992) found increased 5-HT$_2$ receptor binding. PET studies revealed no change (Meyer *et al.*, 1999) or a decrease (Yatham *et al.*, 2000). The decrease, however, could have been caused by previous antidepressant treatment (Yatham *et al.*, 1999). Moreover, different receptor ligands were used.

In blood platelets upregulation of 5-HT$_{2(A)}$ receptors has been frequently observed in depressed patients (Biegon *et al.*, 1990; Pandey *et al.*, 1990), particularly in suicidal depressed patients (Hrdina *et al.*, 1993) and in assaultive personality disordered individuals (Coccaro *et al.*, 1997). However negative reports have also been published (Cowen *et al.*, 1987). The same is true for studies of 5HT$_{2A}$ receptors in the brains of depressed patients, in vivo or postmortem. Signs of both up- and downregulation have been reported (Audenaert *et al.*, 2001).

In rats subjected to chronic unpredictable stress (leading to 'animal depression') 5HT$_{2A}$ receptor density in the brain increases (Ossowska *et al.*, 2001). In animal models of depression, moreover, some 5-HT$_2$ receptor antagonists and inverse agonists have been shown to possess antidepressant potential (Bromidge *et al.*, 2000; Yamada & Sugimoto, 2001).

5-HT receptors and therapeutic activity of present-day antidepressants

It is generally assumed that 5-HT receptors are involved in the therapeutic actions of antidepressants, particularly the receptors discussed above. Long-term administration of TCAs enhances hormonal responses to a fenfluramine or tryptophan challenge (Ressler & Nemeroff, 2000), suggesting an increased responsiveness of postsynaptic 5-HT receptors. By repeated administration of SSRIs and MAOIs inhibitory somatodendritic 5-HT$_{1A}$ and terminal 5-HT$_{1D}$ autoreceptors are desensitized (Bonhomme & Esposito, 1998). Inhibition of these autoreceptors leads to an increase in firing rate and of 5-HT release, respectively, and hence to enhanced 5-HT ergic transmission. As mentioned, much evidence suggests that activation of the 5-HT$_{1A}$ receptor system plays a key role in generating antidepressant as well as anxiolytic and anti-aggressive effects (Blier & de Montigny, 1994; Blier *et al.*, 1997, Dremencov *et al.*, 2002).

The significance of the 5-HT$_2$ receptor for antidepressant activity is unclear. Long-term treatment with TCAs leads to downregulation of the cortical 5-HT$_{2A}$ receptor (Marsden, 1996). This is also true for some of the newer antidepressants, like nefazadone (Ellingrod & Perry, 1995; Eison & Mullins, 1996). 'Knocking-out' this receptor in mice, moreover, leads to antidepressant effects in the forced swimming test (Sibelle *et al.*, 1997). The effects of SSRIs on 5-HT$_{2A}$ receptor density, however, are inconsistent (Cadogan *et al.*, 1993) and electro-convulsive therapy (ECT) actually increases 5-HT$_{2A}$ receptor density. Generally speaking, downregulation of the 5-HT$_{2A}$ receptor would seem to make sense, since it leads to upregulation of the 5-HT$_{1A}$ receptor (Zhang *et al.*, 2001), and, as indicated, quite a lot of evidence implicates hyporesponsivity of the 5-HT$_{1A}$ receptor in the pathophysiology of depression.

The significance of the 5-HT$_{2C}$ receptor for antidepressant activity is also uncertain. Chronic treatment with SSRIs attenuates 5-HT$_{2C}$ receptor-mediated behaviour (Jenck *et al.*, 1992; Kennett *et al.*, 1994a,b). On the other hand, fluoxetine, but not paroxetine (Quested *et al.*, 1997), reportedly potentiates hormonal responses to 5-HT$_{2C}$ receptor agonists. Both agonists and antagonists of the 5-HT$_{2C}$ receptor are active in animal models of anxiety and depression respectively (Stephaniski & Goldberg, 1997; Martin *et al.*, 1998; Yamada & Sugimoto, 2001). These observations are hard to explain.

Involvement in antidepressant action has, so far, been quite conclusively demonstrated only for the 5-HT$_{1A}$ receptor.

5-HT transporter

The uptake of 5-HT in blood platelets and in the presynaptic nerve terminals is considered to proceed via an identical mechanism, using the so-called 5-HT transporter. Several groups have found a reduced density of 5-HT transporter sites both on platelets (Ellis & Salmond, 1994) as well as in the hippocampus and occipital cortex of depressed patients (Perry *et al.*, 1983). In a large multicentre trial the platelet data have not been confirmed (WHO Collaborative Study, 1990). In vivo SPECT studies, on the other hand, have confirmed reduced density of 5-HT transporter binding sites in the midbrain of depressed patients (Malison *et al.*, 1998).

Reduced re-uptake of 5-HT (leading to increased availability of 5-HT in the synapse) might be a compensatory mechanism to counteract transmission deficits in some 5-HT ergic systems.

7.2.4 Postmortem receptor studies

Postmortem studies of patients with major depression have not provided unequivocal support for the 5-HT hypothesis of depression. This is true for measurements of 5-HT and 5-HIAA concentrations in the brainstem as well as for receptor studies. The number of 5-HT uptake sites (5-HT transporter) was found to be reduced by some and unchanged by other authors. The same is true for 5-HT$_{1A}$ receptors. 5-HT$_2$ receptors have been reported to be increased in several cortical regions, but negative results have also appeared (for a review see Stockmeier et al., 1997; Cryan & Leonard, 2000; Rosel et al., 2000). No relationships were found between 5-HT$_{1D}$ receptor-binding indices or genotypes and major depression or suicide (Huang et al., 1999).

The inconsistency of the results comes as no surprise. On different levels, post-mortem studies are fraught with difficulties. Previous medications may have influenced the results and also comorbid somatic disorders. Quite often different brain areas were studied and dissimilar ligands used. Moreover, postmortem diagnoses are difficult to verify and the impact of suicidal behaviour per se and depression is hard to disentangle. Finally, depression is, in all likelihood, a heterogeneous construct and if so, one cannot expect a certain biological aberration to present itself across the board. This latter notion is more often than not ignored.

7.2.5 Genetic studies

Genetic studies, investigating possible association between polymorphisms of 5-HT-related genes and (components of) the depressive syndrome, have been disappointingly contradictory.

Association between polymorphisms of the tryptophan hydroxylase gene and suicidal behaviour as such (Abbar et al., 2001), suicidal behaviour in depressed patients (Mann et al., 1997), anger- and aggression-related traits (Manuck et al., 1999) and manic-depressive illness (Bellivier et al., 1998) have been reported as well as refuted (Kirov et al., 1999; Kunugi et al., 1999; McQuillin et al., 1999).

Likewise, associations between polymorphisms of the 5-HT transporter gene and susceptibility for depression (Ogilvie et al., 1996) as well as for anxiety-related personality traits (Lesch et al., 1996) and suicide (Mann et al., 2000) have been found, but other groups have failed to confirm those (Little et al., 1997; Mazzanti et al., 1998; Serretti et al., 1999a).

Du et al. (2000a,b) reported an association between the 102 T/C polymorphism in the 5-HT$_{2A}$ receptor gene and suicidal behaviour in patients with major depression, observations that could not be confirmed by Geijer et al. (2000). The same polymorphism has been found in schizophrenia by some, though not all authors (Williams et al., 1997). In bipolar patients the findings were negative (Massot et al., 2000). No associations were found between variants of the 5-HT$_{2A}$, 5-HT$_{2C}$ and 5-HT$_{1A}$ receptor genes and various psychopathological features of mood disorders (Frisch et al., 1999; Serretti et al., 2000).

Some data suggest a relationship between certain genetic polymorphisms of the 5-HT$_{2C}$ receptor and particularly personality features. Ebstein *et al.* (1997) reported an association with reward dependence, a finding that could not be replicated by Kuhn *et al.* (1999). Another group found an association with impulsiveness in individuals treated for deliberate self-harm (Evans *et al.*, 2000). The low activity (or short) allele of the 5-HT transporter gene has been reported as associated with violent suicidal behaviour (Bondy *et al.*, 2000; Courtet *et al.*, 2001), findings that could not be confirmed by Fitch *et al.* (2001). A susceptibility locus on chromosome 18 in patient with bipolar disorder has been claimed by some groups (Berrettini *et al.*, 1994; De Bruyn *et al.*, 1996), while others reported negative findings (Mynett-Johnson *et al.*, 1997).

These discrepancies have often been attributed to differences in the way patients were sampled and to variations in genetic techniques. The notion that the depression categories we presently distinguish are utterly heterogeneous in almost every respect – symptoms, severity, duration, course and treatment response – and that in heterogeneous populations one cannot expect to find uniform distribution of biological variables, received scarce attention (see Chapter 1). Yet it seems to be an important source of confusion in biological psychiatry (Van Praag, 1997, 2000).

The most important genetic data pertaining to depression so far, concern the gene expressing the 5-HT transporter protein (5-HTT) (Caspi *et al.*, 2003). This gene shows a functional polymorphism in the promoter region; that is, it exists with a long (l) and a short (s) allele in the promoter region. Individuals may carry two copies of the l-allele, two of the s-allele or one copy of each. They can be, in other words, homozygous or heterozygous for this length variation. The s-promoter is less active than the l-promoter, resulting in lower levels of 5-HT uptake.

Mice with one or two copies of the s-allele show more intense fearful reactions to stressors than their counterparts with the l-allele (s) (Murphy *et al.*, 2001). Monkeys with the s-allele show decreased levels of CSF 5-HIAA, but only if they were reared in stressful conditions. This phenomenon was absent in normally raised monkeys (Bennett *et al.*, 2002). Humans with one or two copies of the s-allele, if stressed, show more intense activation of the amygdala than individuals with two l-alleles (Hariri *et al.*, 2002).

The tentative conclusion drawn from these data, that polymorphisms of the 5-HTT gene determine in some manner the strength of the stress response, was notably strengthened by the data of Caspi *et al.* (2003). In a prospective study, they showed that individuals with one or two copies of the short allele exhibited more depressive symptoms, more 'case-depression', and more suicidality than individuals homozygous for the l-allele. Moreover, they found that abuse as a child predicted depression after the age of 18 only in those individuals with at least one s-allele.

Supporting the conclusions of Caspi *et al.* (2003) is the observation that the ss and sl alleles are over-represented in individuals who had committed (violent) suicide attempts. The highest rates were found in those who also had a history of major depression (Courtet *et al.*, 2001).

The study of Caspi *et al.* (2003) is important for two reasons. It provides additional evidence for the involvement of the 5-HT system in the pathophysiology of depression. Secondly, it demonstrates most elegantly, that the impact of environmental stimuli, i.e. adversity, is modulated by genetic factors, i.e. polymorphisms of the 5-HTT gene.

7.2.6 Conclusions

Several lines of evidence suggest the occurrence of disturbances in 5-HT metabolism in depression. These disturbances persist after remission, whereas increasing 5-HT metabolism and release is an antidepressant intervention. Hence the 5-HT disturbances probably precede the depression, and have pathogenetic significance rather than being its consequences.

Furthermore, disturbances in 5-HT receptor functioning have been established. The $5\text{-}HT_{1A}$ receptor is probably downregulated, while the state of the $5\text{-}HT_2$ system is unclear. Both signs of hyper- and hyporesponsivity have been reported, possibly indicating that $5\text{-}HT_2$ disturbances vary locally. The density of 5-HT transporter binding sites may be reduced. Dysfunctioning of the 5-HT transporter is possibly related to stress-sensitivity. Other 5-HT receptors have not yet been studied sufficiently in depression, due to lack of specific ligands.

It should be emphasized that the 5-HT disturbances mentioned are not characteristic for depression as such, but for a *subgroup* of depressions. The question arises whether it is possible to recognize this subgroup in psychopathological terms. This question will be discussed in Section 7.5 and in Chapter 9.

7.3 Noradrenaline and depression

The relationship between NA and depression (Schildkraut, 1965) and that between 5-HT and depression (Van Praag, 1962; Coppen, 1967) has been studied simultaneously and mostly in a parallel fashion, though initially NA occupied a preferential position. Both metabolic indices and NA ergic receptors have been extensively studied.

7.3.1 Localization

The cell bodies of NA ergic neurons are for the most part located in the locus coeruleus (LC), positioned in the rostral pons, on the floor of the fourth vertricle. Their axonal projections fan out over many areas of both brain and spinal cord. In addition the brain contains smaller collections of NA ergic neurons, located in the

Table 7.4. Data indicative of disturbed NA ergic functioning in (a subgroup of) depression.

Data indicative of NA ergic hypofunctioning	Data indicative of NA ergic hyperfunctioning
↓Urinary MHPG in some patients	↑Plasma concentration NA and adrenalin
CA depletion may cause depressive symptoms	↑Urinary excretion NA and NA metabolites
CA depletion may cause recurrence in remitted depressed patients	↑CSF NA concentration around the clock
↓Arterio-venous NA gradient	
↓Responsivity of the beta-adrenergic receptor	

lateral tegmental area, the axons of which remain more localized. Most NA ergic terminals make contact with other neurons. Some do not, and seem to secrete NA in the way endocrine organs secrete hormones. NA thus released will have a much more generalized effect.

The LC is very sensitive for influences from without. It is kept informed about the internal and external environment via a number of transmitter systems among which are the MA ergic, gabaminergic and glutaminergic pathways. Reciprocal connections exist between the LC and CRH containing neurons located in the hypothalamus and elsewhere in the brain.

7.3.2 Noradrenaline metabolism

The NA hypothesis of depression postulated a NA deficiency to be a component of the pathophysiology of depression (Schildkraut, 1965). In fact, subsequent studies showed that most data point to an *increase* of catecholamine (CA) metabolism in depression, rather than to a decrease, at least in the periphery (Table 7.4). The sympatho-adrenal system – comprising the adrenal medulla and the sympathetic nervous system – often shows signs of hyperactivity, such as increased plasma concentration of adrenalin and NA, increased urinary excretion of NA, 3-methoxy-4-hydroxyphenylglycol (MHPG) and other NA metabolites and around-the-clock increases in NA concentration in CSF (Potter *et al.*, 1993; Wong *et al.*, 2000). Adrenalin in plasma is derived from the adrenal medulla; plasma NA for the most part from the sympathetic nerve terminals and for a small part from the adrenal medulla and extra-adrenal chromaffin cells. MHPG is the major NA metabolite in the CNS; in the periphery NA is for the most part degraded to vanillylmandelic acid (VMA).

Elevation of plasma NA is greatest in melancholic patients and in those with signs of hyperactivity of the HPA axis (dexamethasone non-supression) (Roy *et al.*, 1985). Bipolar patients show greater elevation of plasma NA and greater urinary NA excretion in manic than in depressed episodes, and, when manic, greater elevations if the episode was precipitated by external stressors than when it appears to arise 'out of the blue' (Swann *et al.*, 1990).

Sympatho-adrenal activation is an integral component of Cannon's (1929) 'fight and flight reaction' and the 'general adaptation syndrome' described by Seyle (1936). It occurs in many conditions threatening homeostasis, physical (intensive motor activity; illness, such as a myocardial infarction) or mental (stress) in nature. In the case of depression it is an important but unresolved question whether it relates to depression as such or rather to the emotional turmoil the depression leads to or that preceded the depression (see Chapter 8).

A possible decrease in NA metabolism in depression has largely been studied by determining urinary MHPG excretion, assuming this variable to reflect the metabolism of NA in the CNS. In unipolar depression urinary MHPG concentration varies over a wide range of values. In bipolar I depressed patients urinary MHPG was found to be reduced, compared with unipolar and bipolar II patients. The low MHPG patients may respond better to antidepressants than patients with high urinary MHPG excretion (Schildkraut, 1978a,b; Maas *et al.*, 1984). These findings, however, have not been uniformly confirmed (Janicak *et al.*, 1986).

The supposition that urinary MHPG reliably reflects central NA metabolism, moreover, was challenged by Blomberg *et al.* (1980) who calculated that actually no more than 20% of urinary MHPG is derived from the CNS.

CSF MHPG studies have likewise produced equivocal results. Not surprisingly, because MHPG in lumbar CSF stems mainly from the spinal cord, and only to a minor degree from the brain.

CA depletion studies do provide evidence for the involvement of CA in the action mechanism of antidepressants. α-Methyl-paratyrosine (AMPT), an inhibitor of tyrosine hydroxylase – the enzyme that catalyses the first step in CA synthesis – administered to depressed patients in remission, caused recurrence in those treated with NA reuptake inhibitors (Figure 7.7). This was not the case in those who had responded to SSRIs (Miller *et al.*, 1996a).

CA depletion studies also provide some evidence for reduced CA availability as a pathogenic factor in depression. Neither in normals nor in depressives did CA depletion cause any (increase in) depressive symptoms (Miller *et al.*, 1996b). Euthymic, medication–free subjects, with a history of major depression, however, did show depressive symptoms after administration of AMPT (Berman *et al.*, 1999) (Figure 7.8).

The approaches mentioned so far have produced little evidence that NA metabolism is indeed reduced in depression. A recent study by Lambert *et al.* (2000) threw new light on this issue. They used a new strategy: determining the arterio-venous NA gradient between the vena jugularis interna and the arteria brachialis in depressed patients. They found this gradient to be decreased in depression

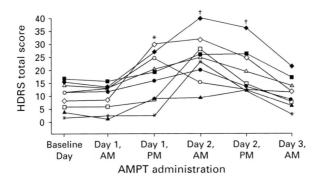

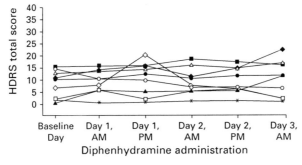

Figure 7.7.   Hamilton Depression Rating Scale (HDRS) scores of depressed patients in remission on
desipramine hydrochloride and tested with AMPT or diphenhydramine (an antihistamine,
used as an active placebo for AMPT, a compound that causes considerable sedation). AMPT
produced a robust increase in depressive symptoms; diphenhydramine did not. Each patient
is represented by a different symbol (Miller *et al.*, 1996a) * P < 0.05, † 0.01.

(Figure 7.9). This is a strong indication for reduced NA turnover in the CNS.
This observation awaits confirmation.

7.3.3 Noradrenaline receptor studies

NA receptors are subdivided into 3 groups, i.e. α_1, α_2 and β-adrenergic receptors.
The α_1 and α_2 groups are subdivided into 4 subtypes, named α_{1A} up to α_{1D} receptors,
and α_{2A} up to α_{2D} receptors. The group of β-adrenergic receptors is subdivided
into 3 subgroups, i.e. β_1–β_3 adrenergic receptors.

As far as the adrenergic receptor system is concerned the α_2 and the β-adrenergic
receptors have been the main focus of research in depression. α_2-Adrenergic receptors are located both pre- and postsynaptically. The presynaptic receptor mediates
a negative feedback system: when stimulated NA release is diminished. The β-
receptor is predominantly localized on postsynaptic sites.

The growth hormone response to clonidine has been used to study the functionality of the α_2 receptor. Clonidine is an α_2-receptor agonist, which in the higher

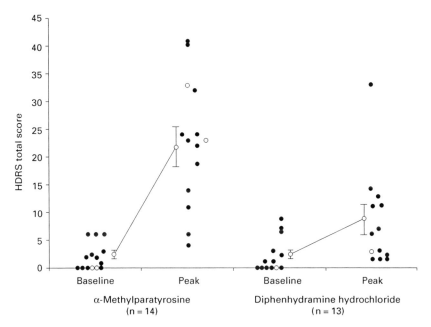

Figure 7.8. Euthymic, medication-free subjects with a history of major depression demonstrated significant depressive symptoms, measured with the Hamilton Depression Rating Scale (HDRS), after AMPT, not after diphenhydramine. Open circles represent patients who completed only one testing condition (Berman *et al.*, 1999).

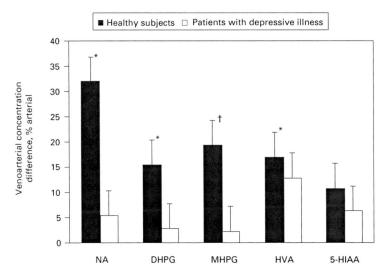

Figure 7.9. Internal jugular venous plasma concentration gradients of noradrenaline (NA) and its principal central nervous system-occurring metabolites, dihydroxyphenylglycol (DHPG) and 3-methoxy-4-hydroxyphenylglycol (MHPG), the dopamine metabolite homovanillic acid (HVA), and the 5-HT metabolite 5-HIAA in healthy subjects and patients with major depression. Catecholamine (metabolite) concentrations were reduced in major depression. * $P < 0.05$, [†] $P < 0.01$. (Lambert *et al.*, 2000).

dose range predominantly activates the postsynaptic α_2-receptor. Blunting of the growth hormone response, therefore, is understood to be a sign of downregulation of the α_2 receptor system. This phenomenon was found to occur in depression (Matussek et al., 1980) and seemed to be trait-related (Siever et al., 1992), i.e. not to disappear after lifting of the depression. However, it has been demonstrated that the growth hormone response is diminished after various monoamine (MA) agonists, such as apomorphine, a dopamine (DA) agonist; amphetamine, a DA and NA agonist, and MCPP, a 5-HT agonist (Asnis et al., 1992; Schatzberg & Schildkraut, 1995). Blunting of the growth hormone response, thus, seems to point to a defect in the growth hormone production or release rather than to a specific NA receptor defect.

In low doses clonidine is thought to stimulate predominantly the presynaptic α_2-adrenergic receptor, leading to reduction of NA release. In normal conditions low doses of clonidine lower plasma MHPG levels; in depression the decrease is greater than normal. This phenomenon has been interpreted as an indication of hypersensitivity of the presynaptic α_2 receptor. Such condition would lead to a decreased efficiency of NA ergic transmission. It has, however, not been consistently confirmed (Anand & Charney, 1997).

α_2-Receptor activation, furthermore, leads to inhibition of adenylate cyclase, thus to a diminished production of cyclic adenosine monophosphate (cAMP) followed by induction of platelet aggregation. Garcia-Sevilla et al. (1990), measuring inhibition of adenylate cyclase in blood platelets and platelet aggregation, before and after α_2-receptor agonists in depressed patients, found this receptor to be hypersensitive. If the platelet α_2-receptor is an appropriate model for the presynaptic α_2-receptor this would mean an exaggerated negative feedback and thus reduced NA release. Other authors, however, using this model, found contradictory evidence, pointing towards desensitization of the α_2 system (Karege et al., 1992).

Direct measurement of the α_2-receptor, too, produced contradictory results. Some investigators found an increased density of this receptor on blood platelets (Piletz et al., 1986) and in the brains of suicidal victims (Callado et al., 1998); others have failed to confirm these findings (Anand & Charney, 1997).

The status of the β-adrenergic receptor system in the brain of depressed patients is equally uncertain. Most antidepressants, chronically administered, produce a downregulation of β-receptors (Hosada & Duman, 1993). Electroconvulsive treatment has the same effect. Some SSRIs, however, defy this rule (Palvimaki et al., 1994). The inference based on these observations, that in depression the β-adrenergic receptor system might be upregulated, has not been substantiated. The relevant data are controversial. Postmortem studies of suicide victims yielded contradictory results (Crow et al., 1984; Mann et al., 1986) and the same is true for measuring

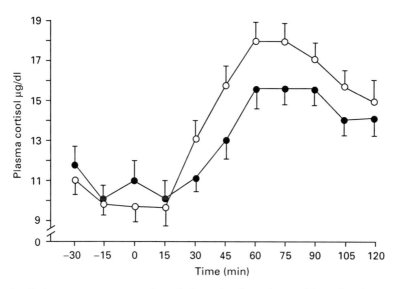

Figure 7.10. Cortisol response to 75 mg i.m. desipramine in patients with major depression (•) and normal control subjects (○). The cortisol response is significantly blunted in the depressed group (Asnis *et al.*, 1992).

β-receptors on blood platelets and lymphocytes (Extein *et al.*, 1979; Healy *et al.*, 1985).

The cortisol response to the NA reuptake inhibitor desipramine is, at least in part, mediated via β-adrenergic receptors. This response has been found to be blunted in depression (Asnis *et al.*, 1986, 1992), a sign of diminished responsivity of the β-receptor (Figure 7.10). The nocturnal increase in melatonin secretion – considered to be a β-receptor mediated effect because it is blocked by β-blockers – is likewise blunted (Frazer *et al.*, 1986). It cannot be excluded, however, that β-receptor downregulation is a phenomenon secondary to stress-induced increase of plasma NA.

Downregulation of the β-receptor system in depression is hard to reconcile with the findings that most antidepressants downregulate the β-receptor system, assuming that this effect forms part of their mechanism of action.

Be this as it may, different strategies resulted in different conclusions regarding the state of the β-adrenergic receptor system in depression.

7.3.4 Conclusions

It is clear that NA metabolism may be disturbed in depression. Most data, however, point to an *increase*, conceivably stress-induced; a *decrease* in NA metabolism has not been convincingly demonstrated, though subgroup-specificity hidden by calculating overall measures for major depression (an utterly heterogeneous construct, as discussed in Chapter 1), remains a distinct possibility. The study by Lambert *et al.* (2000), reporting reduced arterio-venous NA gradient in depressed individuals, is a notable exception, in that it does suggest reduced NA utilization in the CNS of depressed individuals.

If a NA ergic deficit would indeed play a role in the pathogenesis of depression, one would expect antidepressants to facilitate NA-ergic transmission. It is, however, by no means clear that this happens. NA reuptake inhibition by tricyclic antidepressants (TCAs) and inhibition of NA degradation through MAO I indeed lead to a rapid increase of NA availability in NA ergic synapses. This, however, cannot be a crucial mechanism because therapeutic effects of antidepressants do not generally occur before 2–4 weeks of treatment. The effect of most antidepressants and of ECT on adrenergic receptors is one of downregulation. This holds both for β-receptors and for α_2-receptors. This suggests reduced, rather than increased efficiency of NA-ergic transmission. Receptor downregulation may be an adaptation to increased NA availability, rather than a primary component of the action mechanism of antidepressants. CA depletion studies provided strong evidence that CA do indeed play a role in the therapeutic activity of antidepressants, at least in those with specific actions on the NA-ergic system.

The conclusion can only be that the role of NA in the pathogenesis of depression is not clear.

7.4 Dopamine and depression

7.4.1 Localization

Most dopaminergic (DA ergic) cell bodies are located in the ventral mesencephalon, and project to the corpus striatum (nigrostriatal DA system), to limbic areas (mesolimbic DA system) and to the cortex cerebri (mesocortical DA system). In addition DA ergic neurons are found in the nucleus arcuatus. They send their axons to the hypothalamus and pituitary (tuberoinfundibular and tuberohypophysial DA system). The mesocortical and mesolimbic DA systems play a pivotal role in reward experiences and in bringing about goal-directed behaviour. Both behavioural features are diminished in (certain types of) depression, and thus disturbances in the DA system could conceivably be expected to occur in depression.

Just as 5-HT and NA, DA functions as an 'endproduct-inhibitor'. DA receptors are located both pre- and postsynaptically. Stimulation of the presynaptic receptor leads to diminution of DA release and thus to inhibition of DA ergic transmission.

7.4.2 Dopamine metabolism

In humans, homovanillic acid (HVA) is the main degradation product of DA. Most HVA in lumbar CSF originates from the nigrostriatal DA pathways and to a

Table 7.5. Data indicative of disturbed DA ergic functioning in (a subgroup of) depression.

Lowered CSF HVA
Decreased uptake of DA precursors in CNS
Increased hormonal response to D_2 agonists
SPECT study revealed increased number of D_2 receptors
Increased spontaneous eye blinking (suggesting supersensitivity of D_2 receptors)

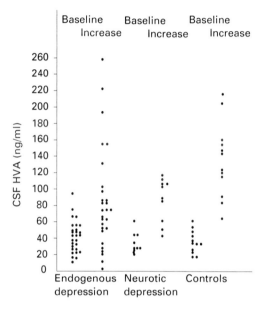

Figure 7.11. Baseline and post-probenecid HVA concentration in CSF in patients with endogenous and neurotic depression and controls. In 11 patients with endogenous depression (major depression, melancholic type) and 3 with neurotic depression (dysthymia) the HVA response to probenecid was below the lower limit of the range of values in the control group. All these patients showed signs of motor retardation (Van Praag et al., 1973).

much lesser extent from the mesocorticolimbic DA system and the spinal cord. The explanation is, that the caudate nucleus is a large, DA-rich structure located close to the ventricles.

Several investigators found CSF HVA concentration to be lowered in a subgroup of depressed patients (Table 7.5). This appeared to be so for both baseline values and for post-probenecid concentrations (see Section 7.2.2) (Van Praag & Korf, 1971a,b; Van Praag et al., 1973; Willner, 1983) (Figure 7.11). In mania, levels of CSF HVA were found to be increased (Willner, 1995). The same is true for delusional melancholic depression (Gjerris et al., 1987). Tremblay et al. (2002) found the rewarding effects of dextra-amphetamine to be increased in depression patients, relative to controls. They hypothesized the enhanced response to reflect decreased DA ergic output resulting in secondary upregulation of DA receptors.

The high incidence of depression in Parkinson's disease has been considered evidence of a causal association between DA deficiency and depression (Willner, 1995). This is not a strong argument, because the DA system is by no means the only transmitter system damaged in Parkinson patients. There is widespread degeneration of 5-HT-, NA-, acetylcholine- and some peptidergic neurons as well (Jellinger, 1991), while depression in Parkinson's disease does not usually respond well to DA-enhancing medications (Anand & Charney, 1997).

7.4.3 DA receptor studies

DA receptors are divided into two groups: the DA_1 (D_1) and DA_2 (D_2) receptors. The D_1 group is subdivided in two subgroups: the D_1 and D_5 receptors; the D_2 group in 3 subgroups: the D_2, D_3 and D_4 receptors. D_3 and D_5 receptors are richly represented in the limbic domain; the D_4 receptor is concentrated in the frontal cortex, midbrain and amygdala. Agonists are available for the D_1 and the D_2 group, not for each receptor subtype separately. This holds for animal work. For human studies selective D_1 and D_2 agonists are not yet available.

The D_1 and D_2 receptors were reported to exert opposite effects on reward systems (Self et al., 1996). In animals, D_1 receptor agonists attenuate and D_2 receptor agonists augment reward-seeking behaviour. Disturbances in reward experiences (translated into the human situation: anhedonia) could conceivably be related to increased D_1 receptor activity or to hypoactivity of the D_2 receptor system.

The results of DA receptor studies in depression have not been unequivocal. The growth hormone (GH) response to apomorphine in major depression was reported to be blunted (Ansseau et al., 1988), but these findings were contradicted by earlier reports (Meltzer et al., 1984). Since apomorphine stimulates both pre- and postsynaptic DA receptors (mostly the D_2 type), results with this test are hard to interpret. Challenge tests with other DA agonists, particularly the DA precursor l-DOPA, bromocriptine and amphetamine, did not reveal differences between depressed patients and control subjects (Matussek, 1988). Sulpiride, a D_2 receptor antagonist, reportedly caused a significantly greater rise in plasma prolactin levels in depression as compared with controls (Verbeeck et al., 2001); possibly an indication of receptor hypersensitivity secondary to DA deficiency (Table 7.5). In a SPECT study with the $D_{2/3}$ ligand ^{123}I-IBZM, Shah et al. (1997) indeed found indications of increased IBZM binding.

Spontaneous eye blinking – a phenomenon mediated by D_2 receptors – was found to be increased in depressed patients with seasonal affective disorder (Depue et al., 1990). The supersensitivity of D_2 receptors that this phenomenon suggests, might be secondary to a central DA deficit. In accordance with these findings D'Haenen & Bossuyt (1994) and Ebert *et al.* (1996), using SPECT methodology, reported a bilateral increase in D_2 receptors in the basal ganglia. In PET studies this finding could not be reproduced (Klimek *et al.*, 1999). Using SPECT methodology, Laasonen-Balk *et al.* (1999) found the density of the DA transporter in the striatum significantly higher in depressed patients than in controls. It was hypothesized that this is a primary phenomenon leading to DA deficiency. The finding that the uptake of DA precursors in the CNS is diminished in depression (Agren & Reibring, 1994), also points to a DA shortage. Lowered DA transporter binding potential, however, has also been reported in depression (Meyer *et al.*, 2001).

No relationships have been established between polymorphisms of the genes coding for DA receptors and major depression (Frisch *et al.*, 1999; Serretti *et al.*, 1999b). Postmortem studies did not reveal consistent abnormalities in number or affinity of DA receptors in the brains of suicide victims.

7.4.4 DA and antidepressant action

The role of DA in the therapeutic actions of antidepressants is insufficiently known. Some SSRIs do increase DA release in the striatum but others do not (Tiihonen *et al.*, 1996). Nomifensine inhibits DA reuptake and has significant antidepressant activity, particularly so in patients with low CSF HVA (Van Scheyen *et al.*, 1977). However, this drug also inhibits NA reuptake. It was removed from the market because of the appearance of the Guillain–Barré syndrome in some patients.

L-DOPA administered in depression exerts activating effects but does not improve mood significantly (Goodwin & Sack, 1974; Van Praag, 1974).

Amphetamine affects mood only transiently. DA agonists like piribedil and bromocriptine have some, but rather weak, antidepressant effects (Willner, 1995). According to Willner (1995), TCAs and SSRIs do sensitize D_2 and D_3 receptors in the mesolimbic system, but conclusive evidence that this effect plays a substantial role in mood elevation is lacking. Amfebutamone (bupropion) is considered to be a 'DA ergic antidepressant' and is an active therapeutic. However, it potentiates, just like nomifensine, NA activity as well (Rampello *et al.*, 2000). Amineptine is a rather selective inhibitor of DA reuptake and an enhancer of DA release. The first studies show it to have antidepressant potential (Rampello *et al.*, 2000). Further data have to be awaited.

7.4.5 Conclusions

CSF HVA, an indicator of DA metabolism in the (nigrostriatal) DA system, may be reduced in depression. The evidence for that is quite firm. Receptor studies, on the other hand, are controversial and no conclusive evidence exists of disturbed DA receptor function in depression. One has to take into account, however, that

Table 7.6. *Behavioural correlates of MA ergic disturbances in depression.*

	↑(Auto) aggressivity	Anxiety	↑Vigilance	Apathy	Motor-retardation	Cognitive disturbances
↓5-HT$_{1A}$	X	X				X
↑5-HT$_{2C}$		X				
↓DA metabolism				X	X	
↓NA metabolism				X	X	X
↑NA metabolism		X	X			

selective agonists for the various subtypes of DA receptors are wanting and that D$_1$ and D$_2$ receptors supposedly exert opposite effects, at least in the mesolimbic and mesocortical systems. Hence one has to dispose of truly selective receptor agonists to sort out whether and which DA receptors might be dysfunctional in depression.

Data recently published by Laasonen-Balk *et al.* (1999), indicating hyperfunctioning of the DA transporter in depression, are intriguing but have not been confirmed (Meyer *et al.*, 2001).

Present-day antidepressants seem to lack pronounced effects on DA ergic transmission. Hence they cannot provide evidence in favour or against involvement of the DA system in the pathophysiology of depression.

7.5 Behavioural correlates of the monoaminergic disturbances in depression

In the previous sections it was emphasized that the disturbances in MA metabolism and MA receptor functioning were by no means characteristic for depression as such, but only demonstrable in subgroups of depression. It became apparent that these subgroups do not coincide with any of the depressive subcategories being distinguished in the present DSM classification nor with any syndromal category presently distinguished (Van Praag *et al.*, 1987, 1990).

Much evidence indicates that MA ergic disturbances are not so much associated with syndromes or categorically defined disorders, but with disturbances in the regulation of particular psychic functions (Table 7.6). In other words they were shown to be *functionally specific* rather than nosologically or syndromally specific (Van Praag *et al.*, 1987). Low CSF 5-HIAA, an indicator of diminished central 5-HT metabolism, appeared to be correlated with *heightened anxiety* as well as with *disturbed aggression regulation* (Figures 7.12, 7.13 and 7.14; Table 7.7). The latter may become manifest in suicidal behaviour and/or in various manifestations

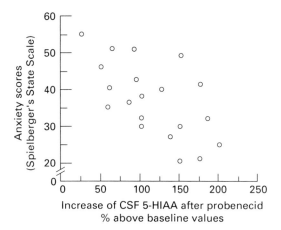

Figure 7.12. Post-probenecid CSF 5-HIAA concentration in patients with major depression, melancholic type. This variable correlates negatively with trait anxiety scores (Van Praag, 1988).

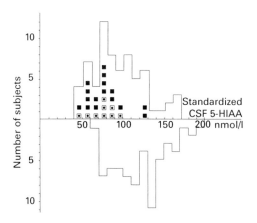

Figure 7.13. Standardized concentrations of CSF 5-HIAA in patients who have attempted suicide (Upward) and healthy volunteer control subjects (Downward). ■: Suicide attempts by a violent method (any method other than a drug overdose, taken by mouth, or a single wrist cut). ▣: a subject who subsequently died from suicide, in all cases but one within 1 year after the lumbar puncture (Åsberg et al., 1976),

of increased outward directed aggression such as irritability, anger outbursts and violence against others (Åsberg et al., 1976; Linnoila et al., 1983; Van Praag et al., 1987; Coccaro, 1992; Virkkunen et al., 1994). These relationships were not only demonstrable in depression but in other diagnostic categories as well. They seemed to occur independent of nosological diagnosis (Van Praag et al., 1987). Oquendo et al. (2003) studied regional brain 5-HT ergic function using PET in depressed patients with a history of high-lethality suicide attempts. They found glucose uptake

Table 7.7. Low 5-HIAA depressives compared with normal 5-HIAA depressives-source behaviours present (Van Praag, 1988).

Finding	P
More suicide attempts	<0.01
Greater number of contacts with police	<0.05
Increased arguments with	
relatives	<0.05
spouse	<0.01
colleagues	<0.05
friends	<0.05
More hostility at interview	<0.05
Impaired employment history (arguments)	<0.05

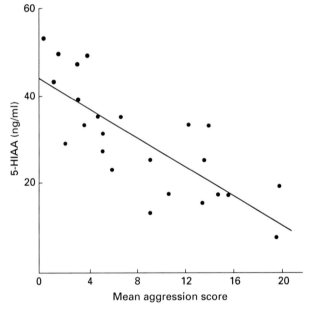

Figure 7.14. CSF 5-HIAA concentration in young male subjects with a variety of personality deviations. This variable correlates negatively with life-time signs of increased aggression (Brown *et al.*, 1979).

to be decreased in the (ventromedial) prefrontal cortex, relative to controls and low-lethality depressed suicide attempters. This effect was most pronounced after administration of fenfluramine, a compound facilitating 5-HT release and inhibiting its reuptake.

Tryptophan depletion in normal individuals provokes aggressive impulses in those who had high aggression scores to begin with (Cleare & Bond, 1995).

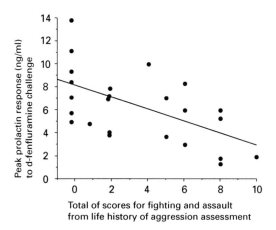

Figure 7.15. Peak prolactin response to d-fenfluramine in subjects with a variety of personality deviations. This variable correlates negatively with scores for life time history of aggression (Cocarro, 1992).

Tryptophan administration, on the other hand, enhances the ability to participate productively in group-related tasks, to display, in other words, affiliative behaviours (Moskowitz *et al.*, 2001).

The blunting of the prolactin response to d-fenfluramine in depression is significantly correlated with the patient's level of state anxiety and life-time aggression, not with the severity of the depression (O'Keane & Dinan, 1991) (Figure 7.15). A significant correlation has also been established between blunting of the prolactin response to fenfluramine and suicidal behaviour (Corrêa *et al.*, 2000) (Figure 7.16). In depressed patients a positive correlation has been found between cortex 5-HT$_2$ receptor binding potential (a variable proportional to receptor density and affinity) and dysfunctional attitudes (Meyer *et al.*, 2003). Dysfunctional attitudes were defined as negatively biased views of oneself, the world and the future.

Lowered CSF HVA, an indicator of reduced DA metabolism in (at least certain parts of) the CNS, was shown to correlate with *motor retardation* (Van Praag & Korf, 1971b) (Figure 7.11). Increased IBZM binding in the striatum as observed in depression was also correlated with signs of motor retardation (Shah *et al.*, 1997). PET studies revealed a decrease of [^{18}F] DOPA in the caudate nucleus in retarded depression, particularly on the left side, observations likewise suggestive for a link between DA hypofunction and psychomotor retardation.

Low CSF HVA appeared not to be restricted to retarded depression but to occur also in other diagnostic categories with motor retardation, such as in Parkinson's disease and certain forms of schizophrenia (Van Praag & Korf, 1971a,b; Van Praag *et al.*, 1973; Willner, 1995). In accordance with these observations, l-DOPA administered in depression exerted activating effects, particularly in low CSF HVA patients, while mood was not significantly altered (Van Praag, 1974). Antidepressants with

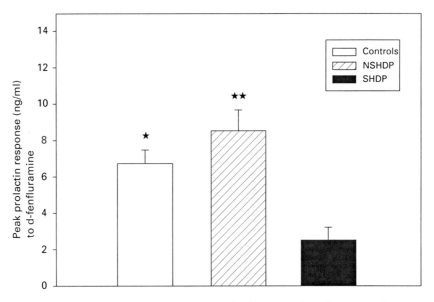

Figure 7.16. Peak prolactin response to d-fenfluramine in healthy controls and a group of patients with major depression with or without a history of suicide attempts. The prolactin response was blunted in the suicidal depressed group (SHDP) relative to the nonsuicidal depressed group (NSHDP) and the control group (Corrêa *et al.*, 2000).

pronounced DA potentiating effects, moreover, are most potent in retarded depression (Brown & Gerston, 1993).

A relationship between low CSF HVA and anhedonia has not been demonstrated. This is not surprising because HVA concentration in lumbar CSF is largely a reflection of DA metabolism in the nigrostriatal DA system (a predominantly motor-regulating system) and not of activity in the mesolimbic and mesocortical DA system, which are considered to be involved in affective pathology.

The behavioural correlates of the NA ergic disturbances are complex. Hyperactivity of this system leads first of all to arousal, increased vigilance and ultimately to *anxiety*. In addition *cognitive changes* appear. Hippocampal function is switched from a state of lowered memory formation to a state of enhanced stimulus detection and encoding when aroused with novelty or stressed with aversion (Ressler & Nemeroff, 2000). NA ergic overactivity, thus, will result in excess hippocampal functioning in the stressed/aroused state, with enhanced or oversensitive memory to aversive stimuli (Mongeau *et al.*, 1997). The NA system, moreover, facilitates the relay of adverse memories from temporary to long-term storage.

NA ergic hypoactivity, as seems likely to occur in some depressed patients, has been hypothesized to be linked to deficits in '*emotional memory*' (Van Praag *et al.*, 1990). Perception in these patients is undisturbed but they are unable to link perceptions to the corresponding emotions. For instance, a patient goes to church, but it does not touch him anymore, while previously such visits used to evoke a sense of devotion. These hypotheses are supported by the studies of O'Carroll *et al.* (1999), demonstrating that, in humans, stimulation of the NA ergic system results in enhancement, and blockade of this system in a reduction of recall and recognition of emotional material.

The cognitive effects of 5-HT ergic stimulation are opposite to those of NA ergic activation. It leads to decreased learning of aversive stimuli and an increase in tolerance toward aversive experiences (Mongeau *et al.*, 1997). A deficit in 5-HT ergic 'tone' will thus reinforce the anxiety/frustration proneness resulting from NA ergic overactivity. Since LC and raphe nuclei are anatomically interconnected and on a functional level mutually inhibitory, activation of the LC system will induce inhibition of the raphe system, thus further enhancing the cognitive effects of NA ergic dominance.

All in all, MA ergic disturbances seem to be *function-specific.* Since psychic dysfunctions are seldom specific for a particular syndrome or nosological entity, it is understandable that the corresponding biological variables, too, are nosologically and syndromally nonspecific. By the same token it is explicable that MA ergic disturbances are demonstrable only in some depressive patients, for the corresponding behavioural variables can be pronounced in one patient and subordinate in the other. In the former case, the MA ergic disturbances are expected to be present, in the latter case to be absent.

7.6 Some animal data on 5-HT ergic regulation of anxiety and aggression

Human and animal data on 5-HT ergic regulation of anxiety and aggression show a remarkable parallelism. In subhuman primates CSF 5-HIAA correlates negatively with aggression and impulse control (Higley *et al.*, 1992; Mehlman *et al.*, 1994). Monkeys with low CSF 5-HIAA show severe aggression, impulsive risk-taking behaviour and violence leading to trauma and early mortality (Westergaard *et al.*, 1999) (Figure 7.17). The level of 5-HIAA in CSF in monkeys is a quite stable variable, probably largely genetically determined and probably linked to particular components of the behavioural repertoire. The prolactin response to the indirect 5-HT agonist fenfluramine is likewise negatively correlated with aggressive behaviours (Kyes *et al.*, 1995) (Figure 7.18).

Drugs decreasing 5-HT functioning increase aggression and vice versa. Similarly, increasing or decreasing dietary tryptophan produced decrease and increase of aggressivity, respectively (Higley *et al.*, 1992). On the other hand, CSF 5-HIAA is positively correlated with social competence, a concept referring to the total time an animal spent in grooming and being groomed and the time spent in close proximity

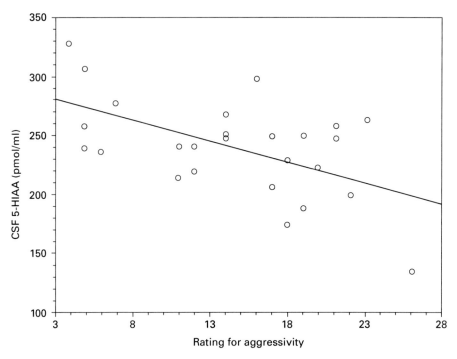

Figure 7.17. Correlation of CSF 5-HIAA concentration and ratings of aggressivity in free-ranging rhesus monkeys (Higley *et al.*, 1992).

to others (Raleigh *et al.*, 1985; Mehlman *et al.*, 1995; Higley *et al.*, 1996). Indirect 5-HT agonists such as tryptophan and fluoxetine increase affiliative behaviours and decrease aggressive behaviours, while 5-HT antagonists such as cyproheptadine have the opposite effect (Raleigh *et al.*, 1991).

In male monkeys affiliative behaviour and dominance are correlated. Individuals that eventually become dominant are more likely to engage in affiliative behaviour with females than are males that will not become dominant (De Waal, 1986; Raleigh *et al.*, 1991). Raleigh *et al.* (1991) remark that monkeys 'attaining male dominance may be less dependent on individual fighting ability than on the ability to establish affiliative relationships with females and recruit allies during aggressive encounters'. The 5-HT ergic system may thus mediate behaviours increasing the chance that the animal will acquire higher dominance status (Bonson *et al.*, 1994).

Interestingly, Knutson *et al.* (1998) demonstrated that in normal volunteers SSRIs facilitate affiliative behaviour as well (Figure 7.19), suggesting that central 5-HT ergic systems modulate functions involved in inter-individual communication both in humans and subhuman primates.

Animal data furthermore indicate the 5-HT$_{1A}$ and 5HT$_2$ receptor system to be involved in *aggression* and *anxiety regulation*. Activation of 5-HT$_{1A}$ receptors

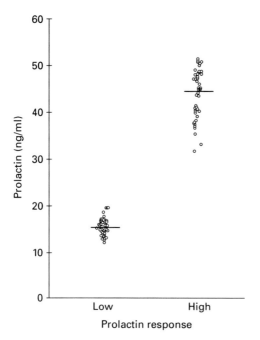

Figure 7.18. Prolactin response to fenfluramine in cynomolgus macaque monkeys. The horizontal bar represents the mean prolactin response. The prolactin responses were distributed bimodally. High: high overt aggression scores, low: low overt aggression scores. Low prolactin responders had a significantly higher index of overt aggression (Botchin *et al.*, 1993).

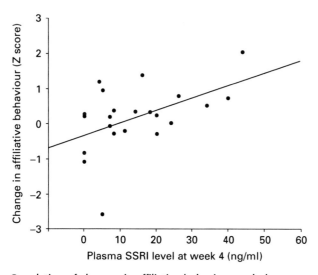

Figure 7.19. Correlation of changes in affiliative behaviour and plasma paroxetine levels in normal volunteers having received 20 mg/day paroxetine for 4 weeks (Knutson *et al.*, 1998).

with 5-HT$_{1A}$ agonists produces anxiolytic effects. The acute effects are possibly related to activation of the 5-HT$_{1A}$ autoreceptors, located on the 5-HT cell bodies and dendrites in the raphe nuclei, resulting in inhibition of the firing of all 5-HT neurons (Schreiber & de Vrij, 1993a,b; Andrews *et al.*, 1994). Chronic anxiolytic effects produced by 5-HT$_{1A}$ agonists are probably mediated via postsynaptic 5-HT$_{1A}$ receptors located in the limbic areas (Przegalinski *et al.*, 1992; Bell & Hobson, 1994). The postsynaptic 5-HT$_{1A}$ effects are probably decisive since the presynaptic 5-HT$_{1A}$ receptor, in contrast to its postsynaptic equivalent, desensitizes rapidly (Chaput *et al.*, 1986; Jolas *et al.*, 1995), while the anxiolytic effects improve over time (Schefke *et al.*, 1989). One has to bear in mind that by stimulation of the postsynaptic 5-HT$_{1A}$ receptor the neuron is hyperpolarized, and the electrical activity of the cell where these receptors are located is reduced (Araneda & Andrade, 1991; Andrade, 1992). This can be more easily understood as an anxiolytic mechanism and as an adaptive stress response (Deakin, 1993) than increased electrical activity. If the (postsynaptic) 5-HT$_{1A}$ receptor is downregulated, as occurs in conditions of sustained stress, depolarization is facilitated, electrical activity in the system increases and anxiety gathers strength.

5-HT$_2$ receptors are likewise involved in anxiety regulation, in particular the 2C subtype. mCPP increases anxiety, probably via activation of the 5-HT$_{2C}$ receptor (Kennett & Curzon, 1988; Gibson *et al.*, 1994). Blockade of that receptor, on the other hand, reduces anxiety (Kennett *et al.*, 1994a).

Most studies have found that enhancement of 5-HT ergic transmission results in attenuation of aggressive behaviours, more particularly of predatory aggression, while inhibition of the 5-HT system furthers aggression. Not only do postsynaptic 5-HT$_{1A}$ receptors seem to be involved but likewise 5HT$_2$ and postsynaptic 5-HT$_{1B/D}$ receptors (Olivier & Mos, 1992; Bell & Hobson, 1993).

Selective activation of the 5-HT$_{1A}$ receptor reduces aggression (Olivier & Mos, 1992, 1994) – particularly offensive aggression (De Almeida & Lucion, 1994; De Boer *et al.*, 1999). Social exploration and motor activity remained uninfluenced. Behavioural inhibition, thus, could not explain the aggression-inhibiting effects. Selective 5-HT$_{1A}$ antagonists obliterate the anti-aggressive effects (De Boer *et al.*, 1999). It has not been excluded that the anti-aggressive effects are secondary to alterations in anxiety. In wild (and more aggressive) rats, as compared with domesticated rats, 5-HT$_{1A}$ receptor binding is decreased (Hammer *et al.*, 1992; Hmer *et al.*, 1992). The excessive aggressiveness and impulsivity of male mice lacking neuronal nitric oxide synthase is caused by selective decrements in 5-HT turnover and deficient 5-HT$_{1A}$ and 5-HT$_{1B}$ receptor function (Chiavegatto *et al.*, 2001).

Decreased activity of the 5-HT$_2$ system, likewise enhances aggressive behaviours in animals (White *et al.*, 1991; Albonetti *et al.*, 1994) as well as possibly in humans (Blumensohn *et al.*, 1995). The 5-HT$_{1B/D}$ receptor is another subtype of 5-HT receptor with a profound effect on aggression. Knock-out of the 5-HT$_{1B}$ receptor gene in mice resulted in increased aggression (Sandou *et al.*, 1994). Postsynaptic 5-HT$_{1B/D}$ receptor agonists have strong aggression-reducing properties (De Almeida & Miczek, 2002).

A notable exception to the general notion that reduced 5-HT synthesis and reduced 5-HT$_{1A}$ receptor functioning promotes aggression, is a study by Korte *et al.* (1996). The starting point was the observation that in wild animal populations individuals with extreme differences in stress reaction coexist. The extremes, they remark, display in response to a threat either an active behavioural response or a passive one. The former group fights the threat or flees if the threat seems unsurmountable. The latter group tends to respond with withdrawal and immobility. The active behavioural response pattern is associated with high sympathetic activity and low corticosteroid levels, the passive response with high parasympathetic activity and high corticosteroid levels.

Korte *et al.* (1996) studied mice genetically selected for either high or low aggression in a resident–intruder paradigm. The high-aggression group was considered to represent the active responders to threat, the low aggression group the passive cohort. The high-aggression group showed increased numbers of postsynaptic 5-HT$_{1A}$ receptor in limbic and cortical regions, as compared with the low-aggression mice.

Possible explanations for these discrepant findings are the following: (1) In this model 5-HT$_{1A}$ receptor density and level of offensive aggression are not related; (2) The increase in the 5-HT$_{1A}$ receptor density is a secondary phenomenon, compensating for a primary reduced sensitivity of 5-HT$_{1A}$ receptors; (3) The relationship between the 5-HT(1A) system and aggression is restricted to a particular manifestation of aggression (still to be investigated). The latter possibility is intriguing and might turn out to be of considerable importance in human aggression research too.

In conclusion, data from animal research strongly suggest the 5-HT$_1$ and 5-HT$_2$ receptor systems to be involved in the regulation of both anxiety and aggression.

7.7 Conclusions

Various disturbances in MA ergic functioning have been ascertained in mood disorders. Broadly speaking, data pertaining to 5-HT and DA point to functional deficits, while those related to the NA ergic system are mixed. Some indicate NA ergic overdrive, while others are suggestive of hypoactivity of that system. As to the 5-HT system, both metabolic and receptor disturbances have been ascertained. The 5-HT$_1$ and 5-HT$_2$ receptor systems seem to be particularly involved. Since (1) the 5-HT disturbances precede a depressive episode and (2) pharmacological interventions geared towards amelioration of the 5-HT disturbances produce antidepressant effects, it seems likely that the 5-HT disturbances may play a role in the pathophysiology of depression. It has been hypothesized that they represent vulnerability factors increasing the risk of affective disturbances in times of mounting stress.

The disturbances in the catecholamine systems are more likely to be state-related, but available evidence is insufficient for definitive statements.

MA ergic disturbances are not a universal phenomenon in depression. They occur in particular subgroups, that do not coincide with the present nosological or syndromal groupings of mood disorders. Much evidence indicates that the MA ergic disturbances are functionally specific, being associated with particular psychic dysfunctions, irrespective of categorical or syndromal diagnosis.

Stress triggers CRH release and activation of both the HPA system and the NA ergic system. The question arises whether (chronic) stress syndromes and (certain) mood disorders share biological characteristics. Formulated more pointedly: can (chronic) stress disturb MA ergic functioning in the brain in a way demonstrated to occur in (certain forms of) depression. If so, this would strongly suggest that stress can indeed *cause* (certain forms of) depression. This issue is the subject matter of the next chapter.

REFERENCES

Abbar, M., Courtet, P., Bellivier, F. *et al.* (2001). Suicide attempts and the tryptophan hydroxylase gene. *Molec. Psychiatry*, 6, 268–73.

Abe, M., Nakai, H., Tabata, R., Saito, K. & Egawa, M. (1998). Effects of 5-{3-[((2S)-1, 4-Benzodioxan-2-ylmethyl)amino]propoxy}-1, 3-benzodioxole HC1 (MKC-242), a novel 5-HT$_{1A}$-receptor agonist, on aggressive behavior and marble burying behavior in mice. *Jpn. J. Pharmacol.*, 76, 297–304.

Agren, H. & Reibring, L. (1994). PET studies of presynaptic monoamine metabolism in depressed patients and healthy volunteers. *Pharmacopsychiatry*, 27, 2–6.

Agren, H., Reibring, L., Hartvig, P. *et al.* (1991). Low brain uptake of L [^{11}C]5-hydroxytryptophan in major depression: a position emission tomography study on patients and healthy volunteers. *Acta Psychiatr. Scand.*, 83, 449–55.

Albonetti, M. E, Gonzalez, M. I., Wilson, C. A. & Farabollini, F. (1994). Effects of neonatal treatment with 1-(2,5-dimethoxy-4-iodophenyl)-2 aminopropane HCI (DOI) and ritanserin on agonistic behavior in adult male and female rats. *Aggressive Behav.*, 20, 235–42.

Anand, A. & Charney, D. S. (1997). Catecholamines in depression. In *Depression. Neurobiological, Psychopathological and Therapeutic Advances*, ed. A. Honig & H. M. van Praag. Chichester: John Wiley & Sons.

Andrade, R. (1992). Electrophysiology of 5-HT1a in rat hippocampus and cortex. *Drug Rev. Res.*, 2, 275–86.

Andrews, N., Hogg, S., Gonzalez, L. E. & File, S. E. (1994). 5-HT1a receptors in the median raphe nucleus and dorsal hippocampus may mediate anxiolytic and anxiogenic behaviours respectively. *Eur. J. Pharmacol.*, **264**, 259–64.

Ansseau, M. (1997). Hormonal disturbances in depression. In *Depression. Neurobiological, Psychopathological and Therapeutic Advances*, ed. A. Honig & H. M. van Praag. Chichester: John Wiley & Sons.

Ansseau, M., Von Frenckell, R., Cerfontaine, J. L. *et al.* (1988). Blunted response of growth hormone to clonidine and apomorphine in endogenous depression. *Br. J. Psychiatry*, **153**, 65–71.

Araneda, R. & Andrade, R. (1991). 5-Hydroxytryptamine 2 and 5- hydroxytryptamine 1A receptors mediate opposing responses on membrane excitability in rat association cortex. *Neuroscience*, **40**, 399–401.

Åsberg, M., Thorén, P., Träskman, L., Bertilsson, L. & Ringbergen, V. (1976). Serotonin depression – a biochemical subgroup within the affective disorders? *Science*, **191**, 478–80.

Asnis, G. M., Halbreich, U., Rabinovich, H. *et al.* (1986). The cortisol response to desipramine in endogenous depressives and normal controls: preliminary findings. *Psychiatr. Res.*, **14**, 225–33.

Asnis, G. M., Wetzler, S., Sanderson, W. C., Kahn, R. S. & van Praag, H. M. (1992). Functional interrelationship of serotonin and norepinephrine: cortisol response to MCPP and DMI in patients with panic disorder, patients with depression, and normal control subjects. *Psychiatr. Res.*, **43**, 65–76.

Audenaert, K., Van Laere, K., Dumont, F. *et al.* (2001). Decreased frontal serotonin 5-HT$_{2A}$ receptor binding index in deliberate self-harm patients. *Eur. J. Nucl. Med.*, **28**, 175–82.

Bell, R. & Hobson, H. (1993). Effects of pindobind 5-hydroxytryptamine$_{1A}$ (5-HT1A, a novel and potent 5-HT$_{1A}$ antagonist), on social and agonistic behaviour in male albino mice. *Pharmacol. Biochem. Behav.*, **46**, 67–72.

(1994). 5-HT1a receptor influences on rodent social and agonistic behavior: a review and empirical study. *Neurosci. Behav. Rev.*, **18**, 325–38.

Bellivier, F., Leboyer, M., Courtet, P. *et al.* (1998). Association between the tryptophan hydroxylase gene and manic-depressive illness. *Arch. Gen. Psychiatry*, **55**, 33–7.

Benkelfat, C., Ellenbogen, M., Dean, P., Palmour, R. & Young, S. (1994). Mood-lowering effect of tryptophan depletion. Enhanced susceptibility in young men at genetic risk for major affective disorders. *Arch. Gen. Psychiatry*, **51**, 687–97.

Benkelfat, C., Young, S. N., Leyton, M. & Diksie, M. (2002). Impulsivity: serotonergic mechanisms. *Int. J. Neuropsychopharm.*, **5** (Suppl. I) S13.

Bennett, A. J., Lesch, K. P., Heils, A. *et al.* (2002). Early experience and serotonin transporter gene variation interact to influence primate CNS function. *Mol. Psychiatry*, **7**, 118–22.

Berman, R. M., Darnell, A. M., Miller, H. L., Anand, R. A. & Charney, P. S. (1997). Effect of pindolol in hastening response to fluoxetine in the treatment of major depression: a double blind, placebo controlled trial. *Am. J. Psychiatry*, **154**, 37–43.

Berman, R. M., Narasimhan, M., Miller, H. L. *et al.* (1999). Transient depressive relapse induced by catecholamine depletion. *Arch. Gen. Psychiatry*, **56**, 395–403.

Berrettini, W. H., Ferraro, T. N., Goldin, L. R. *et al.* (1994). Chromosome 18 DNA markers and manic-depressive illness: evidence for susceptibility gene. *Proc. Natl. Acad. Sci. USA*, **91**, 689–96.

Bhagwagar, Z., Whale, R. & Cowen, P. J. (2002). State and trait abnormalities in serotonin function in major depression. *Br. J. Psychiatry*, **180**, 24–8.

Biegon, A., Grinspoon, A., Blumenfeld, B., Bleich, A., Apter, A. & Mester, R. (1990). Increased serotonin 5-HT2 receptor binding on blood platelets of suicidal men. *Psychopharmacology*, **100**, 165–7.

Blier, P. & Bergeron, R. (1998). The use of pindolol to potentiate antidepressant medication. *J. Clin. Psychiatry*, **59**, 16–23.

Blier, P. & de Montigny, C. (1994). Current advances and trends in the treatment of depression. *Trends Pharm. Sci.*, **15**, 220–6.

Blier, P., Bergeron, R. & de Montigny, C. (1997). Selective activation of postsynaptic 5-HT$_{1A}$ receptors induces rapid antidepressant response. *Neuropsychopharmacology*, **16**, 333–8.

Blomberg, P. A., Kopin, I. J., Gordon, E. K., Markey, S. P. & Ebert, M. H. (1980). Conversion of MHPG to vanillylmandelic acid. *Arch. Gen. Psychiatry*, **37**, 1095–8.

Blumensohn, R., Ratzoni, G., Weizman, A. *et al.* (1995). Reduction in serotonin 5HT2 receptor binding on platelets of delinquent adolescents. *Psychopharmacology*, **118**, 354–6.

Bondy, B., Erfurth, A., de Jonge, S., Krüger, M. & Meyer, H. (2000). Possible association of the short allele of the serotonin transporter gene polymorphism (5-HTTLPR) with violent suicide. *Mol. Psychiatry*, **5**, 193–5.

Bonhomme, N. & Esposito, E. (1998). Involvement of serotonin and dopamine in the mechanism of action of novel antidepressant drugs: a review. *J. Clin. Psychopharm.*, **18**, 447–54.

Bonson, K. R., Johnson, R. G., Fiorella, D., Rabin R. A. & Winter, J. C. (1994). Serotonergic control of androgen-induced dominance. *Pharmacol. Biochem. Behav.*, **49**, 313–22.

Borsini, F., Brambilla, A., Grippa, N. & Pitsikas, N. (1999). Behavioral effects of flibanserin (BIMT 17). *Pharmacol. Biochem. Behav.*, **64**, 137–46.

Botchin, M., Kaplan, J., Manuck, S. & Mann, J. (1993). Low versus high prolactin responders to fenfluramine challenge: marker of behavioral differences in adult male cynomolgus macaques. *Neuropsychopharmacology*, **9**, 93–9.

Bromidge, S. M., Dabbs, S., Davies, D. T. *et al.* (2000). Biarylcarbamoylinodolines are novel and selective 5-HT2C receptor inverse agonists: identification of 5-methyl-1-[[2-[(2-methyl-3-pyridyl)oxy]-5-pyridyl]carbamoyl]-6-trifluoromethylindoline (SB-243213) as a potential antidepressant/anxiolytic agent. *J. Med. Chem.*, **43**, 1123–34.

Brown A. S. & Gerston, S. (1993). Dopamine and depression. *J. Neural Transm.*, **91**, 75–109.

Brown, G., Goodwin, F., Ballenger, J., Goyer, P. & Major, L. (1979). Aggression in humans correlates with cerebrospinal fluid amine metabolites. *Psychiatr. Res.*, **1**, 131–9.

Cadogan, A. K., Marsden, C. A., Tulloch, I. & Kendall, D. A. (1993). Evidence that administration of paroxetine or fluoxetine enhances 5-HT$_2$ receptor function in the brain of the guinea-pig. *Neuropharmacology*, **32**, 249–56.

Callado, L. F., Meana, J. J., Grijalba, B., Pazos, A., Sastre, M. & García-Sevilla, J. A. (1998). Selective increase of α_{2A}-adrenoceptor agonist binding sites in brains of depressed suicide victims. *J. Neurochem.*, **70**, 1114–23.

Cannon, W. B. (1929). *Body Changes in Pain, Hunger, Fear, and Rage.* New York: Appleton.

Carroll, B. J., Curtis, G. C. & Mendels, J. (1976). Neuroendocrine regulation in depression: discrimination of depressed from nondepressed patients. *Arch. Gen. Psychiatry*, **33**, 1051–8.

Caspi, A., Sugden, K., Moffitt, T. *et al.* (2003). Influence of life stress on depression: moderation by a polymorphism in the 5-HTT gene. *Science*, **301**, 386–9.

Chaput, Y., de Montigny, C. & Blier, P. (1986). Effect of a selective 5-HT reuptake blocker, citalopram on the sensitivity of 5-HT autoreceptors: electrophysiological studies in the rat brain. *Naunyn Schmiederbergs Arch. Pharmacol.*, **333**, 342–8.

Chiavegatto, S., Dawson, V. L., Mamounas, L. A., Koliatsos, V. E., Dawson, T. & Nelson, R. J. (2001). Brain serotonin dysfunction accounts for aggression in male mice lacking neuronal nitric oxide synthase. *Proc. Natl. Acad. Sci. USA*, **98**, 1277–81.

Chugani, D. C. & Muzig, O. (2000). α-[^{11}C]Methyl-l-tryptophan PET maps brain serotonin synthesis and kynurenine pathway metabolism. *J. Cereb. Blood Flow Metab.*, **20**, 2–9.

Cleare, A. J. & Bond, A. J. (1995). The effect of tryptophan depletion and enhancement on subjective and behavioural aggression in normal male subjects. *Psychopharmacology*, **118**, 72–81.

Coccaro, E. F. (1992). Impulsive aggression and central serotonergic system function in humans; an example of a dimensional brain–behavior relationship. *Intern Clin. Psychopharm.*, **7**, 3–12.

Coccaro, E. F., Kavoussi, R. J., Sheline, Y. I., Berman, M. E. & Csernansky, J. G. (1997). Impulsive aggression in personality disorder correlates with platelet 5-HT$_{2A}$ receptor binding. *Neuropsychopharmacology*, **16**, 211–16.

Coppen, A. J. (1967). The biochemistry of affective disorders. *Br. J. Psychiatry*, **113**, 1237–64.

Corrêa, H., Duval, F., Mokrani, M.-C. *et al.* (2000). Prolactin response to D-fenfluramine and suicidal behavior in depressed patients. *Psychiatry Res.*, **93**, 189–99.

Courtet, P., Baud, P., Abbar, M. *et al.* (2001). Association between violent suicidal behavior and the low activity allele of the serotonin transporter gene. *Mol. Psychiatry*, **6**, 338–41.

Cowen, P. J., Charig, E. M., Fraser, S. & Elliot, J. M. (1987). Platelet 5HT receptor binding during depressive illness and tricyclic anti-depressant treatment. *J. Affect. Disord.*, **13**, 45–50.

Cowen, P. J., Power, A. C., Ware, C. J. & Anderson, I. M. (1994). 5-HT$_{1A}$ receptor sensitivity in major depression. A neuroendocrine study with buspirone. *Br. J. Psychiatry*, **164**, 372–9.

Crow, T. J., Cross, A. J., Cooper, S. J. *et al.* (1984). Neurotransmitter receptors and monoamine metabolites in the brains of patients with Alzheimer-type dementia and depression, and suicides. *Neuropharmacology*, **23**, 1561–9,

Cryan, J. F. & Leonard, B. E. (2000). 5-HT$_{1A}$ and beyond: the role of serotonin and its receptors in depression and the antidepressant response. *Hum. Psychopharm. Clin. Exp.*, **15**, 113–35.

De Almeida, R. M. M. & Lucion, A. B. (1994). Effects of intracerebroventricular administration of 5-HT receptor agonist on the maternal aggression of rats. *Eur. J. Pharmacol.*, **264**, 445–8.

De Almeida, R. M. M. & Miczek, K. A. (2002). Aggression escalated by social instigation or by discontinuation of reinforcement ('frustration') in mice: inhibition by anpirtoline: a 5-HT$_{1B}$ receptor agonist. *Neuropsychopharmacology*, **27**, 171–81.

De Boer, S. F., Lesourd, M., Mocaer, E. & Koolhaas, J. M. (1999). Selective antiaggressive effects of alnespirone in resident-intruder test are mediated via 5-hydroxytryptamine$_{1A}$ receptors:

a comparative pharmacological study with 8-hydroxy-2-dipropylaminotetralin, ipsapirone, buspirone, eltopraxine, and WAY-100635. *J. Pharmacol. Exp. Ther.*, **288**, 1125–33.

De Bruyn, A., Souery, D., Mendelbaum, K., Mendlewicz, J. & van Broeckhoven, C. (1996). Linkage analysis of families with bipolar illness and chromosome 18 markers. *Biol. Psychiatry*, **39**, 679–88.

De Vrij, J. (1995). 5-HT$_{1A}$ agonists: recent developments and controversial issues. *Psychopharmacology*, **121**, 1–32.

De Waal, F. B. M. (1986). The integration of dominance and social bonding in primates. *Q. Rev. Biol.*, **61**, 459–79.

Deakin, J. F. W. (1993). A review of clinical efficacy of 5-HT$_{1A}$ agonists in anxiety and depression. *J. Psychopharm.*, **7**, 283–9.

Deakin, J. F. W., Pennell, I., Upaxhyaya, A. J. *et al.* (1990). A neuroendocrine study of 5-HT function in depression: evidence for biological mechanisms of endogenous and psychosocial causation. *Psychopharmacology (Berlin)*, **101**, 85–92.

Delgado, P. & Moreno, F. (2000). Role of norepinephrine in depression. *J. Clin. Psychiatry*, **61** (suppl), 5–12.

Delgado, P. L., Charney, D. S., Price, L. H., Landis, H. & Heninger, G. R. (1990). Neuroendocrine and behavioral effects of dietary tryptophan restriction in healthy subjects. *Life Sci.*, **45**, 2323–32.

Depue, R. A., Arbisi, P., Krauss, S. *et al.* (1990). Seasonal independence of low prolactin concentration and high spontaneous eye blink rates in unipolar and bipolar II seasonal affective disorder. *Arch. Gen. Psychiatry*, **47**, 356–64.

D'Haenen, H. & Bossuyt, A. (1994). Dopamine D2 receptors in the brain measured with SPECT. *Biol. Psychiatry*, **35**, 128–32.

D'Haenen, H., Bossuyt, A., Mertens J. *et al.* (1992). SPECT imaging of serotonin$_2$ receptors in depression. *Psychiatr. Res. Neuroimaging*, **45**, 227–37.

Diksic, M., Nagahiro, S., Sourkes, T. L. & Yamamoto, Y. L. (1990). A new method to measure brain serotonin synthesis in vivo, I: theory and basic data for a biological model. *J. Cereb. Blood Flow Metab.*, **10**, 1–12.

Dremencov, E., Gur, E., Lerer, B. & Newman, M. E. (2002). Effects of chronic antidepressants and electroconvulsive shock on serotonergic neurotransmission in the rat hypothalamus. *Prog. Neuro-Psychopharmacol. Biol. Psychiatry*, **26**, 1029–34.

Drevets, W. C., Frank, E., Price, J. C. *et al.* (1999). PET imaging of serotonin 1A receptor binding in depression. *Biol. Psychiatry*, **46**, 1375–87.

Du, L., Bakish, D., Lapierre, Y. D., Ravindran, A. V. & Hrdina, P. D. (2000a). Association of polymorphism of serotonin 2A receptor gene with suicidal ideation in major depressive disorder. *Am. J. Med. Genet.*, **96**, 56–60.

Du, L., Faludi, G., Palkovits, M., Bakish, D. & Hrdina, P. D. (2000b). Tryptophan hydroxylase gene 218A/C polymorphism is not associated with depressed suicide. *Intern. J. Neuropsychopharm.*, **3**, 215–20.

Ebert, D., Feistel, H., Loew, T. & Pirner, A. (1996). Dopamine and depression – striatal dopamine D$_2$ receptor SPECT before and after antidepressant therapy. *Psychopharmacology*, **126**, 91–4.

Ebstein, R. P., Segman, R., Benjamin, J., Osher, Y., Nemanov, L. & Belmaker, R. H. (1997). 5-HT2c (HTR2C) serotonin receptor gene polymorphism associated with the human personality trait of reward dependence: interaction with dopamine D4 receptor (D4DR) and dopamine D3 receptor (D3DR) polymorphisms. *Am. J. Med. Genet. (Neuropsychiatr. Genet.)*, **74**, 65–72.

Eison, A. S. & Mullins, U. L. (1996). Regulation of central 5-HT$_{2A}$ receptors: a review of in vivo studies. *Behav. Brain Res.*, **73**, 177–81.

Ellingrod, V. L. & Perry, P. J. (1995). Nefazodone: a new antidepressant. *Am. J. Health-Systems Pharm.*, **52**, 2799–812.

Ellis, P. & Salmond, C. (1994). Is platelet imipramine binding reduced in depression? A meta-analysis. *Biol. Psychiatr.*, **36**, 292–9.

Evans, J., Reeves, B., Platt, H. *et al.* (2000). Impulsiveness, serotonin genes and repetition of deliberate self-harm (DSH). *Psychol. Med.*, **30**, 1327–34.

Extein, I., Tallman, J., Smith, C. C. & Goodwin, F. K. (1979). Changes in lymphocyte beta-adrenergic receptors in depression and mania. *Psychiatry Res.*, **1**, 191–7.

Fitch, D., Lesage, A., Seguin, M. *et al.* (2001). Suicide and the serotonin transporter gene. *Mol. Psychiatry*, **6**, 127–8.

Florey, J. D., Mann, J. J., Manuck, S. B. & Muldoon, M. F. (1998). Recovery from major depression is not associated with normalisation of serotonergic function. *Biol. Psychiatry*, **43**, 320–6.

Frazer, A., Brown, R., Koesis, J. *et al.* (1986). Patterns of melatonin rhythms in depression. *J. Neural Transm.*, **67**, 215–24.

Frisch, A., Postilnick, D., Rockah, R. *et al.* (1999). Association of unipolar major depressive disorder with genes of the serotonergic and dopaminergic pathways. *Mol. Psychiat.*, **4**, 389–92.

Garcia-Sevilla, J. A., Padro, D., Giralt, T., Guimon, J. & Areso, P. (1990). Alpha-2 adrenoceptor-mediated inhibition of platelet adenyl cyclase and induction of aggregation in major depression. *Arch. Gen. Psychiatry*, **47**, 125–32.

Geijer, T., Frisch, A,. Persson, M.-L. *et al.* (2000). Search for association between suicide attempt and serotonergic polymorphisms. *Psychiatr. Genet.*, **10**, 19–26.

Germine, M., Goddard, A. W., Woods, C. W., Charney, D. S. & Heninger, G. R. (1992). Anger and anxiety responses to m-chlorophenylpiperazine in generalized anxiety disorder. *Biol. Psychiatry*, **32**, 457–61.

Gibson, E. L., Barnfield, A. M. C. & Curzon, G. (1994). Evidence that mCPP-induced anxiety in the plus-maze is mediated by postsynaptic 5-HT2c receptors but not by sympathomimetic effects. *Neuropharmacology*, **33**, 457–65.

Gjerris, A., Werdelin, L., Rafaelson, O. J., Ailing, C. & Christensen, N. J. (1987). CSF dopamine increased in depression: CSF dopamine, noradrenalin and their metabolites in depressed patients and in controls. *J. Affect. Disord.*, **13**, 279–86.

Golden, R. N., Durr Heine, A., Ekstrom, R. D., Bebchuk, J. M., Leatherman, M. E. & Garbutt, J. C. (2002). A longitudinal study of serotonergic function in depression. *Neuropsychopharmacology*, **26**, 653–9.

Goodwin, F. K. & Sack, R. L. (1974). Central dopamine function in affective illness: evidence from precursors, enzyme inhibitors, and studies of central dopamine turnover. In *Neuropharmacology of Monoamines and their Regulatory Enzymes*, ed. E. Usdin. New York: Raven Press.

Gross, C., Zhuang, X., Stark, K. et al. (2002). Serotonin$_{1A}$ receptor acts during development to establish normal anxiety-like behavior in the adult. *Nature*, **416**, 396–400.

Haddjeri, N., Szabo, S., De Montigny, C. & Blier, P. (2000). Increased tonic activation of rat forebrain 5-HT$_{1A}$ receptors by lithium addition to antidepressant treatments. *Neuropsychopharmacology*, **22**, 346–56.

Hammer, R. P., Hori, K. M., Blanchard, R. J. & Blanchard, D. C. (1992). Domestication alters 5-HT$_{1A}$ receptor binding in rat brain. *Pharmacol. Biochem. Behav.*, **42**, 25–8.

Hariri, A. R., Mattay, V. S., Tessitore, A. et al. (2002). Serotonin transporter genetic variation and the response of the human amygdala. *Science*, **297**, 400–3.

Healy, D., Carney, P. A., O'Halloran, A. & Leonard, B. E. (1985). Peripheral adrenoceptors and serotonin receptors in depression: changes associated with response to treatment with trazodone or amitriptyline. *J. Affect. Disord.*, **9**, 285–96.

Heiser, J., & Wilcox, Ch. S. (1998). Serotonin 5-HT$_{1a}$ receptor agonists as antidepressants. *CNS-Drugs*, **10**, 343–53.

Heninger, G. R., Charney, D. S. & Sternberg, D. E. (1984). Serotonergic function in depression. *Arch. Gen. Psychiatry*, **41**, 398–402.

Higley, J. D., Mehlman, P. T., Taub, D. M. et al. (1992). Cerebrospinal fluid monoamine and adrenal correlates of aggression in free-ranging rhesus monkeys. *Arch. Gen. Psychiatry*, **49**, 436–41.

Higley, J. D., King, S. T., Hasert, M. F., Champoux, M., Suomi, S. J. & Linnoila, M. (1996). Stability of interindividual differences in serotonin function and its relationship to severe aggression and competent social behavior in rhesus macaque females. *Neuropsychopharmacology*, **14**, 67–76.

Hmer, R. P., Hori, K. M., Blanchard, R. J. & Blanchard, D. C. (1992). Domestication alters 5-HT1a receptor binding in rat brain. *Pharmacol. Biochem. Behav.*, **42**, 25–8.

Holsboer, F. (2000). Current theories of the pathophysiology of mood disorders. In *Pharmacotherapy for Mood, Anxiety and Cognitive Disorders*, ed. U. Halbreich & S. A. Montgomery. Washington, DC: American Psychiatric Press.

Honig, A. & van Praag, H. M. (ed.) (1997). *Depression. Neurobiological, Psychopathological and Therapeutic Advances*. Chichester: John Wiley & Sons.

Hosada, K. & Duman, R. S. (1993). Regulation of beta 1-adrenergic receptor mRNA and ligand binding by antidepressant treatment and norepinephrine depletion in rat frontal cortex. *J. Neurochem.*, **60**, 1335–43.

Hrdina, P. D., Demeter, E., Vu, T. B., Sotonyi, P., & Palkovits, M. (1993). 5-HT uptake sites and 5-HT$_2$ receptors in brain of antidepressant-free suicide victims/depressives: increase in 5-HT$_2$ sites in cortex and amygdala. *Brain Res.*, **614**, 37–44.

Huang, Y., Grailhe, R., Arango, V., Hen, R. & Mann, J. J. (1999). Relationship of psychopathology to the human serotonin$_{1B}$ genotype and receptor binding kinetics in postmortem brain tissue. *Neuropsychopharmacology*, **21**, 238–46.

Janicak, P. G., Davis, J. M., Chan, C., Altman, E. & Hedeker, D. (1986). Failure of urinary MHPG levels to predict treatment response in patients with unipolar depression. *Am. J. Psychiatry*, **143**, 1398–402.

Jellinger, K. (1991). Overview of morphological changes in Parkinson's disease. *Adv. Neurol.*, **45**, 1–18.

Jenck, F., Perrin, S., Mutel, V. & Martin, J. R. (1992). 5-HT$_{1C}$ receptor antagonism is a major component of the effects of some antidepressants on the serotonergic system. *Clin. Neuropharm.*, **15**, 422.

Jolas, T., Schreiber, R., Laporte, A. M. *et al.* (1995). Are postsynaptic 5-HT1A receptors involved in the anxiolytic effects of 5-HT1A receptor agonists and in their inhibitory effects on the firing of serotonergic neurons in the rat? *J. Pharmacol. Exp.*, **272**, 920–9.

Kahn, R. S., Wetzler, S., Van Praag, H. M., Asnis, G. M. & Strauman, T. (1988). Behavioral indications for serotonin receptor hypersensitivity in panic disorder. *Psychiatr. Res.*, **25**, 101–4.

Kahn, R. S., Wetzler, S., Asnis, G. M., Papolos, D. & van Praag, H. M. (1990). Serotonin receptor sensitivity in major depression. *Biol. Psychiatry*, **28**, 358–62.

Karege, F., Bovier, P., Widmer, J., Gaillard, J. M. & Tissot, R. (1992). Platelet membrane alpha-2-adrenergic receptors in depression. *Psychiatr. Res.*, **43**, 243–52.

Kennett, G. A. & Curzon, G. (1988). Evidence that mCPP may have behavioral effects mediated by central 5-HT1c receptors. *Br. J. Pharmacol.*, **94**, 137–47.

Kennett, G. A., Lightowler, S., De Biasi, V. *et al.* (1994a). Effect of chronic administration of selective 5-hydroxytryptamine and noradrenaline uptake inhibitors on a putative index of 5-HT$_{2C/2B}$ receptor function. *Neuropharmacology*, **33**, 1581–8.

Kennett, G. A., Pittaway, K. & Blackburn, T. P. (1994b). Evidence that 5-HT2c receptor antagonists are anxiolytic in the rat Geller–Seifter model of anxiety. *Psychopharmacology*, **114**, 90–6.

Kim, S. W., Park, S. Y. & Hwang, O. (2002). Up-regulation of tryptophan hydroxylase expression and serotonin synthesis by sertraline. *Mol. Pharmacol.*, **61**, 778–85.

Kirov, G., Owen, M. J., Jones, I., McCandless, F. & Craddock, N. (1999). Tryptophan hydroxylase gene and manic-depressive illness. *Arch. Gen. Psychiatry*, **56**, 98–9.

Klaassen, T., Riedel, W. J., Van Someren, A., Deutz, N. E. P., Honig, A. & Van Praag, H. M. (1999a). Mood effects of 24-hour tryptophan depletion in healthy first-degree relatives of patients with affective disorders. *Biol. Psychiatry*, **46**, 489–97.

Klaassen, T., Riedel, W. J., Deutz, N. E. P., van Someren, A., & van Praag, H. M. (1999). Specificity of the tryptophan depletion method. *Psychopharmacology*, **141**, 279–86.

Klaassen, T., Riedel, W. J., Van Praag, H. M., Menheere, P. P. C. A. & Griez, E. (2002). Neuroendocrine response to mCPP and ipsapirone in relation to anxiety and aggression. *Psychiatry Res.*, **113**, 29–40.

Klimek, V., Rajkowska, G., Luker, B. S. *et al.* (1999). Brain noradrenergic receptors in major depression and schizophrenia. *Neuropsychopharmacology*, **21**, 69–81.

Knutson, B, Wolkowitz, O., Cole, S. *et al.* (1998). Selective alteration of personality and social behavior by serotonergic intervention. *Am. J. Psychiatry*, **155**, 373–9.

Korf, J. & van Praag, H. M. (1971). Amine metabolism in the human brain: further evaluation of the probenecid test. *Brain Res.*, **35**, 221–30.

Korte, S. M., Meijer, O. C., de Kloet, E. R. *et al.* (1996). Enhanced 5-HT$_{1A}$ receptor expression in forebrain regions of aggressive house mice. *Brain Res.*, **736**, 338–43.

Kuhn, K. U., Meyer, K., Nothen, M. M., Gansicke, M., Papassotiropoulos, A. & Maier, W. (1999). Allelic variants of dopamine D4 (DRD4) and serotonin receptor 5-HT2c (HTR2c) and temperament factors: replication tests. *Am. J. Med. Genet.*, **88**, 168–72.

Kunugi, H., Ishida, S., Kato, T. *et al.* (1999). No evidence for an association of polymorphisms of the tryptophan hydroxylase gene with affective disorders or attempted suicide among Japanese patients. *Am. J. Psychiatry*, **156**, 774–6.

Kyes, R. C., Botchin, M. B., Kaplan, J. R., Manuck, S. B. & Mann, J. J. (1995). Aggression and brain serotonergic responsivity: response to slides in male macaques. *Physiol. Behav.*, **57**, 205–8.

Laasonen-Balk, T., Kuikka, J., Viinamäki, H., Husso-Saastamoinen, M., Lehtonen, J. & Tiihonen, J. (1999). Striatal dopamine transporter density in major depression. *Psychopharmacology*, **144**, 282–5.

Lambert, G., Johansson, M., Ågren, H. & Firberg, P. (2000). Reduced brain norepinephrine and dopamine release in treatment-refractory depressive illness. *Arch. Gen. Psychiatry*, **57**, 787–93.

Lesch, K. P., Mayer, S., Disselkamp-Tietze, J. *et al.* (1990). 5-HT$_{1a}$ receptor responsivity in unipolar depression evaluation of ipsapirone-induced ACTH and cortisol secretion in patients and controls. *Biol. Psychiatry*, **28**, 620–8.

Lesch, K. P., Bengel, D., Heils, A. *et al.* (1996). Association of anxiety-related traits with a polymorphism in the serotonin transporter gene regulatory region. *Science*, **274**, 1527–31.

Leyton, M., Okazawa, H., Diksic, M. *et al.* (2001). Brain regional α-[^{11}C]Methyl-l-tryptophan trapping in impulsive subjects with borderline personality disorder. *Am. J. Psychiatry*, **158**, 775–82.

Linnoila, M., Virkkunen, M. Scheinin, M., Nuutila, A., Rimon, R. & Goodwin, F. K. (1983). Low cerebrospinal fluid 5-hydroxyindoleacetic acid concentration differentiates impulsive from nonimpulsive violent behavior. *Life Sci.*, **33**, 2609–19.

Little, K. Y., McLauglin, D. P., Ranc, J. *et al.* (1997). Serotonin transporter binding sites and mRNA levels in depressed persons committing suicide. *Biol. Psychiatry*, **41**, 1156–64.

Maas, J. W., Koslow, S. H., Katz, M. M. *et al.* (1984). Pretreatment neurotransmitter metabolite levels and response to tricyclic antidepressant drugs. *Am. J. Psychiatry*, **141**, 1159–71.

Maes, M., Jacobs, M. P., Suy, E. *et al.* (1990). Suppressant effects of dexamethasone on the availability of plasma l-tryptophan and tyrosine in healthy controls and in depressed patients. *Acta Psychiatr. Scand.*, **81**, 19–23.

Malison, R. T., Price, L. H., Berman, R. *et al.* (1998). Reduced brain serotonin transporter availability in major depression as measured by [^{123}I]-2β-carbomethyoxy-3β-(4-iodophenyl)tropane and single photon emission computed tomography. *Biol. Psychiatry*, **44**, 1090–8.

Mann, J. J., Stanley, M., McBride, P. A. & McEwen, B. S. (1986). Increased serotonin 2 and β-adrenergic receptor binding in the frontal cortices of suicide victims. *Arch. Gen. Psychiatry*, **43**, 954–9.

Mann, J. J., Malone, K. M., Nielsen, D. A., Goldman, D., Erdos, J. & Gelernter, J. (1997). Possible association of a polymorphism of the tryptophan hydroxylase gene with suicidal behavior in depressed patients. *Am. J. Psychiatry*, **155**, 1451–3.

Mann, J. J., Huang, Y.-Y., Underwood, M. D. *et al.* (2000). A serotonin transporter gene promotor polymorphism (5-HTTLPR) and prefrontal cortical binding in major depression and suicide. *Arch. Gen. Psychiatry*, **57**, 729–38.

Manuck, S. B., Flory, J. D., Deut, K. M., Mann, J. J. & Muldon, M. F. (1999). Aggression and anger-related traits associated with a polymorphism of the tryptophan hydroxylase gene. *Biol. Psychiatry*, **45**, 603–614.

Marsden, C. A. (1996). The neuropharmacology of serotonin in the central nervous system. In *Selective Serotonin Re-uptake Inhibitors: Advances in Basic Research and Clinical Practice*, ed. J. P. Feighner & W. F. Boyer. Chichester: John Wiley & Sons.

Martin, J. R., Bos, M., Moreau, J.-L. *et al.* (1998). 5-HT$_{2C}$ receptor agonists: pharmacological characteristics and therapeutic potential. *J. Pharmacol. Exp. Ther.*, **286**, 913–24.

Massot, I., Souery, D., Lipp, O. *et al.* (2000). A European multicenter association study of *HTR2A* receptor polymorphism in bipolar affective disorder. *Am. J. Med. Genet. (Neuropsychiatr. Genet.)*, **96**, 136–40.

Matussek, N. (1988). Catecholamines and mood: neuroendocrine aspects. *Curr. Topics Neuroendocrinol.*, **8**, 145–82.

Matussek, N., Ackenheil, M., Hippius, H. *et al.* (1980). Effects of clonidine on growth hormone release in psychiatric patients and controls. *Psychiatry Res.*, **2**, 25–36.

Mayorga, A., Dalvi, A., Page, M., Zimov-Levinson, S., Hen, R. & Lucki, I. (2001). Antidepressant-like behavioral effects in 5-hydroxytryptamine$_{1A}$ and 5-hydroxytryptamine$_{1B}$ receptor mutant mice. *J. Pharmacol. Exper. Ther.*, **298**, 1101–7.

Mazzanti, C. M., Lappalainen, J., Long, J. C. *et al.* (1998). Role of the serotonin transporter promoter polymorphism in anxiety-related traits. *Arch. Gen. Psychiatry*, **55**, 936–40.

McQuillin, A., Lawrence, J., Kalsi, G., Chen, A. & Gurling, H. (1999). No allelic association between bipolar affective disorder and the tryptophan hydroxylase gene. *Arch. Gen. Psychiatry*, **56**, 99–100.

Mehlman, P. T., Higley, J. D., Faucher, I. *et al.* (1994). Low CSF 5-HIAA concentrations and severe aggression and impaired impulse control in nonhuman primates. *Am. J. Psychiatry*, **151**, 1485–91.

Mehlman, P. T., Higley, J. D., Faucher, I. *et al.* (1995). Correlation of CSF 5-HIAA concentration with sociality and the timing of emigration in free-ranging primates. *Am. J. Psychiatry*, **152**, 907–13.

Meltzer, H. Y., Kolakowska, T., Fang, V. S. *et al.* (1984). Growth hormone and prolactin response to apomorphine in schizophrenia and major affective disorders: relation to duration of illness and affective symptoms. *Arch. Gen. Psychiatry*, **41**, 512–19.

Meyer, J. H., Kapur, S., Houle, S. *et al.* (1999). Prefrontal cortex 5-HT$_2$ receptors in depression: an [^{18}F]Setoperone PET imaging study. *Am. J. Psychiatry*, **156**, 1029–34.

Meyer, J. H., Krüger, S., Wilson, A. A. *et al.* (2001). Lower dopamine transporter binding potential in striatum during depression. *Neuroreport*, **12**, 4121–5.

Meyer, J. H., McMain, S., Kennedy, S. H. *et al.* (2003). Dysfunctional attitudes and 5-HT$_2$ receptors during depression and self-harm. *Am. J. Psychiatry*, **160**, 90–9.

Mignot, E., Seffano, A., Laude, D., Elghozi, J. L., Dedek, J. & Scatton, B. (1985). Measurement of 5-HIAA levels in ventricular CSF (by LCEC) and in striatum (by in vivo voltametry) during pharmacological modification of serotonin metabolism in the rat. *J. Neural Transm.*, **62**, 117–24.

Miller, H. L., Delgado, P. L., Salomon, R. M., Heninger, G. R. & Charney, D. S. (1996a). Clinical and biochemical effects of catecholamine depletion on antidepressant-induced remission of depression. *Arch. Gen. Psychiatry*, **53**, 117–28.

(1996b). Effects of AMPT in drug free depressed patients. *Neuropsychopharmacology*, **14**, 151–7.

Moja, E., Cipolla, P., Castoldi, D. & Tofanetti, O. (1989). Dose-response decrease in plasma tryptophan and in brain tryptophan and serotonin after tryptophan-free amino acid mixtures in rats. *Life Sci.*, **44**, 971–6.

Mongeau, R., Blier, P. & de Montigny, C. (1997). The serotonergic and noradrenergic systems of the hippocampus: their interactions and the effects of antidepressant treatments. *Brain Res. Rev.*, **23**, 145–95.

Moreno, F. A., Heninger, G. R., McGahuey, C. A. & Delgado, P. L. (2000). Tryptophan depletion and risk of depression relapse: a prospective study of tryptophan depletion as a potential predictor of depressive episodes. *Biol. Psychiatry*, **48**, 327–9.

Moskowitz, D. S., Pinard, G., Zaroff, D. C., Annable, L. & Young, S. H. (2001). The effect of tryptophan on social interaction in everyday life: a placebo-controlled study. *Neuropsychopharmacology*, **25**, 277–89.

Muñoz, C. & Papp, M. (1999). Alnespirone (S 20499), an agonist of 5-HT$_{1A}$ receptors, and imipramine have similar activity in a chronic mild stress model of depression. *Pharmacol. Biochem. Behav.*, **63**, 647–53.

Murphy, D. L., Li, Q., Engel, S. *et al.* (2001). Genetic perspectives on the serotonin transporter. *Brain Res. Bull.*, **56**, 487–94.

Mynett-Johnson, L. A., Murphy, V. E., Manley, P., Schields, D. C. & McKeon, P. (1997). Lack of evidence for a major locus for bipolar disorders in the pericentromeric region of chromosome 18 in Irish pedigrees. *Biol. Psychiatry*, **42**, 486–94.

Newman, M. E., Shapira, B. & Lerer, B. (1998). Evaluation of central serotonergic function in affective and related disorders by the fenfluramine challenge test: a critical review. *Int. J. Neuropsychopharmacology*, **1**, 49–69.

O'Carroll, R. E., Drysdale, E., Cahill, L., Shajahan, P. & Ebmeier, K. P. (1999). Stimulation of the noradrenergic system enhances and blockade reduces memory for emotional material in man. *Psychol. Med.*, **29**, 1083–8.

Ogilvie, A. D., Battersby, S., Bubb, V. J. *et al.* (1996). Polymorphism in serotonin transporter gene associated with susceptibility to major depression. *Lancet*, **347**, 731–3.

O'Keane, V. & Dinan, T. G. (1991). Prolactin and cortisol responses to *d*-Fenfluramine in major depression: evidence for diminished responsivity of central serotonergic function. *Am. J. Psychiatry*, **148**, 1009–15.

Olivier, B. & Mos, J. (1992). Rodent models of agressive behavior and serotonergic drugs. *Prog. Neuropsychopharmacol. Biol. Psychiat.*, **16**, 847–70.

(1994). Serotonin receptor subtypes and aggressive behaviour. *Neuropsychopharmacology*, **10**, 944s.

Olivier, B., Soudijn, W. & van Wijngaarden, I. (1999). The 5-HT$_{1A}$ receptor and its ligands: structure and function. *Progress in Drug Research*, **52**, 104–65.

Oquendo, M. A., Placidi, G. P. A., Malone, K. M. *et al.* (2003). Positron emission tomography of regional brain metabolic responses to a serotonergic challenge and lethality of suicide attempts in major depression. *Arch. Gen. Psychiatry*, **60**, 14–22.

Ossowska, G., Nowak, G., Kata, R., Klenk-Majewska, B., Danilczuk, Z. & Zebrowska-Lupina, I. (2001). Brain monoamine receptors in a chronic unpredictable stress model in rats. *J. Neural Transm.*, **108**, 311–19.

Palvimaki, E. P., Laakso, A., Kuoppamaki, M., Sylvalahti, E. & Hietala, J. (1994). Up-regulation of beta-1-adrenergic receptors in rat brain after chronic citalopram and fluoxetine treatments. *Psychopharmacology*, **115**, 543–6.

Pandey, G. N., Pandey, S. C., Janicak, P. G., Marks, R. C. & Davis, J. M. (1990). Platelet serotonin receptor binding sites in depression and suicide. *Biol. Psychiatry*, **28**, 215–22.

Parks, C., Robinson, P., Sibille, E., Shenk, Th. & Toth, M. (1998). Increased anxiety of mice lacking the serotonin1A receptor. *Proc. Natl. Acad. Sci. USA*, **95**, 10734–9.

Pecknold, J. C. (1994). Serotonin 5-HT$_{1A}$ agonists – a comparative review. *CNS Drugs*, **2**, 235–51.

Perry, E. K., Marshall, E. F., Blessed, G., Tomlinson, B. E. & Perry, R. H. (1983). Decreased imipramine binding in the brains of patients with depressive illness. *Br. J. Psychiatry*, **142**, 188–92.

Piletz, J. E., Schuberg, D. S. P. & Halaris, A. (1986). Evaluation of studies on platelet α_2 adrenoreceptors in depressive illness. *Life Sci.*, **39**, 1589–616.

Potter, W. Z., Grossman, F. & Rudorfer, M. V. (1993). Noradrenergic function in depressive disorders. In *Biology of Depressive Disorders, Part A: A Systems Perspective*, ed. J. J. Mann & D. J. Jupter. New York: Plenum Press.

Przegalinski, E. Chojnacka-Wojcik, E. & Filip, M. (1992). Stimulation of postsynaptic 5-HT1a receptors is responsible for the anticonflict effect of ipsapirone in rats. *J. Pharmacol.*, **44**, 780–2.

Quested, D. J., Sargent, P. A. & Cowen, P. J. (1997). SSRI treatment decreases prolactin and hyperthermic responses to mCPP. *Psychopharmacology*, **133**, 305–8.

Rabiner, E. A., Bhagwagar, Z., Gunn, R. N. *et al.* (2001). Pindolol augmentation of selective serotonin reuptake inhibitors: PET evidence that the dose used in clinical trials is too low. *Am. J. Psychiatry*, **158**, 2080–2.

Raleigh, M. J., Brammer, G. L., McGuire, M. T. & Yuwiler, A. (1985). Dominant social status facilitates the behavioral effects of serotonergic agonists. *Brain Res.*, **348**, 274–82.

Raleigh, M. J., McGuire, M. T., Brammer, G. L., Pollack, D. B. & Yuwiler, A. (1991). Serotonergic mechanisms promote dominance acquisition in adult male vervet monkeys. *Brain Res.*, **559**, 181–90.

Rampello, L., Nicoletti, F. & Nicoletti, F. (2000). Dopamine and depression. Therapeutic implications. *CSN Drugs*, **13**, 35–45.

Redrobe, J. P., MacSweeney, C. P. & Bourin, M. (1996). The role of 5-HT$_{1A}$ and 5-HT$_{1B}$ receptors in antidepressant drug actions in the mouse forced swimming test. *Eur. J. Pharmacol.*, **318**, 213–30.

Ressler, K. J. & Nemeroff, Ch. B. (2000). Role of serotonergic and noradrenergic systems in the pathophysiology of depression and anxiety disorders. *Depression and Anxiety*, **12** suppl. 1, 2–19.

Rosel, P., Arranz, B., San, L. *et al.* (2000). Altered 5-HT$_{2A}$ binding sites and second messenger triphosphate (IP$_3$) levels in hippocampus but not in frontal cortex from depressed suicide victims. *Psychiatr. Res.*, **99**, 173–82.

Roy, A., Pickar, D., Linnoila, M. & Potter, W. Z. (1985). Plasma norepinephrine level in affective disorders. Relationship to melancholia. *Arch. Gen. Psychiatry*, **42**, 1181–5.

Sachar, E. J., Hellman, L., Roffwarg, H. P., Halpern, F. S., Fukushima, D. K. & Gallagher, T. F. (1973). Disrupted 24-hour patterns of cortisol secretion in psychotic depression. *Arch. Gen. Psychiatry*, **28**, 19–24.

Sandou, F., Aimara, D. A., Dierick, A. *et al.* (1994). Enhanced aggressive behavior in mice lacking 5-HT$_{1B}$ receptors. *Science*, **265**, 1875–8.

Sargent, P. A., Husted Kjaer, K., Bench, Chr. J. *et al.* (2000). Brain serotonin $_{1A}$ receptor binding measured by positron emission tomography with [^{11}C]WAY-100635. Effects of depression and antidepressant treatment. *Arch. Gen. Psychiatry*, **57**, 174–80.

Schatzberg, A. F. & Schildkraut, J. J. (1995). Recent studies on norepinephrine systems in mood disorders. In *Psychopharmacology: the Fourth Generation of Progress*, ed. F. E. Bloom & D. J. Kupfer. New York: Raven Press.

Schefke, D. M., Fontana, D. J. & Commissaris, R. L. (1989). Anti-conflict efficacy of buspirone following acute vs chronic treatment. *Psychopharmacology*, **99**, 427–9.

Schildkraut, J. J. (1965). The catecholamine hypothesis of affective disorders: a review of supporting evidence. *Am. J. Psychiatry*, **122**, 509–22.

Schildkraut, J. J., Orsulak, P. J., LaBrie, R. A. *et al.* (1978a). Toward a biochemical classification of depressive disorders, II: application of multivariate discriminant function analysis to data on urinary catecholamines and metabolites. *Arch. Gen. Psychiatry*, **35**, 1436–9.

Schildkraut, J. J., Orsulak, P. J., Schatzberg, A. F. *et al.* (1978b). Toward a biochemical classification of depressive disorders, I: differences in urinary excretion of MHPG and other catecholamine metabolites in clinically defined subtypes of depression. *Arch. Gen. Psychiatry*, **35**, 1427–33.

Schreiber, R. & de Vrij, J. (1993a). Neuronal circuits involved in the anxiolytic effects of the 5-HT1a receptor agonists 8-OH-DPAT, ipsapirone and buspirone in the rat. *Eur. J. Pharmacol.*, **249**, 341–51.

(1993b). Neuroanatomical basis for the antidepressant-like effects of the 5-HT1a receptor agonists 8-OH-DPAT and ipsapirone in the rat forced swimming test. *Behav. Pharmacol.*, **4**, 625–36.

Self, D. W., Barnhart, W. J., Lehman, D. A. & Nestler, E. J. (1996). Opposite modulation of cocaine-seeking behavior by D$_1$- and D$_2$-like dopamine receptor agonist. *Science*, **271**, 1586–9.

Serretti, A., Cusin, C., Lattuada, E., Di Bella, D., Catalano, M. & Smeraldi E. (1999a). Serotonin transporter gene (5-HTTLPR) is not associated with depressive symptomatology in mood disorders. *Mol. Psychiat.*, **4**, 280–3.

Serretti, A., Lattuada, E., Cusin, C., Lilli, R., Lorenzi, C. & Smeraldi, E. (1999b). Dopamine D3 receptor gene not associated with symptomatology of major psychoses. *Am. J. Med. Genet. (Neuropsychiatr. Genet.)*, **88**, 476–80.

Serretti, A., Lilli, R., Lorenzi, C., Lattuada, E. & Smeraldi, E. (2000). Serotonin-2C and serotonin-1A receptor genes are not associated with psychotic symptomatology of mood disorders. *Am. J. Med. Genet. (Neuropsychiatr. Genet.)*, **96**, 161–6.

Seyle, H. (1936). Syndrome produced by nocuous agents. *Nature*, **138**, 32.

Shah, P. J., Ogilvie, A. D., Goodwin, G. M. & Ebmeier, K. P. (1997). Clinical and psychometric correlates of dopamine D_2 binding in depression. *Psychol. Med.*, **27**, 1247–56.

Sibelle, E., Sarnyai, Z., Benjamin, D., Gal, J., Baker, H. & Toth, M. (1997). Antisense inhibition of 5-Hydroxytryptamine$_{2A}$ receptor induces an antidepressant-like effect in mice. *J. Pharmacol. Exp. Ther.*, **52**, 1056–63.

Siever, L. J., Trestman, R. L., Coccaro, E. F. *et al.* (1992). The growth hormone response to clonidine in acute and remitted depressed male patients. *Neuropsychopharmacology*, **6**, 165–77.

Stanley, M., Traskman, L. & Dorovine, K. (1985). Correlation between aminergic metabolites simultaneously obtained from human CSF and brain. *Life Sci.*, **37**, 1279–86.

Stephaniski, R. & Goldberg, S. R. (1997). Serotonin 5-HT$_2$ receptor antagonist potential in the treatment of psychiatric disorders. *CNS Drugs*, **7**, 388–409.

Stockmeier, C. A., Dilley, G. E., Shapiro, A., Overholser, J. C., Thompson, P. A. & Meltzer, H. Y. (1997). Serotonin receptors in suicide victims with major depression. *Neuropsychopharmacology*, **16**, 162–73.

Strickland, P., Deakin, J., Percival, C., Dixon, J., Gater, R. & Goldberg, D. (2002). Bio-social origins of depression in the community. *Br. J. Psychiatry*, **180**, 168–73.

Suwabe, A., Kubota, M., Niwa, M., Kobayashi, K. & Kanba, S. (2000). Effect of a 5-HT$_{1A}$ receptor agonist, flesinoxan, on the extracellular noradrenaline level in the hippocampus and on the locomotor activity of rats. *Brain Res.*, **858**, 393–401.

Swann, A. C., Secunda, S. K., Stokes, P. E. *et al.* (1990). Stress, depression and mania; relationship between perceived role of stressful events and clinical and biochemical characteristics. *Acta Psychiatr. Scand.*, **81**, 389–97.

Tiihonen, J., Kuoppamäki, M., Någren, K. *et al.* (1996). Serotonergic modulation of striatal D_2 dopamine receptor binding in humans measured with positron emission tomography. *Psychopharmacology*, **126**, 277–80.

Träskman-Bendz, L., Åsberg, M., Bertilsson, L. & Thorén, P. (1984). CSF monoamine metabolites of depressed patients during illness and after recovery. *Acta Psychiatr. Scand.*, **69**, 333–42.

Tremblay, L. K., Naranjo, C. A., Cardenas, L., Herrmann, N. & Busto, U. E. (2002). Probing brain reward system function in major depressive disorder. *Arch. Gen. Psychiatry*, **59**, 409–16.

Van Praag, H. M. (1962). A critical investigation of the significance of monoamine oxidase inhibition as a therapeutic principle in the treatment of depression. Thesis, University of Utrecht.

(1974). Towards a biochemical typology of depressions. *Pharmacopsychiatry*, **7**, 281–92.

(1977a). *Depression and Schizophrenia. A Contribution on their Chemical Pathologies.* New York: Spectrum Publications.

(1977b). Significance of biochemical parameters in the diagnosis, treatment and prevention of depressive disorders. *Biol. Psychiatry*, **12**, 101–31.

(1982). Depression, suicide and the metabolism of serotonin in the brain. *J. Affect. Disord.*, **4**, 275–90.

(1988). Serotonergic mechanisms and suicidal behavior. *Psychiatr. Psychobiol.*, **3**, 335–46.

(1992). About the centrality of mood lowering in mood disorders. *Eur. Neuropsychopharmacol.*, **2**, 393–404.

(1996). Faulty cortisol/serotonin interplay, psychopathological and biological characterisation of a new hypothetical depression subtype (SeCa depression). *Psychiatr. Res.*, **65**, 143–57.

(1997). Over the mainstream: diagnostic requirements for biological psychiatric research, *Psychiatr. Res.*, **72**, 201–12.

(2000). Nosologomania, a disorder of psychiatry. *World J. Biol. Psychiat.*, **1**, 151–8.

Van Praag, H. M. & de Haan, S. (1980a). Central serotonin deficiency. A factor which increases depression vulnerability? *Acta Psychiatr. Scand.*, **61**, 89–95.

(1980b). Depression vulnerability and 5-hydroxy-tryptophan prophylaxis. *Psychiatr. Res.*, **3**, 75–83.

Van Praag, H. M. & Korf, J. (1971a). Endogenous depressions with and without disturbances in the 5-hydroxytryptamine metabolism: a biochemical classification? *Psychopharmacology*, **19**, 148–52.

(1971b). Retarded depression and the dopamine metabolism. *Psychopharmacology*, **19**, 199–203.

Van Praag, H. M., Korf, J. & Puite, J. (1970). 5-Hydroxindoleacetic acid levels in the cerebrospinal fluid of depressive patients treated with probenecid. *Nature*, **225**, 1259–60.

Van Praag, H. M., Korf, J. & Schut, T. (1973). Cerebral monoamines and depression. An investigation with the probenecid technique. *Arch. Gen. Psychiatry*, **28**, 827–31.

Van Praag, H. M., Kahn, R., Asnis, G. M. *et al.* (1987). Denosologization of biological psychiatry or the specificity of 5-HT disturbances in psychiatric disorders. *J. Affect. Disord.*, **13**, 1–8.

Van Praag, H. M., Asnis, G. M., Kahn, R. S. *et al.* (1990). Monoamines and abnormal behavior. A multi-aminergic perspective. *Br. J. Psychiatry*, **157**, 723–34.

Van Scheyen, J. D., van Praag, H. M. & Korf, J. (1977). A controlled study comparing nomifensine and clomipramine in unipolar depression, using the probenecid technique. *Br. J. Clin. Pharmacol.*, **4**, 179S–84S.

Verbeeck, W. J. C., Berk, M., Paiker, J. & Jersky, B. (2001). The prolactin response to sulpiride in major depression: the role of the D_2 receptor in depression. *Eur. Neuropsychopharmacol.*, **11**, 215–20.

Virkkunen, M., Rawlings, R., Tokola, R. *et al.* (1994). CSF biochemistries, glucose metabolism and diurnal activity rhythms in alcoholic violent offenders, fire setters and healthy volunteers. *Arch. Gen. Psychiatry*, **51**, 20–7.

Westergaard, G. C., Suomi, S. J., Higley, J. D. & Mehlman, P. T. (1999). CSF 5-HIAA and aggression in female macaque monkeys: species and interindividual differences. *Psychopharmacology*, **146**, 440–6.

Whale, R., Clifford, E. M., Bhagwagas, Z. & Cowen, Ph. J. (2001). Decreased sensitivity of 5-HT$_{1D}$ receptors in melancholic depression. *Br. J. Psychiatry*, **178**, 454–7.

White, S. M., Kucharik. R. F. & Moyer, J. A. (1991). Effects of serotonergic agents on isolation-induced aggression. *Pharmacol. Biochem. Behav.*, **39**, 729–36.

Williams, J., McGuffin, P., Nothen, M. & Owen, M. J. (1997). Meta-analysis of association between the 5-HT2a receptor T102C polymorphism and schizophrenia. European Multicentre Association Study of Schizophrenia (EMASS Group). *Lancet*, **26**, 1221.

Williams, W. A., Shoaf, S. E., Hommer, D., Rawlings, R. & Linnoila, M. (1999). Effects of acute tryptophan depletion on plasma and cerebrospinal fluid tryptophan and 5-hydroxyindoleacetic acid in normal volunteers. *J. Neurochem.*, **72**, 1641–7.

Willner, P. (1983). Dopamine and depression: a review of recent evidence. *Brain Res. Rev.*, **6**, 211–46.

Willner, P. (1995). Dopaminergic mechanism in depression and mania. In *Psychopharmacology – The Fourth Generation of Progress*, ed. F. E. Bloom & D. J. Kupfer. New York: Raven Press.

World Health Organization Collaborative Study (1990). Validity of imipramine platelet binding sites as a biological marker for depression. *Pharmacopsychiatry*, **23**, 113–17.

Wong, M. H., Saam, J. R., Stappenbeck, T. S., Rexer, C. H. & Gordon, J. I. (2000). Genetic mosaic analysis based on Cre recombinase and navigated laser capture microdissection. *Proc. Natl. Acad. Sci. USA*, **97**, 12601–6.

Yamada, J. & Sugimoto, Y. (2001). Effects of 5-HT$_2$ receptor antagonists on the anti-immobility effects of imipramine in the forced swimming test with mice. *Eur. J. Pharmacol.*, **427**, 221–25.

Yatham, L. N., Liddle, P. F., Dennie J. L. *et al.* (1999). Decrease in brain serotonin 2 receptor binding in patients with major depression following desipramine treatment. *Arch. Gen. Psychiatry*, **56**, 705–11.

Yatham, L. N., Liddle, P. F., Shiah, I.-S. *et al.* (2000). Brain serotonin$_2$ receptors in major depression. A positron emission tomography study. *Arch. Gen. Psychiatry*, **57**, 850–8.

Young, S., Smith, S., Pihl, R. & Ervin, F. (1985). Tryptophan depletion causes a rapid lowering of mood in normal males. *Psychopharmacol. (Berlin)*, **87**, 173–7.

Zhang, Y., D'Souza, D., Raap, D. K. *et al.* (2001). Characterization of the functional heterologous desensitization of hypothalamic 5-HT$_{1A}$ receptors after 1-HT$_{2A}$ receptor activation. *J. Neurosci.*, **15**, 7919–27.

Stress hormones and depression

8.1 Stress and stress response

Human beings, like any other living organism, strive towards a state of dynamic equilibrium, the regulation of a setpoint, called *homeostasis*. The continuance of this state can be threatened by a variety of variables originating from within or without, biological or psychological in nature. Psychological stimuli or stressors are evaluated as to their destabilizing potential. Dependent on the outcome of the appraisal the organism will marshall a set of adaptive responses to maintain or re-establish equilibrium. They are partly biological, partly behavioural in nature, and collectively named the *stress-response*, or in short stress. The latter term, thus, refers to the state evoked by the stressor. The limbic brain, e.g. hippocampus, amygdala and frontal cortex serve as an interface between the appraisal process and the appropriate biological and psychological responses to the incoming information.

The physiological components of the stress response are geared towards activation of functions needed for survival. For instance, the availability of energy increases through enhancement of gluconeogenesis, protein catabolism and lipolysis. Oxygen supply is stepped up by increasing respiratory rate, heart rate and blood pressure. Functions not of immediate survival value, such as digestive functions, appetite, growth, reproductive behaviour and immune functions are downregulated. On the behavioural level, alertness, vigilance, focused attention and cognition surge. In animals 'risk assessment' is stimulated, i.e. information-gathering behaviours displayed in potentially threatening situations, the function of which is to optimize adaptive behavioural strategies (Rodgers *et al.*, 1999).

The ability to re-establish homeostasis through change has been called *allostasis* (Sterling & Eyer, 1981). Successful allostasis means that the systems involved are turned on when needed, and turned off when homeostasis has been achieved. In principle these changes are adaptive, self-preservative and short-lasting. Responses, however, may be inadequate, excessive or prolonged, and the cost to maintain

Table 8.1. CRH_1 and CRH_2 receptor systems drive in anti-parallel fashion the sympathetic and parasympathetic components of the stress response system. Mineralocorticoid receptors (MR) control higher brain functions involved in control of sensitivity and/or threshold, while glucocorticoid receptors (GR) facilitate termination of the stress response.

Stress	Adaptation
CRH	Stresscopin
CRH_1 receptor	CRH_2 receptor
Sympathetic immediate fight–flight	Parasympathetic late sustained coping
MR	GR

homeostasis may become too high. They then lead to wear and tear and ultimately to disease (Selye, 1936). The wear and tear has been named *allostatic load* (McEwen & Stellar, 1993; Schulkin *et al.*, 1998). On a *behavioural level*, for instance, depression may be interpreted as a consequence of sustained *hyper*activity of the stress-system due to CRH overdrive, hyperactivity of the adrenergic system, and excess circulating glucocorticoid hormones. This will be discussed in the following sections. Chronic *hypo*activity of the stress system may lead to inertia, excessive fatigue and amotivational syndromes.

Examples of *bodily damage* induced by dysfunctional stress responses are loss of bone mass, hippocampal atrophy and acceleration of ageing, due probably to prolonged increase of glucocorticoid levels. If cortisol does not increase in response to a stressor, secretion of inflammatory cytokines (normally counter-regulated by cortisol) increases and this produces other types of wear and tear. Failed control of stress or defence reactions presumably is an important pathogenic mechanism in mood and anxiety disorders.

8.2 Stress and the HPA system

8.2.1 The stress response

The key CNS systems generating the stress response have two modes of operation (Table 8.1). These two modes involve the fast, CRH-driven, neuroendocrine/sympathetic 'fight–flight' response mediated by CRH_1 receptors and a slower system promoting recovery and adaptation which is activated by the recently discovered urocortins acting via CRH_2 receptors (Hsu & Hsueh, 2001; Reul & Holsboer, 2002). The CRH-mediated systems are discussed in Section 8.4.3. These two modes are superimposed over the pulsatile activity of the HPA axis with about 20 secretory bursts over 24 hours. The amplitude and frequency of the pulses vary during the circadian rhythm and the stress response. Neither the identity of the pulse generator nor the effect of cortisol pulsatility is known.

The fast stress-responding system includes CRH-producing neurons located in the parvocellular division of the paraventricular nucleus (PVN) of the hypothalamus as well as beyond (see Section 8.4.3), and the NA ergic neurons located in the locus coeruleus (LC) and adjacent areas in pons and medulla oblongata. In the periphery the adrenal cortex producing, amongst others, cortisol and the adrenal medulla secreting catecholamines (CA), particularly adrenalin, are the principal pacemakers. The fast response mediated by CRH_1 receptors located in pituitary and brain depends on a permissive glucocorticoid action (see Section 8.2.3).

The other, the late responding and slower operating system driven by urocortin II (stresscopin-related) and urocortin III (stresscopin) peptides has a neuroanatomical organization distinct from that of the CRH peptides (Li et al., 2002). The urocortins II and III were identified as selective high affinity ligands for the CRH_2 receptor system (Hsu & Hsueh, 2001; Lewis et al., 2001; Reyes et al., 2001). Urocortin I is synthesized in a discrete region in the midbrain, the eddinger westphal nucleus, and binds to both CRH receptor sites. Urocortin II is expressed in PVN and LC and urocortin III in the hypothalamic area rostral of the PVN, the preoptic nucleus and medial amygdala, but not in cerebellum, cerebral cortex or pituitary. Their terminal fields innervate hypothalamic and brain stem areas matching CRH_2 receptor distribution (Li et al., 2002). The CRH_2 receptor system is thought to be prominent in the late recovery phase of the stress response facilitating processes underlying coping and behavioural adaptation. Administration of the urocortins II and III evokes anxiolytic responses as opposed to the anxiogenic activity of CRH (Hsu & Hsueh, 2001).

This finding has led to the concept that the urocortin II/III system operates in balance with the classical CRH system. Since not much is known of the urocortin/CRH_2 system, it will not further be discussed. However, glucocorticoids have a key role in the control of both stress system modes because of their permissive role in the fast response and their slow feedback action.

8.2.2 The hypothalamic–pituitary–adrenal response

The fast, CRH-driven stress response to adverse stimuli is a complex one, encompassing behavioural, endocrine, autonomic and immunological components. The CRH system is considered to integrate it all. Thus exogenous CRH evokes sympathetic responses with their behavioural expressions of fear and anxiety. CRH also triggers the neuroendocrine cascade known as the hypothalamic–pituitary–adrenal (HPA) axis (Figure 8.1). The activation of the HPA axis is initiated from the neurosecretory cells of the parvocellular division of the PVN that produce CRH. Via the projections of these cells CRH is transported to the median eminence and from the nerve terminals into the hypothalamo-hypophyseal portal system.

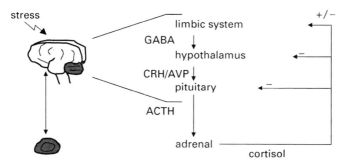

Figure 8.1. Organization of the hypothalamic-pituitary-adrenal axis. Cortisol released in secretory bursts from the adrenals coordinates daily activity and sleep related events, and mediates the animal's ability to cope with stress – indicates negative feedback, + indicates positive feedback.

Via these vessels CRH is transported to the anterior pituitary, where it binds to CRH_1 receptors on ACTH-producing cells (corticotropes). Via a number of intermediary steps, this leads to increased production of pro-opiomelanocortin, the precursor molecule of peptides such as β-endorphin and ACTH. ACTH is released into the systemic circulation and triggers the release of the glucocorticoid cortisol (in humans, and corticosterone in rodents) by the adrenal cortex. In addition, the adrenal cortex produces mineralocorticoids, particularly aldosterone and androgens such as testosterone and dehydroepiandrosterone.

CRH neurons in the parvocellular PVN synthesize both CRH and arginine vasopressin (AVP), while the PVN magnocellular neurons produce AVP only. The proportion of cells that produce both peptides increases during stress (Chrousos, 1998). The release of CRH is accompanied by AVP release. AVP by itself stimulates ACTH release only weakly, but it potentiates the effect of CRH on ACTH release. Long-term stress leads eventually to downregulation of CRH_1 receptors at the pituitary, but under those circumstances the AVP receptors are upregulated. In this way the increased release of ACTH is sustained (Antoni, 1996; Scott & Dinan, 1998).

A number of other peptides are present in the PVN and co-stored with CRH. These include neurotensin, neuropeptide Y, cholecystokinin and some endogenous opioids such as dynorphin. Most of them have only weak activity on ACTH release. Their role in the occurrence of stress responses is largely unknown. It is thought that in response to different stressors the cocktail of these ACTH secretagogues can change in composition with resultant changes in dynamics of pituitary ACTH release (Romero & Sapolsky, 1996).

CRH neurons are activated by numerous inputs from many brain regions utilizing a variety of neurotransmitters, amongst others 5-HT, NA and peptides such as neuropeptide Y. Inhibitory inputs include the 3-γaminobutyric acid (GABA)/benzodiazepine (BZ), and the opioid peptide systems (Chrousos & Gold,

1992). These distinct afferent neurotransmitter and neuropeptide pathways convey stressor-specific information to the PVN. A global distinction can be made between physical stressors, which activate directly monosynaptic inputs to the CRH neurons, and psychological stressors. The latter require complex processing of information involving polysynaptic transmission from limbic-cortical regions to the CRH neurons.

Physical stimuli evoked by pain, infection, inflammation, toxic agents, hypoglycaemia and blood pressure changes enter the CNS by autonomic efferents. Their first synaptic relay is the n. tractus solitarii from where the A2 noradrenergic neurons arise that stimulate the hypothalamic CRH cells through long mono-synaptic axons (Palkovits, 1999). Another pathway directly innervating the hypothalamic CRH neurons stems from the circumventricular organs, that monitor osmotic and volume changes in the circulation (Kovacs & Sawchenko, 1993).

Psychological stimuli evoked by processing of complex environmental information activate neurons of the limbic-cortical circuitry subserving functions with nociceptive, emotional and cognitive components. Prominent are circuits in the central amygdala, hippocampus and frontal cortex that project to a GABA ergic network surrounding the PVN, which exerts inhibitory control over the CRH neurons. The input to this hypothalamic GABA ergic network varies. It can be activated – thus becoming more inhibitory to CRH – by an excitatory input from the hippocampus. The GABA neurons also can be inhibited – resulting in a disinhibition of CRH – by the inhibitory input from the amygdala (Herman & Cullinan, 1997). In addition, a direct excitatory CRH tract projects from the central amygdala to the parvocellular PVN. Circuits in hippocampus, amygdala and frontal cortex also have polysynaptic contacts among each other and play a role in processing the cognitive and emotional content of stressful information. One network that has received much attention is the bi-directional amygdala-locus coeruleus connection activated by sympathetic arousal. All these afferent limbic-cortical and brain stem neuronal projections to the HPA axis are targets for the stress hormones involved in expression of CRH and corticosteroid receptors (Dallman *et al.*, 2002).

In summary, afferent inputs to the CRH neurons convey stressor-specific information to the HPA axis, and are the ultimate determinants of the sets of physiological and behavioural adaptations to be elicited by the stressor. They determine the specificity of the stress response.

8.2.3 Cortisol: permissive, feedback and preparatory actions

In response to stress ACTH stimulates the secretion of cortisol from the adrenals. The sensitivity of the adrenals to ACTH is regulated by many factors including a nervous input from the hypothalamus which is most active during the circadian surge of cortisol in the morning (Buijs *et al.*, 1999; Dallman *et al.*, 2002).

Table 8.2. Short-term effects and long-term consequences
of cortisol action.

Physiology: short-term effects of acute exposure
  Mobilization of energy
  Control of stress reactions
  Increased vascular tone
  Suppression of growth
  Suppression of bone recalcification
  Suppression of reproduction
  Suppression of immunity, anti-inflammatory

Pathophysiology: long-term consequences of chronic exposure
  Myopathy, fatigue, risk of steroid diabetes
  Hypertension
  Osteoporosis
  Amenorrhoea, impotency
  Impaired immune defences
  Affective and eating disorders, addiction
  Neurotoxicity

See also Sapolsky, 1992.

Three modes of cortisol action can be distinguished. Firstly, the hormone acts permissively in energy metabolism, stress responsiveness and information processing (Table 8.2). Secondly, the hormone prepares for future needs by disposition of glycogen and by facilitating the storage of information. Thirdly, the hormone restrains stress reactions to prevent them from overshooting to become damaging themselves. For instance, immune response to infection, inflammatory reaction to tissue damage and neurochemical reaction to a psychosocial stressor are all suppressed (Munck et al., 1984; Sapolsky et al., 2000). As a consequence inputs driving the CRH neurons are attenuated, leading at last to termination of the stress-induced HPA response.

This control exerted by cortisol on the afferent inputs to CRH neurons is distinct from cortisol feedback regulation in the core of the HPA axis, i.e. the suppression of hypothalamic CRH and AVP, and pituitary ACTH synthesis and release. The permissive, regulatory and preparatory modes of action of cortisol control the various pathways that innervate the CRH neurons either directly or indirectly via an inhibitory GABA-ergic network surrounding these neurons (Cullinan et al., 1995). Ascending aminergic pathways directly innervate the PVN and mediate the effect of somatic stressors. Indirect pathways stem from the amygdala-locus coeruleus network driven by emotions. Other trans-synaptic inputs from hippocampus and frontal cortex are activated by cognitive aspects of the stress response. The action of cortisol therefore has an enormous diversity. These actions are mediated by nuclear

Table 8.3. Properties of mineralocorticoid (MR or type I) and glucocorticoid (GR or type II) receptors in the brain.

Mineralocorticoid receptor	Glucocorticoid receptor
Corticosterone, cortisol (aldosterone)	Corticosterone, cortisol (dexamethasone, RU486)
High affinity	Low affinity
Almost always occupied	Occupied after stress
Limbic system (hippocampus)	Ubiquitous

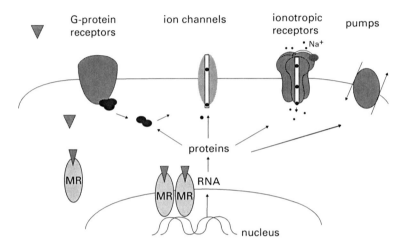

Figure 8.2.   Action mechanism of corticosteroids. MR, mineralocorticoid receptor; GR, glucocorticoid receptor; triangle, agonist cortisol. Note that MR and GR bind to hormone response elements on DNA to influence gene transcription. Gene products are translated in proteins that serve functions in signalization on the level of the cell membrane. This includes ion pumps, ion channels, G protein coupled and ionotropic receptors that respond to neurotransmitters and neuropeptides.

receptors that either directly modulate gene transcription or that interact with other transcription factors in control of genomic functions.

8.2.4 Brain corticosteroid receptors

The modes of action of cortisol are mediated by two types of nuclear corticosteroid receptors, i.e. mineralocorticoid receptors (MR) or type I and the already mentioned GR or type II receptors (De Kloet *et al.*, 1998), that have distinctly different functions in the response to stress (Figure 8.2; Table 8.3). The high affinity MRs have an almost exclusive localization in the limbic system, e.g. hippocampus, amygdala and frontal cortex. They are largely occupied under normal conditions, control basal HPA activity and determine the sensitivity or threshold of the

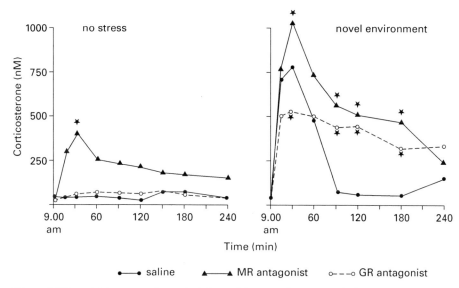

Figure 8.3. Effect of MR and GR antagonists administered intracerebroventricularly (icv) in rats under basal conditions and prior to exposure to a novelty stressor. Note that MR antagonist increases basal and stress-induced corticosterone concentrations. Acute GR antagonist is not active under basal conditions, but flattens the corticosterone response to novelty (Ratka *et al.*, 1989).

CRH-driven stress system. Compelling evidence came from experiments in which minute amounts of an MR antagonist were administered intracerebroventricularly. Blockade of the central MRs enhanced basal and stress-induced HPA activity. Via a similar experimental approach it was revealed that the MR controls autonomic outflow (Van den Berg *et al.*, 1990, 1994; Van den Buuse *et al.*, 2002), facilitates the conservation/withdrawal response if animals are exposed to a severe stressor (Korte, 2001) and enhances aggressive behaviour of a resident mouse to an intruder (Haller *et al.*, 2000). In the cognitive realm the MR activates a gene pattern underlying a neural network involved in interpretation of environmental information and selection of the appropriate behavioural strategy to deal with the stressor. Experimental evidence for this thesis comes from experiments in rats. The administration of a few ng mineralocorticoid antagonist intracerebroventricularly immediately before testing altered the search strategy for an escape route from a maze (Oitzl & De Kloet, 1992).

The lower-affinity GRs have a widespread distribution in the brain with abundant expression in stress regulation centres such as pituitary corticotropes, PVN and hippocampus and ascending MA neurons. When cortisol levels rise the GRs become more and more occupied, and provide the signal for reduction of CRH and ACTH release in the HPA core (Figure 8.3). In the afferent inputs the increasing GR activity mediates numerous changes in metabolism, structural plasticity and

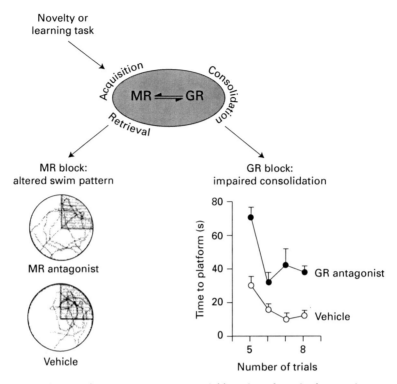

Figure 8.4. Effect of MR and GR antagonists on spatial learning of rats in the Morris maze. Blockade of GR interferes with consolidation of learned information as derived from the latency to find the hidden platform as an escape route from the water maze the next day. Blockade of MR alters retrieval of information (the antagonist is given briefly prior to the test), because the rat changes its search pattern for the escape route from the water maze (De Kloet *et al.*, 1999).

neurotransmission that are induced by stress. These actions serve behavioural adaptations and help to store information useful to cope with upcoming events. Blockade of brain GR impairs the storage of new information (Oitzl & De Kloet, 1992). A glucocorticoid antagonist administered around the time of learning in the hippocampus impaired the consolidation of newly acquired information (Figure 8.4). As a consequence 24 hours later, the rat is unable to retrieve the information that was learned the previous day and has to learn the maze problem all over again. Likewise, mutant mice with a point mutation in the GR which obliterates binding to DNA are unable to store learned information (Oitzl *et al.*, 2001). Such mutants lack the direct activation of glucocorticoid responsive genes, but still have a GR that can interact with other transcription factors. Transgenic mice with downregulated GRs (knock-down) also show cognitive defects and elevated plasma ACTH and corticosterone concentrations in response to stress. After treatment with an antidepressant GRs are increased in concentration and the mice simultaneously show behavioural and hormonal corrections (Montkowski *et al.*, 1995).

How do these MR- and GR-mediated effects on cognition relate to emotional behaviour? This can be illustrated in the following experiment measuring an anxiety paradigm. After exposure to a stressor, activation of GR-dependent mechanisms promotes storage of newly acquired information (Korte, 2001). This memory is helpful to predict the nature of upcoming events if the animal is exposed to the same place and context. During subsequent visits to the same 'stressful' situation the individual's initial response is triggered by the previous experience. It depends on MR, because this behavioural repertoire is blocked by an MR-antagonist given just before behavioural testing suggesting anxiolytic activity of such antagonists. It is also blocked by exogenous GR antagonists prior to the initial stressful event the day before. One day later memory to the previous stressful experience is extinguished. Obviously, blockade of brain GR interferes with cognitive aspects of fear and anxiety.

The above studies were all performed with acute administration of the antagonists in the context of the learning experience. Two aspects deserve further attention. Firstly, only a few ngs are active after intracerebroventricular administration, while systemic administration requires mg amounts: this is a million times higher dose. The reason for this enormous difference in effective dosage regime is probably the P glycoprotein pump which extrudes synthetic compounds and therefore also limits access of the antagonists to the brain, while facilitating the entrance of cortisol (Meijer *et al.*, 1998; Karssen *et al.*, 2001). Also, the current antagonists are rapidly cleared from the systemic circulation.

Secondly, the acute effects changed completely when the antagonists were administered chronically. In that case, chronic administration of the GR antagonist actually improved cognitive performance (Oitzl *et al.*, 1998). It also increased the amplitude in the circadian variation of corticosterone in that peak levels increased, while trough levels became even lower (van Haarst *et al.*, 1996). The latter finding has implications for therapy of depression with the GR antagonists. The circadian pattern in cortisol is flattened during depression and chronic GR antagonists will facilitate recovery of the reactive circadian pattern in circulating corticosterone levels.

In summary, animal studies have revealed that the naturally occurring glucocorticoids cortisol and corticosterone operate through a binary receptor system, MR and GR. These receptors respond to different levels of circulating glucocorticoid and have different, sometimes opposite functions (Table 8.4). Via the MR, corticosterone maintains stability on the neuronal and neuroendocrine level. On the behavioural level activation of MR helps to select the most appropriate behavioural response to achieve this stability and to maintain homeostasis. High levels of

Table 8.4. Function of mineralocorticoid (MR) and glucocorticoid (GR) receptors in the brain.

Mineralocorticoid receptors (Type I)
   Prevent disturbance of cellular homeostasis
   Control sensitivity stress response system
   Help to select behavioural response

Glucocorticoid receptors (Type II)
   Control energy metabolism
   Facilitate recovery of cellular homeostasis
   Restrain stress-induced responses
   Promote information storage
   Promote behavioural adaptation

corticosterone activate GR, and its function is to facilitate recovery from disturbances induced by the stressor. Corticosterone stores energy via GR for future needs. In the behavioural realm corticosterone and cortisol promote storage of information to be used at a later date for coping with a similar encounter. Thus, MR prevents disturbance of homeostasis, while GR promotes its recovery and prepares for future events. It is hypothesized that once the balance in MR- and GR-mediated effects is disturbed, the individual loses the ability to maintain homeostasis, if challenged by an adverse event. This leads to a conditon of neuroendocrine dysregulation and impaired behavioural adaptation, which may precipitate stress-related disorders such as depression in genetically predisposed individuals (De Kloet *et al.*, 1998).

8.2.5 Heterogeneity of the stress response

The previous discussion implies that the HPA response to physical and psychological stressors in normal subjects cannot be expected to be homogeneous, and in fact it is not. There are, for instance, high and low responders both in animals and humans (Petrides *et al.*, 1997; Singh *et al.*, 1999). These high and low HPA responders represent individuals that coexist in a normal population with the extremes displaying either an active fight-flight or a passive conservation-withdrawal response to a psychosocial challenge (Henry & Stephens, 1977). Active animals rely on stable living conditions, show impaired adaptation to a changing environment, display territorial aggression and flee after defeat. Their sympathetic response pattern dominates. Passive animals thrive better on changing conditions and they seem to be more dominated by parasympathetic activity and have high circulating glucocorticoid levels after stress.

The setpoint of the HPA system, defined as the balance between the CRH_1/MR and CRH_2/GR driven stress systems, is probably determined by genetic factors, but it can be reset to a lower or higher level by acquired variables such as adverse early experiences. Over the years a great variety of genetically selected mouse and rat lines have been selected by criteria based on behavioural and endocrine response patterns to psychosocial challenges (Benus *et al.*, 1991; Keck *et al.*, 2001) or on responses to pharmacological agents such as apomorphine (Cools *et al.*, 1990).

8.2.6 The pacemaker

The key pacemaker of the stress responses is not known with certainty. Generally, increased release of CRH is considered as the key organizer of the behavioural, autonomic and endocrine stress responses. As was discussed in Section 8.2.2, there are numerous stressor-specific convergent neuro-anatomical pathways which control in an integrated fashion the activity of the CRH neurons. Under conditions of psychosocial challenge, however, the NA ergic cells in the locus coeruleus seem to dominate as a trigger for the CRH response. The two systems are highly intertwined. CRH and NA neurons stimulate each other while autoregulatory negative feedback loops are present in both the PVN and the locus coeruleus. In addition both the PVN and the locus coeruleus receive stimulatory input (amongst others 5-HT ergic and cholinergic in nature) and inhibitory input (amongst others GABA ergic in nature) from several other regions (Chrousos & Gold, 1992). It will be a tall order to identify the prime mover.

8.3 Depression and the HPA system

Since the introduction of the antidepressants, monoamines (MA) have been a major focus of biological depression research (Chapter 7). A second line of intense investigation relates to the HPA axis. It received its major impetus from the work of Sachar *et al.* (1970), showing that in depression around the clock elevation of plasma cortisol concentration may occur as well as an altered circadian pattern of cortisol secretion (Figure 8.5). In the latter case, both the frequency, duration and magnitude of secretory bursts are increased. The usual dip between 20.00 and 2.00 h disappears and instead cortisol hypersecretion continues. Sachar and his group were not the first to report on hypercortisolaemia in depression (Board *et al.*, 1956), but it was the first detailed 24-hour study. Self-report measures of anxiety, negative mood states and daily hassles all were found to be accompanied by increased salivary cortisol (Van Eck *et al.*, 1996). High morning salivary cortisol, moreover, was shown to be a possible risk factor for depression (Harris *et al.*, 2000). Conversely, in a large epidemiological study it was established that persons taking corticosteroids had a higher rate of major depression than nonexposed individuals (Patten, 2000). Interestingly, in animals, low concentrations of glucocorticoids have rewarding, i.e. positive reinforcing effects, probably mediated via stimulation of mesencephalic DA ergic transmission. Possibly in this way, the aversive, anxiety-provoking 'load' of threatening stimuli is diminished and coping ability

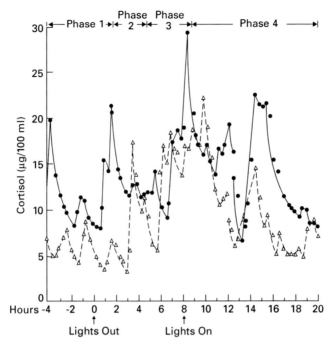

Figure 8.5.   24-h plasma concentrations of cortisol in a depressed patient (•——•) and a normal control (△ . . . . . . △) (Sachar et al., 1970).

strengthened. It is through higher concentrations that anxiety- and depression-like features become manifest (Piazza & Le Moal, 1997).

Depressed patients with high resting plasma cortisol, still show a substantial cortisol response to physiological or psychological stressors. Failure to limit the stress-induced cortisol response will thus result in greater overall exposure to cortisol. Assuming excess cortisol to be related to changes in mood and cognition, a vicious circle will therefore be initiated (Young et al., 2000). In chronic depression HPA axis function tends to normalize (Watson et al., 2002).

Normally, approximately 90% of glucocorticoids are bound to corticosteroid-binding globulin (CBG). It binds cortisol with high affinity but with rather low capacity. Bound cortisol cannot reach many target tissues and is not able to bind to receptors. Under stressful conditions when the demand for glucocorticoids increases CBG levels decrease, making more free cortisol available for coping with the stressor. This at least is the case in animals (Spencer et al., 1996). In depressed individuals Deuschle et al. (1996) found the CBG concentration unchanged.

Many additional data indicate that the *HPA system may be hyperactive* in depression (Table 8.5). Pertinent are the following observations (for reviews see Musselman et al., 1998; Arborelius et al., 1999; Holsboer, 2000).

Table 8.5. Major disturbances in the functioning of the HPA axis in (a subtype of) depression.

Clinical findings	Challenge tests	Postmortem findings
↑ CSF CRH	Dexamethasone (Dex) nonsuppression of cortisol	↑ Number CRH neurons in hypothalamus
↑ Plasma ACTH		
↑ Plasma cortisol	Blunting ACTH response to CRH	↑ CRH messenger RNA in hypothalamus
↑ Urinary cortisol		
↓ GR binding on blood platelets	Dex/CRH challenge: increased ACTH response	↑ Number vasopressin neurons in hypothalamus
Enlargement pituitary and adrenal cortex		↓ GR binding in brain

1 Increased levels of circulating ACTH (Deuschle *et al.*, 1997).

2 Increased urinary cortisol excretion.

3 Increased levels of corticotrophin releasing hormone (CRH) in cerebrospinal fluid (CSF) (Nemeroff *et al.*, 1984; Banki *et al.*, 1987) (Figure 8.6) and an increased number of CRH secreting neurons and CRH messenger RNA in the hypothalamus (Raadsheer *et al.*, 1995). The number of CRH binding sites, on the other hand, is reduced, possibly consequent to elevation of CRH availability.

4 The number of neurons containing both CRH and vasopressin is increased and so is the number of neurons that produce vasopressin or oxytocin only (Purba *et al.*, 1996) (Figure 8.7). Plasma levels of arginine vasopressin were found to be elevated in depression (Van Londen *et al.*, 1997). Both vasopressin and oxytocin potentiate CRH-mediated ACTH release (Gillies *et al.*, 1982; Von Bardeleben *et al.*, 1985).

  CSF concentration of CRH as well as plasma cortisol and ACTH levels tend to normalize on recovery. If not, this might be a harbinger of early relapse (Banki *et al.*, 1992).

5 GR binding on lymphocytes and in postmortem brain is decreased (Dinan, 1994), explaining the observed attenuation of GR-mediated negative feedback in depression (Young & Vazques, 1996; Modell *et al.*, 1997).

  Furthermore, in depression, various *hormonal challenge tests* may reveal disturbed HPA axis regulation.

6 First of all, the suppression of cortisol release that normally follows administration of dexamethasone may be incomplete (Carroll, 1982). Dexamethasone is a synthetic glucocorticoid that, like cortisol, binds to GRs on ACTH-producing cells in the anterior pituitary. In the lower dose range it penetrates the brain poorly

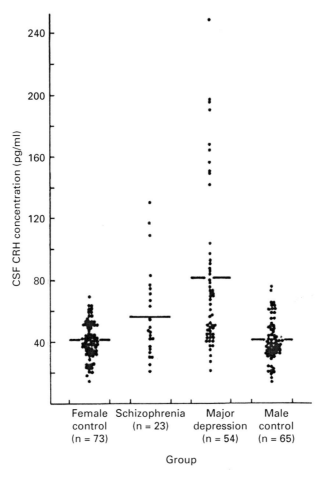

Figure 8.6. CSF CRH-like immunoreactivity in patients with schizophrenia, patients with major depression, and control subjects with various peripheral neurological diseases (Banki *et al.*, 1987).

(Meijer & De Kloet, 1998). The dexamethasone suppression test measures the capacity of GRs on the anterior pituitary to negatively control the ACTH/cortisol release in the face of the CRH/vasopressin overdrive. To achieve the normal degree of cortisol suppression in depressed nonsuppressors, a higher dose of dexamethasone is required (Modell *et al.*, 1997). Apparently, the function of the GRs is reduced (Pariante & Miller, 2001) and, consequently, the negative feedback acting through GRs is changed to a higher setpoint. Possibly as a compensatory mechanism the functional activity of the MR system is increased (Young *et al.*, 2003).

7 The ACTH response to CRH may be blunted, supposedly due to downregulation of CRH receptors on the pituitary gland, secondary to overproduction of CRH (Gold *et al.*, 1986). Blunting of the ACTH response to CRH is positively correlated

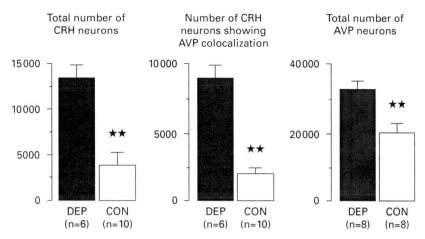

Figure 8.7.   Number of CRH and arginine vasopressin (AVP) neurons in the paraventricular nucleus
(PVN) of depressed patients. Patients with major depression have an increased number
of CRH and AVP neurons and neurons containing both CRH and AVP in the hypothalamic
PVN. Both peptides potentiate their actions on pituitary CRH receptors. DEP, depressed
patients; CON, controls (adapted from Raadsheer *et al.*, 1994; Purba *et al.*, 1996; Holsboer,
1999).

with dexamethasone nonsuppression (Krishnan *et al.*, 1993). The ACTH response
to vasopressin remains normal and so does the ACTH response to a combination
of CRH and vasopressin (Dinan *et al.*, 1999). The cortisol response to a CRH challenge remains normal as well, possibly because the adrenal cortex is hyperactive
and secretes more cortisol per ACTH pulse than normal (Krishnan *et al.*, 1993).
Hyperactivity of the adrenal cortex could also explain why the cortisol response
to an ACTH challenge in depression might be greater than normal (Amsterdam
et al., 1987).

8 After pretreatment with dexamethasone, the ACTH response to CRH is *not*
decreased, as it is in depressed patients not pretreated with dexamethasone,
but rather *increased* (Figure 8.8). This has been explained in the following way
(Holsboer *et al.*, 1987). Dexamethasone (in low doses) does not penetrate the
blood brain barrier well because of a multidrug resistance P-glycoprotein (Meijer
& De Kloet, 1998; Karssen *et al.*, 2001). Its inhibitory effects on the HPA axis are
effected predominantly by inhibiting ACTH release and not via interference with
CRH release (De Kloet *et al.*, 1974, 1975; Cole *et al.*, 2000). ACTH and cortisol
levels are thus reduced. The negative feedback on CRH release by endogenous cortisol diminishes and consequently the release of CRH (and that of other ACTH-
stimulating peptides such as vasopressin) will increase. An additional CRH pulse
will override downregulation of the CRH receptors on the pituitary and produce an increased ACTH response. This effect will be even more pronounced

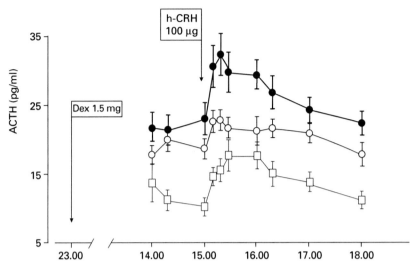

Figure 8.8.   ACTH response to CRH after pretreatment with dexamethasone in depressed patients (•), in depressed patients after remission (o) and in normal controls (□).
Relative to the control group the response in depressed patients is significantly increased. The response in the group of remitted patients is significantly lower than in the depressed phase but still greater than in the control group (after Holsboer-Trachsler *et al.*, 1991).

in depressed patients in whom CRH and ACTH production are already elevated to begin with. Increased ACTH response to CRH after pretreatment with dexamethasone may continue after remission (Holsboer-Trachsler *et al.*, 1991) and is also found in a substantial proportion of first-degree relatives of patients with depression without a history of psychiatric illness or current stressful life events (Modell *et al.*, 1998). Raadsheer *et al.* (1994) reported that hypothalamic CRH cells may remain activated in depressed patients who had been in remission. Apparently, CRH overproduction may continue in spite of hypercortisolaemia, possibly due to GR resistance which might be of genetic origin or acquired.

Reinstatement of a normal HPA setpoint is a prognostic sign. Persistence of abnormalities in the dexamethasone suppression test and the dexamethasone/CRH test is associated with poor treatment response, and predicts increased relapse risk (Ribeiro *et al.*, 1993; Zobel *et al.*, 2001).

9 Possibly in response to hypersecretion of CRH and ACTH respectively, the pituitary gland and the adrenal gland may be enlarged in depression (Krishnan *et al.*, 1991; Nemeroff *et al.*, 1992).

Hypercortisolaemia, if persistent, is not innocuous. It may lead to hippocampal damage (see Sections 8.4.3 and 8.4.5) and furthermore to demineralization of bone tissue, intra-abdominal fat accumulation and increased risk of heart diseases.

It should be emphasized that stress hormone abnormalities are not typical for depression as such, but occur only in a *subgroup of depression*. Indeed, in some depressives signs of hypothalamic CRH deficiency have been observed (Van der Pool et al., 1991; Posener et al., 2000). According to Joyce et al. (1994), personality factors such as dependence are a major determinant of hypercortisolaemia in depression.

Moreover the hormonal abnormalities discussed above, are *not specific for (a subgroup of) depression*. In panic disorder, for instance, the ACTH response to CRH may be blunted (Chalmers et al., 1996), and the dexamethasone/CRH test shows alterations similar to those observed in depression (Schreiber et al., 1996). Alterations of the dexamethasone/CRH test similar to those observed in depression may also be found in schizophrenia (Lammers et al., 1995). In obsessive-compulsive disorder and in posttraumatic stress disorder (PTSD) CSF CRH was found to be increased (Bremner et al., 1997a,b) and in anorexia nervosa a markedly attenuated ACTH response to CRH has been reported (Chalmers et al., 1996).

In summary, depression (at least some types of depression) is characterized by glucocorticoid feedback resistance and enhanced CRH/vasopressin drive. However, the disturbances in the HPA axis are categorically nonspecific and possibly related to disturbances in specific psychic regulation systems, across diagnoses (see also Chapter 9). It is not yet known, however, which regulatory systems might be involved.

8.4 CRH and HPA axis abnormalities: stress-related or depression-related?

8.4.1 How should the question be phrased?

A major issue is whether the increased release of CRH and other hormones produced by the HPA axis are epiphenomenal or pathogenic. Pathogenic means involved in the pathophysiology of depression. Epiphenomenal indicates that the hormonal disturbances are secondary phenomena: the result of anxiety and tension that often accompany depression. In essence this is a derivative question. The pertinent question is what the role of stress is in the causation of depression. Is stress a precursor and pacemaker of (certain types of) depression and a factor sustaining depression, or is stress purely a consequence of depression? In the former case the question arises whether stress hormones are involved in the pathophysiology of depression and if so, in what manner. If the latter is true, the hormonal changes are pretty much inconsequential. The pertinent question is not whether overproduction of stress hormones in depression is epiphenomenal or essential, but whether stress is or is not a dominant aetiological factor in the occurrence of (certain forms of) depression.

Since signs of increased HPA axis hyperactivity continue around the clock, it has been concluded that this is a *primary* phenomenon and *not* the *resultant* of conscious upsetting experiences (Wong et al., 2000). This is not a convincing argument, because depression is often accompanied by frequent and vivid dreaming and such dreams can be pretty alarming. Several lines of evidence, however, point to stress

Table 8.6. The hypothesis that stress and stress hormones play a role in the pathogenesis of (certain types of) depression would gain in strength if the following could be demonstrated.

Antidepressants affect corticosteroid receptor gene expression

CRH administration generates anxiety-like and/or depression-like behavioural changes.

CRH systems were shown to be disturbed in (certain types of) depression

Early adversity (a known risk factor for adult depression) would disturb the development of the CRH system, leading to increased stress reactivity

Stress hormones would generate MA ergic disturbances similar to those found in (certain types of) depression

CRH and cortisol antagonists would exert therapeutic effects in (certain types of) depression

---

and stress hormones as depressogenic variables (Van Praag, 2002): the effect of antidepressants on corticosteroid receptor gene expression; the behavioural seque-lae of CRH administration; CRH disturbances in depression; the impact of early life adversity (a known risk factor for depression) on the development of the CRH sys-tem, on stress reactivity and depression proneness; the inter-relationships of stress hormones and monoaminergic transmission and finally, the therapeutic potential of CRH and cortisol antagonists (Table 8.6). These issues will be discussed in the following sections.

8.4.2 Antidepressants and the HPA axis

Treatment with antidepressants, if effective, leads to normalization of HPA axis activity, including CSF concentrations of CRH and AVP (de Bellis et al., 1993). As such, this is not an argument in support of a primary role of HPA axis overac-tivity in the causation of depression. Even if overdrive of this system were to be a secondary phenomenon one would expect it to normalize after remission. Sev-eral phenomena, however, suggest a primary role of HPA axis overactivity. Various types of antidepressants, including SSRIs, noradrenaline reuptake inhibitors and monoamine oxidase inhibitors, increase: (a) MR and GR mRNA expression, (b) the capacity of brain tissue to bind corticosteroids and (c) steroid receptor immuno-reactivity in the brain. The time course of the actions of antidepressants on corti-costeroid receptor concentration, moreover, follows that of clinical improvement (Seckl & Fink, 1992; Reul et al., 1993, 1994). Transgenic mice with diminished GRs show cognitive defects, reduced anxiety, low plasma corticosterone and elevated plasma ACTH and corticosterone concentrations in response to stress (Contarino et al., 1999). After treatment with antidepressants both the behavioural and the hormonal alterations will disappear (Montkowski et al., 1995).

Rats treated with various types of antidepressants show first an increase of MRs, an effect followed by upregulation of GRs (Reul et al., 1993, 1994).

Antidepressant-induced upregulation of corticosteroid receptors, particularly GRs, leads to strengthening of the negative feedback and consequently to decrease of HPA axis hyperactivity with lowering of CSF CRH concentration, plasma ACTH and cortisol levels and normalization of the dexamethasone suppression test and the dexamethasone/CRH test (Zobel *et al.*, 1999). Several SSRIs, however, do not increase GR mRNA (Seckl & Fink, 1992) and hence upregulation of GRs cannot be considered as a unitary antidepressant mechanism.

The pronounced effects of most, but not all antidepressants on GR gene expression support the view that hyperactivity of the CRH-ACTH-cortisol system in depression is more than just an epiphenomenon, and might be involved in the pathophysiology of (certain types of) depression.

8.4.3 CRH, a depressogenic substance?
CRH localization and CRH receptors

CRH is a 41 amino-acid peptide isolated and structurally characterized by Vale *et al.* (1981). High concentrations of CRH are found in the parvocellular division of the PVN. These cells project to the median eminence. This pathway represents the hypothalamic branch of the HPA system (see Section 8.2).

CRH-containing neurons, however, are not restricted to the PVN but have in addition a wide extra-hypothalamic distribution. They are found, for instance, in the neocortex, the amygdala, the bed nucleus of the stria terminalis, the substantia innominata and also in brainstem nuclei involved in regulation of the autonomic nervous system, such as the raphe nuclei and locus coeruleus, the cradle of 5-HT ergic and NA ergic neurons respectively. A dense network of CRH immunoreactive axons is also found in the mesencephalic DA ergic nuclei (Austin *et al.*, 1997). Extra-hypothalamic CRH is considered to be a putative neurotransmitter, and the extra-hypothalamic CRH system is thought to be responsible for the behavioural and some of the autonomic components of the stress response. The behavioural effects of CRH occur independent of the HPA axis, since they persist after hypophysectomy. CRH in human lumbar CSF is probably mainly of extra-hypothalamic origin (Geracioti *et al.*, 1997).

Glucocorticoids restrain CRH and AVP-producing cells in the PVN steering the HPA axis, by inhibiting CRH and AVP gene expression (Holsboer, 1999). During chronic stress hypothalamic CRH/AVP expression becomes resistant to glucocorticoid suppression. If chronically elevated, glucocorticoids, however, *enhance* CRH activity in the extra-hypothalamic CRH system, most notably in the two regions with predominant CRH-containing neurons, i.e. the central nucleus of the amygdala and the lateral bed nucleus of the stria terminalis. They do so by inducing CRH gene expression. The central nucleus of the amygdala is involved in processing and encoding of emotions. As such, it is an important structure for the retrieval of information that could be relevant for the emotional analysis of a given event or situation that is or might become harmful. This information is necessary for proper appraisal of dangerousness. CRH neurons project directly from this site to the parvocellular division of the PVN. Hyper-responsiveness of the amygdala will render an individual probably fearful and anxiety prone (Schulkin *et al.*, 1998; Heim & Nemeroff, 1999).

The behavioural stress phenomena, thus, are not subject to the cortisol-mediated negative feedback system. On the contrary, extra-hypothalamic CRH and cortisol work together in a mutually reinforcing positive feedback loop, at least under chronic stress conditions. This permissive action of cortisol, under chronic stress conditions, contrasts with the facilitatory role of this hormone in the acute recovery phase of the stress response when it promotes behavioural adaptation (see Section 8.2.3). CRH antagonists, on the other hand, block many behavioural stress phenomena induced by CRH or by adverse stimuli.

In summary, CRH is located in the PVN as well as extra-hypothalamically. The former system regulates the HPA axis, the latter is responsible for the behavioural stress responses. The CRH_1 receptor system is associated with anxiety and depression-like behaviour. CRH_2 receptor trajectories exert anxiolytic effects and use urocortins. Cortisol exerts negative feedback action on hypothalamic CRH, but stimulates in a reverberating positive feedback loop extra-hypothalamic CRH if the elevation is prolonged.

Effects of CRH in animals

Administration of CRH directly into the brain at specific sites, either intraventricularly or intra cerebrally, leads *in rodents* to a wide array of behavioural effects, the character of which depends on dose and on the behavioural state the test animal find itself in (Heinrichs *et al.*, 1995). In animals under low arousal conditions, CRH in moderate doses produces dose-dependent behavioural activation with increased arousal and vigilance. Locomotor activity is increased, and likewise rearing, sniffing and grooming when rats are tested in a familiar environment. These effects remain after hypophysectomy, indicating that they appear independent of the HPA axis (Eaves *et al.*, 1985; Britton *et al.*, 1986).

In higher doses, or administered to stressed animals, the CRH effects are quite different and can be construed as anxiogenic. Heart rate and respiration increase and so do blood pressure, blood sugar level, gluconeogenesis and the acoustic startle response. Exploration of unfamilar environments is decreased; stress-induced freezing is increased, and likewise the responsiveness to sensory stimuli and the conditioned fear response during aversive stimulation. Sexual activity and receptivity are decreased and so is food intake while grooming is increased (Chrousos & Gold, 1992; Koob *et al.*, 1993; Heinrichs *et al.*, 1995). Plasma concentrations of adrenalin, NA, cortisol and ACTH are elevated. Whereas the sympathetic nervous system is obviously activated, the parasympathetic nervous system is inhibited (de Souza, 1995). Rats, selectively bred according to high anxiety, have increased CRH expression in several brain areas (Holsboer, 2001). Transgenic mice overproducing CRH were found to be 'anxious', e.g. to over-respond to novel environments.

In *non-human primates* CRH triggers anxiety/despair-related phenomena such as frequent vocalizations, potentiation of the acoustic startle response, facilitation of fear conditioning, suppression of exploratory behaviour in a novel environment, enhancement of shock-induced freezing and fighting behaviour. The anxiogenic effects of CRH are supposedly mediated via CRH neurons connecting the amygdala and the LC (Owens & Nemeroff, 1991; Koob *et al.*, 1993; Arborelius *et al.*, 1999).

In addition, depression-like phenomena are observed, such as huddling, lying down behaviour (also seen after infant monkeys are separated from their mothers), loss of interest, sleep disturbances, decreased libido and motor hyperactivity (Heim & Nemeroff, 1999). These effects, too, are independent of the effects of CRH on the HPA axis and are abolished or prevented by CRH receptor antagonists or CRH antisense oligodeoxynucleotide (Heinrichs *et al.*, 1995). Apparently the regulatory significance of CRH reaches far beyond the control of the HPA axis.

Which of the CRH receptors mediate the anxiety-like behaviours?

Antisense oligodeoxynucleotides against CRH_1 receptors produce anxiolytic effects in rats; i.e. those animals are less anxious than their wild-type counterparts (Skutella *et al.*, 1994; Timpl *et al.*, 1998). The same is true for CRH_1 receptor antagonists (Koob *et al.*, 1993). Knocking out the CRH_2 receptor does not produce such effects (Liebsch *et al.*, 1999). On the contrary, such mice display anxiety-like behaviour and are hypersensitive to stress, suggesting that its activation might have anxiolytic effects (Bale *et al.*, 2000; Kishimoto *et al.*, 2000).

These data indicate that only activation of the CRH_1 receptor induces anxiety-related behaviour. The CRH_2 receptor seems to have opposite effects (Heinrichs *et al.*, 1997).

As pointed out in Section 8.2.1, the urocortin family is now completed with two splice variants: urocortin II and III which serve as the specific high affinity ligands for the CRH_2 receptors in mammals, while urocortin I binds to both receptor types. Accordingly, an urocortin system exists distinct from the CRH system that exerts its anxiolytic effects by stimulating the CRH_2 receptor but its precise role in stress-related behaviour is unknown. The fact that CRH deficient mice (knockouts) display normal behaviour and normal stress responses, might be due to the fact that in those circumstances urocortin I replaces CRH in activating the CRH_1 receptor (Weninger *et al.*, 1999; Habib *et al.*, 2000).

In summary, CRH in animals leads to a series of stress-like physiological and behavioural phenomena. The behavioural features indicate increased anxiety, while some phenomena are also observed in animal models of depression (e.g. decreased food intake, inhibition of sexual behaviour, sleep disturbances and psychomotor activation). Opposing actions are being recorded for the urocortins II and III and that has led some (Hsu & Hsueh, 2001) to suggest that CRH and urocortin are two *anti-parallel stress systems* that function as organizers of the sympathetic and parasympathetic response, respectively. These data strongly suggest a role for the CRH/urocortin family of peptides in the pathophysiology of states of anxiety and depression.

CRH and depression

In depression CRH overdrive may occur (Nemeroff *et al.*, 1984) as is apparent from a number of observations:

1 Increased CRH concentration in plasma and CSF (Catalán *et al.*, 1998), whereas the level of CSF CRH and dexamethasone nonsuppression are positively correlated (Figure 8.6).

2 Serial CSF samples over 6 hours revealed increased CRH levels at all time points (Baker *et al.*, 1999).

3 In postmortem studies of depressed patients an increase has been observed in brain CRH concentrations, CRH mRNA expression, in the number of AVP and CRH containing neurons and in those that contain both peptides (Raadsheer *et al.*, 1994, 1995; Purba *et al.*, 1996). Possibly secondary to increased CRH production, CRH receptor density was found to be decreased (Nemeroff *et al.*, 1988).

4 Blunted ACTH response to CRH, conceivably due to CRH receptor downregulation on the pituitary, consequent to CRH overproduction.

5 Some authors did report downregulation of CRH receptors and decreased CRH mRNA in the cortex of (depressed) suicide victims. Decreased CRH mRNA was also found in schizophrenia, indicating this phenomenon to be nosologically nonspecific (Webster *et al.*, 1999). Other investigators, however, found the number of CRH receptors and the affinity of CRH receptors in depression to be unchanged (Hucks *et al.*, 1997).

Overproduction of CRH could be a primary phenomenon (enhanced forward drive) (Nemeroff, 1996) or, alternatively, the consequence of impaired GR function, leading to reduced cortisol-mediated negative feedback at the level of the pituitary corticotrope or the hypothalamus (Young *et al.*, 1991). Some data suggest impaired feedback inhibition. Dexamethasone nonsuppression is one case in point (Modell *et al.*, 1997). Furthermore, GRs on lymphocytes have been found to be reduced in depressed patients (Whalley *et al.*, 1986). Accordingly, the fast and early phases of the negative feedback have been reported to be impaired (Young *et al.*, 1991), but negative reports have also been published (Cooney & Dinan, 1996, 2000). The fast feedback refers to the role of hippocampal MR because of the role of this receptor system in the onset of the HPA response to stress. Indeed, a recent study showed that while acute stress increased hippocampal MR expression, MR was downregulated during chronic stress in a CRH-dependent manner (Gesing *et al.*, 2001). Decreased hippocampal MR activity suggests diminished inhibitory control over the HPA axis and thus elevated cortisol. In this way a reverberating positive feedback loop evolves in the hippocampus involving CRH and cortisol (Reul and Holsboer, 2002).

In summary, then, it appears that CRH overdrive might occur in depression, but it is by no means a universal phenomenon in this group of disorders, nor is it specific for depression. Its cause is often surmised to be downregulation or desensitization of MRs and/or GRs and thus escape from feedback inhibition. Quite some evidence supports this view (Pariante & Miller, 2001). Primacy of CRH overdrive remains, however, an arguable standpoint. Interestingly, in some depressed patients CSF CRH levels were found to have *decreased* (Geracioti *et al.*, 1997) again, suggesting that the group of mood disorders is heterogeneous in a biological sense, as much as it is psychopathologically.

Three issues pertinent in this context, have not been discussed in this section. Firstly, is stress the sole condition bringing about hyperactivity of both CRH systems: the hypothalamic and the extra-hypothalamic? Secondly, do both CRH systems always function in parallel or are they basically independent? In other words: is it possible that the extra-hypothalamic system is hyperactive with normal CRH secretion by the PVN and vice versa? Thirdly, how do the CRH and urocortin systems interact in depression? These questions were passed over because of want of answers.

CRH, corticosteroids, depression and brain morphology

Some studies, using in vivo imaging methods, have reported smaller volumes and reduced metabolic activity of hippocampus, amygdala and prefrontal cortex (i.e. subgenual medial prefrontal cortex, mPFC) of depressed patients (Drevets *et al.*, 1997; Sheline *et al.*, 1999; Bremner *et al.*, 2000). These smaller tissue volumes could either be a cause or consequence of the disease. Since the hippocampus plays a role in slowing down the HPA response to adverse stimuli, damage to this part of the brain may play a role in the inability to keep stress responses at bay (Herman & Cullinan, 1997). Hence shrinkage of the hippocampus was initially thought to be due to the hypercorticism associated with depression. In support of this notion reduced hippocampal volume has been found in patients suffering from Cushing's syndrome with sustained hypercortisolaemia (Starkman *et al.*, 1992). Normalization of cortisol levels in those patients restores hippocampal size. However, patients suffering from posttraumatic stress syndrome also have reduced hippocampal size (Bremner *et al.*, 1995), while such patients usually are characterized by hypocortisolaemia.

The hippocampus and amygdala are part of the limbic system, originally indicated as the centre of emotion. Nowadays the amygdala and hippocampus are viewed as operating in different functional modes of emotion. The amygdala is the site where basic emotions like fear, fight and flight are generated before these emotions have been evaluated by the cortical brain regions. Dysregulations in the amygdala are probably the basis of inexplicable feelings of apprehension and aversion. The amygdala triggers the endocrine, autonomic and behavioural stress reactions that make up the initial emotional response to a trauma. The hippocampus is involved in remembering these emotion-laden events and the context, time and place in which they take place (Pugh *et al.*, 1997). Conceivably and hypothetically, disturbances in emotional memory play a role in: (a) failure to properly evaluate the dangerousness of a given situation (McEwen, 1998) and (b) in the ability to link a given perception to an appropriate emotion. The prefrontal cortex (PFC) is able to inhibit the emotionally driven fearful reactions generated by the amygdala and provides reason to emotions. Furthermore, the PFC is important for the selection of an appropriate strategy to cope with a challenge and the facilitation of complex cognitive processes (Lupien *et al.*, 1994; Lupien & McEwen, 1997).

These functions of the hippocampus, amygdala and PFC have been deduced from experiments with patients in whom these brain regions were damaged. A literature is evolving relating neuropsychological impairments in depression, to defective functioning of the hippocampus and the PFC. As mentioned above, high concentrations of cortisol, as may be observed in depression, have been associated with volume changes of these brain regions.

The question can be raised whether the shrinkage of brain tissue in depression can be attributed to neuronal atrophy due to stress hormones. A study by Lucassen *et al.* (2001) and by Müller *et al.* (2001) saw no signs of cell death in postmortem hippocampus of depressed patients. On the other hand, histopathology of the PFC of depressives showed reduced grey matter and glial number, but no equivalent loss of neurons (Drevets *et al.*, 1997). Thus, though the size of these tissues seems to correlate with cognitive performance and the occurrence of depression and PTSD, the evidence that the reduced size of these tissues reflects neuronal atrophy is far from convincing, and neither is it clear whether the effects of cortisol on cognition proceeds through changes in volume and gross anatomical features of hippocampus and PFC.

Yet, in animal studies stress, particularly repeated stress, *does* affect the fine structure of neurons particularly in the hippocampus, a brain region rich in GRs (Figure 8.9). These changes are effected through glucocorticoids (Sapolsky, 1996; Magarinos *et al.*, 1997; McEwen, 1998). Dendrites of pyramidal neurons in the CA3 region retract and this was shown to be reversible if stress is short-lived, and irreversible if stress is long-lasting (Watanabe *et al.*, 1992). Several antidepressants, benzodiazepine agonists and cortisol antagonists prevent stress-induced dendritic atrophy (Kaufman *et al.*, 2000). In the stressed tree shrew, a model for depression, the in vivo cerebral concentration of N-acetyl-aspartate, a marker for neuronal viability,

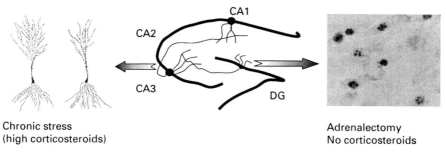

Chronic stress
(high corticosteroids)

Adrenalectomy
No corticosteroids

Figure 8.9.   Cell viability in hippocampus. Chronic stress causes atrophy of the pyramidal neurons in the CA3 pyramidal cell field. Adrenalectomy causes apoptosis and alters the rate of neurogenesis in the dentate gyrus (DG).

was reduced, and so were hippocampal volume and dentate gyrus proliferation. These reductions were counteracted by treatment with the antidepressant tianeptine (Czéh et al., 2002). Collectively, the data provide some but inconclusive evidence for causality between stress-induced dendritic retraction and the reduced hippocampal and PFC volume (Czéh et al., 2002).

Another line of research revealed that in hippocampal CA1 neurons glucocorticoids enhance the vulnerability to neurotoxic agents. According to Sapolsky (1992), the neuronal damage caused by chronic elevated concentrations of glucocorticoids is caused by energy depletion. Glucocorticoids block glucose uptake in the neuron, making it more vulnerable to excitotoxicity, such as effected by glutamate. The excitatory amino acid glutamate is released in excess not only after physical damage, e.g. ischaemia, but also after psychological stress (Moghaddam, 1993). Moreover, glucocorticoids increase extracellular glutamate levels by preventing its reuptake into glia cells (McEwen & Sapolsky, 1995). In this way its extracellular presence is prolonged and the opportunity to bind to NMDA receptors is increased (Virgin et al., 1991). 5-HT$_{1A}$ agonists decrease glutamate release and in this way exert neuroprotective effects. Chronic exposure to glucocorticoids decreases 5-HT$_{1A}$ receptor expression. This may add to the neuronal damage.

Finally, stress and glucocorticoids suppress neurogenesis. In the majority of brain regions production and migration of nerve cells remain restricted to the gestational period. In the hippocampal dentate gyrus region, however, the production of granule neurons continues well into adulthood. Newly generated cells mature into functional neurons in the adult mammalian brain (Van Praag et al., 2002). This has been demonstrated in several species, including humans (Gould, 1999; Gould et al. 1999a, b). This process is not only enhanced by brain-derived neurotrophic factor (BDNF), but also by activation of 5-HT receptors, in particular the 5HT$_{1A}$ receptor, a receptor abundantly present in the dentate gyrus (Yan et al., 1997). Neurogenesis depends on the expression and functioning of MR rather than GR. In MR knock-out mice and in adrenalectomized mice neurogenesis in dentate gyrus is reduced (Gass et al., 2000).

Stress and glucocorticoids reduce mRNA of certain growth factors, particularly of brain-derived neurotrophic factor (BDNF) in the hippocampus which also may contribute to hippocampal damage (Smith, 1996; Schaaf et al., 2001). These substances promote growth of neurons, particularly granule neurons in the dentate gyrus of the hippocampus and in the neocortex (Azmitia, 1999; Gould, 1999; Gould et al., 1999a,b). The actions of BDNF and 5-HT are inter-related. Reduction of BDNF impairs the 5-HT ergic system. 5-HT$_1$ receptor binding in the hippocampus, for instance, is decreased and 5-HT$_2$ receptor binding in the frontal cortex increased. On a behavioural level, BDNF-depleted animals show increased aggressiveness, just as 5-HT depleted do (Lyons et al., 1999). Stressful experiences suppress the formation of new hippocampal granule neurons and it seems likely that suppressed expression of BDNF and 5-HT$_{1A}$ receptors represent causative factors (Gould et al., 1999a; Czéh et al., 2002; Rasmusson et al., 2002). These changes have led to the suggestion that reduced neurogenesis may be responsible for the smaller hippocampus size observed in affective disorders (Fuchs & Gould, 2000).

This suggestion was reinforced by the notion that chronic antidepressant administration increases neurogenesis (Duman et al., 2000). Firmer conclusions, however, must await the functional role of the newborn neurons in the hippocampus.

Collectively, rodent studies suggest that very high levels of glucocorticoids and repeated stress may alter structural features of the hippocampus, while the evidence from primate studies is ambiguous in particular since the studies in man do not allow observations on the ultrastructural level. Moreover, a smaller hippocampus observed with imaging methodology could still reflect both a cause or an effect of depression. Findings in the monkey suggest that small hippocampi reflect (in part) an inherited characteristic of the brain. This inherited variation in hippocampal morphology could contribute to excessive stress responses through diminished inhibitory control over neuroendocrine regulation (Lyons et al., 2001). In support of this reasoning mouse lines genetically selected for profound differences in aggressiveness, coping style and stress regulation also show different structural features in the hippocampus. These mice display under basal conditions profound differences in expression of patterns of cytoskeleton genes such as tubulin and cofilin. These cytoskeleton genes may reflect the size of the hippocampus as one of the determinants in the genetic selection of the endocrine and behavioural traits (Feldker et al., 2003). If these mice were exposed to chronic stress gene patterns underlying plasticity rather than the rigid cytoskeleton genes were affected. These stress-induced gene patterns encode for pathways involving growth factors. Accordingly, the gross anatomy is genetically determined, but its plasticity and ultrastructure can change during stress and steroid exposure. It cannot be excluded therefore that a smaller hippocampal size may be a risk factor in the development of depression (Sullivan et al., 2001), and that the structural plasticity observed in animal experiments has escaped detection in the imaging studies so far.

In summary, current evidence suggests that cognitive dysfunction observed in depression relates to reduced hippocampal size. The smaller hippocampus might very well be genetically determined and constitute a risk factor for depression rather than the consequence. Yet, animal data indicate that very high levels of glucocorticoids can cause atrophy of many tissues including the hippocampus. Such animals show profound changes in cognitive functions and those may be related to cortisol-induced changes in markers for neuronal plasticity of amygdala, hippocampus and PFC.

Fundamental for these effects are interactions of cortisol with monoamines and neuropeptides like CRH in these brain regions. There is evidence that multiple reverberating positive feedback loops of cortisol may evolve in these areas that compromise cognitive and emotional performance, and that over-ride through their afferents to the PVN the autoregulatory negative feedback action exerted by that hormone. The implications of these basic studies for the clinic must await further experimentation.

8.4.4 CRH, corticosteroids and early life stress in animals

Early adversity is a known risk factor for depression in adulthood (see Section 8.4.5). Adversity is stress-generating. If early adversity could be shown to exert a lasting effect on CRH production and stress reactivity this would strengthen the hypothesis that stress indeed may play a causative role in depression. Successively, relevant animal and human data will be discussed.

Early life stress and stressor responsivity

Animal studies on the biological and behavioural effects of being exposed to stress early in life provide the most cogent arguments for an anxiogenic/depressogenic role of overproduction of CRH or hypersensitivity of CRH receptors. Several methods have been used to induce early life stress, most frequently various forms of maternal deprivation. The animals – mostly rodents and monkeys – grow up either motherless, i.e. alone or with peers only, or are separated from their mother during certain time periods. Monkey infants raised under such conditions show signs of desperation: they are anxious, locomotion is decreased, they shun exploring new environments, play less, are socially withdrawn and show disturbances in sleep and food intake and 'anhedonia' (diminished consumption of sweetened solutions). Several of these symptoms persist later in life (McKinney et al., 1984). They tend to respond favourably to antidepressant or electric shock treatment (Lopez et al., 1999).

Table 8.7. The responses of adult rats that had been subjected to daily 6-hour separation from their mother during postnatal days 2–20, compared with rats raised under normal conditions.

Biological	Behavioural
↑ Stress-induced increase of plasma ACTH and corticosterone	Anxious behaviour
↑ CRH in CSF and median eminence	↓ Social interaction
↑ Expression of CRH mRNA in the PVN	↓ Locomotion
↓ CRH binding in pituitary	↓ Exploration of new environments
↑ CRH binding in the extra-hypothalamic CRH system	'Anhedonia' (↓ consumption of sweetened solutions)
↑ Responsiveness of 5-HT$_2$ receptors	↑ Food intake
↓ Responsiveness of 5-HT$_{1A}$ receptors	Sleep disturbances
↑ NA concentratrion in PVN	
↑ Rise of CSF NA in response to stressor	
↓ GABA$_A$ receptor binding	

Those traumatized animals show an increased ACTH/cortisol response to stress; often plasma cortisol levels are permanently above normal (Levine *et al.*, 1997), and CSF CRH is persistently elevated (Coplan *et al.*, 1996). Monkeys raised in social groups that were repeatedly destabilized by changing of group membership showed comparable HPA axis disturbances, as compared with specimens raised in stable groups (Brooke *et al.*, 1994).

Similar observations were made in rats. Adult rats, that had been subjected to daily 6-hour separation from their mother during postnatal days 2–20 showed greater stress-induced increase of plasma ACTH and corticosterone levels, than rats raised under normal conditions. Moreover, CRH concentrations in CSF and in the median eminence were elevated, expression of CRH mRNA in the PVN was increased, CRH binding in the pituitary decreased and that in the extra-hypothalamic CRH system increased (Plotsky & Meaney, 1993; Ladd *et al.*, 1996; Arborelius *et al.*, 1999). The responsiveness of the 5-HT$_{2c}$ receptor increased while that of the 5-HT$_{1a}$ receptor was found to be reduced (McKittrick *et al.*, 1995; Fone *et al.*, 1996). The NA concentration in the PVN rose, and so did the NA concentration in CSF in response to an acute stressor. GABA$_A$ receptor binding was reduced (Kaufman *et al.*, 2000). CRH and NA drive are obviously increased, and the GABA/benzodiazepine 'tone' decreased. Behaviourally these animals are anxious, show decreased social interaction and impaired cognitive functioning (Kaufman *et al.*, 2000) (Table 8.7).

Stressor hypersensitivity remains up to adulthood and can be successfully treated with antidepressants. After discontinuation the abnormalities return.

Total or partial separation from the mother are rather crude laboratory models of neglect, and an imperfect representation of how maternal deprivation manifests itself in the human situation. A model that mimics that situation much better is the unpredictable foraging demand model (Rosenblum & Paully, 1984). Monkey mothers are placed in three different foraging conditions: in the first one food is easily available; in the second they have to work hard for food but it arrives predictably; in the third one, food conditions are unpredictable, i.e. sometimes easy to get, sometimes only at the expense of great efforts. In the latter condition the mother remains available, but she is 'nervous', 'absent-minded' and tends to neglect her children.

Adult monkeys raised in the latter condition show persistent signs of increased anxiety, increased timidity, behavioural inhibition in unfamiliar environments, social subordinance, 'depressive episodes' upon maternal deprivation, increased levels of CRH in CSF and, against expectations, decreased CSF cortisol concentration (Andrews & Rosenblum, 1994; Coplan et al., 2000). In addition animals raised under such stressful conditions show an enhanced endocrine response to the anxiogenic NA agonist yohimbine, while responses to 5-HT agonists are blunted. Furthermore there are indications of less endogenous opioid and GABA/benzodiazepine inhibitory activity (Rosenblum et al., 1994).

The stress of social subordination causes in female cynomolgus monkeys hypersecretion of cortisol and insensitivity to negative feedback. Subordinates engaged less in affiliation, spent more time alone than dominants, and showed more behavioural depression (Shively et al., 1997)

Prenatal stress, too – induced for instance by unexpected events in the maternal environment during gestation – may lead in the offspring to enhanced emotional reactivity, depression-like behaviour, propensity to learn learned-helplessness behaviour, enhanced responsivity of the HPA axis to stress, and impaired glucocorticoid feedback. This has been demonstrated in rodents and monkeys (Weinstock et al., 1988; Clarke et al., 1994; Maccari et al., 1995; Weinstock, 1997, 2001). The same developmental disturbances may occur after acute birth insults, such as those induced by brief periods of hypoxia during labour and birth (Boksa et al., 1996).

Mechanisms underlying immediate and long-term effects of maternal separation

There is ample evidence that the exposure to stressors during pre- and postnatal life programs the stress system for later life, but how do these persistent effects occur in the developing brain? In rats, the first 2 weeks of life are called the stress hyporesponsive period (SHRP) because stressors produce only a minor corticosterone response (Figure 8.10). Only some signals e.g. interleukin-1 and histamine break through the SHRP and stimulate corticosterone secretion. A psychological stimulus as novelty produces a CRH and AVP response, but not of ACTH and

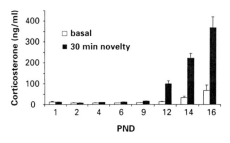

Figure 8.10. The stress hyporesponsive period (SHRP) in the rat. Corticosterone levels do not rise after a mild psychological stress during the first 2 weeks of life. PND, postnatal day.

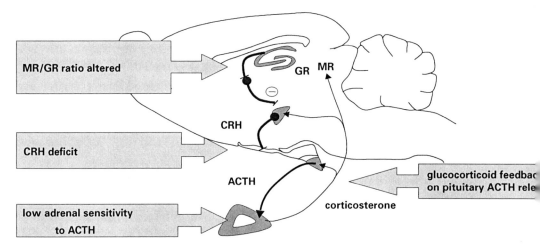

Figure 8.11. The HPA axis during the first 2 weeks of postnatal development: the stress hyporesponsive period (SHRP) (from Schmidt et al., 2003). Note that this so-called stress hyporesponsive period is due to poor CRH signalling, altered MR/GR function, glucocorticoid feedback and adrenal hyporesponsiveness as compared with stress-responsive adult animals. Maternal deprivation i.e. lack of sensory stimulation and feeding activates the otherwise quiescent HPA axis during the SHRP.

corticosterone. Exogenous ACTH is also ineffective in adrenocortical stimulation. However, administration of a glucocorticoid antagonist triggers a pronounced ACTH and corticosterone response during the SHRP. This implies that the most proximal cause of the SHRP lies at the level of the pituitary and that reduced adrenal sensitivity to ACTH is one of the consequences (Levine et al., 2000; Schmidt & De Kloet, unpublished) (Figure 8.11).

During development maternal behaviour ensures a quiescent adrenocortical system in the newborn rat. Myron Hofer (1983) has defined the mother–infant behavioural interactions and referred in this context to 'hidden regulators'. These hidden factors regulate processes underlying mother–infant interactions as well as the physiological and behavioural features of the infant during development.

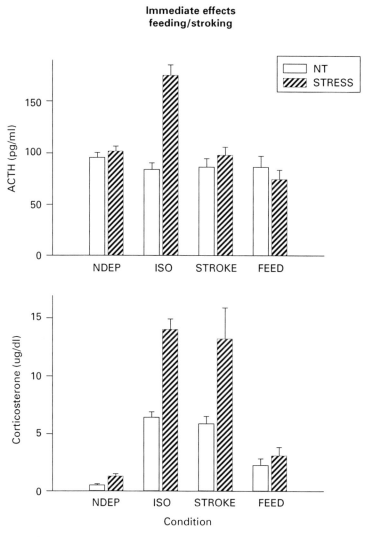

Figure 8.12. Immediate effects of 24-hour maternal deprivation (ISO) on ACTH and corticosterone levels. Stroking and feeding mimic aspects of maternal behaviour. Stroking the rat pup 3 times for 45 seconds every 8 hours normalizes ACTH. Stroking and feeding also normalizes corticos terone (Van Oers *et al.*, 1998). NDEP, not deprived. NT, not treated. Stress is exposure to a novelty stressor.

The hidden regulators cannot be detected by simple observation. The significance of these hidden regulators only becomes apparent after separation of mother and infant (Figure 8.12).

Studies using maternal separation have demonstrated that the mother regulates physiological responses in the infant. These physiological responses slowly develop as a function of time after maternal separation and appear tightly linked to specific aspects of mother–infant interaction. If, for instance, pups are separated from the mother for 24 h there is a 40% decline in heart rate. This decrease results specifically from the absence of milk, as opposed to the lack of maternal contact or other aspects of maternal care. When milk is infused in the infant normal cardiac rate reappears. Growth hormone secretion is also reduced after maternal separation. However, this decline appears due to the lack of tactile stimulation by the mother, instead of deprivation of milk. Stroking of the deprived pup with a moistened brush normalizes growth hormone secretion. Sleep/wake cycles are also disturbed after maternal separation, and this disturbance is corrected by suckling rather than feeding (Hofer, 1983).

While the cardiac response, growth hormone secretion and sleep/wake rhythm were all under the stimulatory influence of maternal care, the presence of the mother suppresses adrenocortical activity of the infant. Maternal deprivation causes small, but significant increases in corticosteroid levels over the course of the separation. Depending on age and duration of separation the effects on HPA activity are of larger magnitude. Thus, a single separation of mother and infant for at least 8 up to 24 h is needed to sensitize the adrenal for response to exogenous ACTH or to novelty stress (Levine et al., 2000). Recently, deprivation-induced changes were found in gene expression levels of MR, GR and CRH in the brain. Stroking pups three times a day with a warm wet brush prevented the rise in ACTH and CRH mRNA and restored MR mRNA levels in the hippocampus. If the animals were also fed, the level of circulating corticosterone and the expression of GR mRNA levels were normalized as well. Thus, mimicking some aspects of maternal behaviour during the time of deprivation prevented all deprivation-induced effects on the HPA axis (Van Oers et al., 1998).

A caregiving environment can also modify the adverse consequences of early stress. Adoption of maltreated pups by caring foster mothers reduces the behavioural and endocrine consequences of early adverse experiences (Maccari et al., 1995). Foster mothers generally provide more attention to the adoptees than do biological mothers (Maccari et al., 1995). Caldji et al. (1998) hypothesized that maternal care during infancy serves to 'program' behavioural responses to stress into the offspring by altering the development of the neural systems that mediate fearfulness.

In summary, deprivation of maternal care results in profound activation of the HPA axis and corticosterone secretion at a time that presence of the mother otherwise ensures a quiescent stress system. This finding in rodent studies predicts that variations in maternal care program brain and behaviour for later life.

Persistent effects of mother–pup interaction

Handling of rats (i.e. daily separation for approximately 15 min from the mother) provides a brief intermezzo in mother–pup interaction, which subsequently results in increased sensory stimulation by intensified maternal care triggering a set of physiological responses. Like adult offspring of high-licking and grooming mother rats, neonatal handling enhances maturation of the HPA circadian rhythm and the glucocorticoid negative feedback response, and thus achieves a reduction in duration of the SHRP. As adults, the neonatally handled animals exhibit reduced fearfulness, since the animals explore a novel environment, in contrast to the nonhandled animals that crouch in a corner. Neonatally handled rats show, as adults, more rapid activation and termination of the adrenocortical responses than their nonhandled littermates. This apparently enhanced inhibition of stress-induced HPA activity seems to be associated with increased numbers of GRs in the hippocampus and frontal cortex. Increased 5-HT activity is possibly involved in raising corticosteroid receptor binding capacity (Meaney *et al.*, 1988; Mitchell *et al.*, 1990). Offspring that had experienced intensified maternal care showed similar changes, and in addition increased synaptogenesis in hippocampus characterized by increased expression of BDNF mRNA, NMDA receptor subunits, cholinergic innervation of the hippocampus and spatial learning (Liu *et al.*, 2000).

During senescence handled animals that had experienced enhanced maternal care, displayed a better performance in a Morris maze test designed to evaluate cognitive functions of the rat. Deprivation from maternal care has a very different effect at senescence. Infant rats of the Brown Norway strain (these animals are usually in excellent health at old age) were maternally deprived for 24 hours at postnatal day 3. Spatial learning ability in the Morris water maze and circulating corticosterone were measured at 3, 12, 24 and 32 months of age. The results show that after maternal deprivation cognitive performance declined until midlife more rapidly in the deprived rats than in the mother-reared control animals. This difference in behaviour was abolished at old age (Figure 8.13). Rather the inter-individual difference in cognitive performance of the deprived animals was enhanced (Figure 8.15). Thus, the majority of the mother-reared senescent animals was partially impaired with few animals either unimpaired or fully impaired. In contrast, maternal deprivation drives spatial learning ability to the extremes, at the expense of the average partially impaired performance characteristic for the controls. The transition to cognitively impaired animals is promoted (about 50% are impaired), while now also 40% of the deprived animals show excellent performance (Oitzl *et al.*, 2000; Workel *et al.*, 2001). The latter successful agers have the highest expression of BDNF in the hippocampus (Schaaf *et al.*, 2001). The high expression of BDNF in the cognitively unimpaired senescent animals supports the concept that this growth factor is implicated in the regulation of synaptic plasticity underlying memory performance.

Maternal deprivation also had life-long consequences for HPA activity of the healthy ageing Brown Norway rats (Figure 8.14). In the mother-reared animals corticosterone concentrations slowly declined during ageing in parallel with the

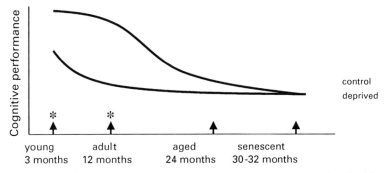

Figure 8.13. Cognitive performance in the water maze: Brown Norway rats that had been maternally deprived once for 24 hours from postnatal day 3–4. Deprived and their non-deprived littermates (control) were tested for their spatial learning and memory abilities in the Morris water maze at 3, 12, 24 and 30–32 months of age. At 3 and 12 months of age, maternally deprived rats had difficulties in acquiring the task (Oitzl et al., 2000).

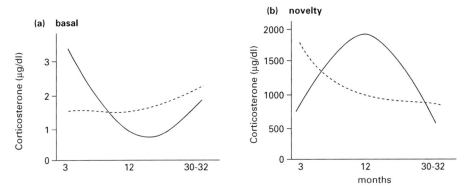

Figure 8.14. Schematic representation of corticosterone concentration in blood plasma (μg/dl) of 3, 12 and 30–32 months old control (----) and maternally deprived (—) Brown Norway rats: (a) under basal resting conditions, at the trough of the circadian rhythm and (b) in response to novelty exposure, accumulated over 120 min (based on Workel et al., 2001).

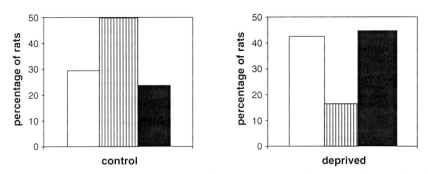

Figure 8.15. Percentage of animals with non-impaired (open bars), partially impaired (striped bars) and impaired (black bars) water maze performance. At senescence, the distribution of the quality of spatial performance differs between control (left, n = 34) and maternally deprived (right, n = 47) animals, respectively. Spatial learning of the maternally deprived animals is impaired at the expense of average performance (i.e. partially impaired).

modest cognitive decline. The pattern in the deprived animals, however, was completely different. At 3 months of age the stress-induced corticosterone level was below that of the control mother-reared animals. Subsequently, corticosterone responses to novelty dramatically increased during midlife reaching values higher than in controls. Then, stress-induced corticosterone concentrations declined reaching lower levels than control mother-reared animals at 32 months of age.

Thus, enhanced sensory stimulation by the mother programs low adrenocortical and emotional reactivity, and an apparent improved cognitive performance. In contrast, adult rats exposed as infants to maternal deprivation display high adrenocortical reactivity and cognitive impairment, while in these deprived animals during the ageing process individual differences in cognitive performance are amplified. These distinct early life programming effects may be related to genetic background or to differences in mother–pup interaction.

Genetic influences are likely. Due to early life experiences particular genes may be turned on, never to be switched off. Moreover, genetic influences may modify the susceptibility for the effects of early adversities. For instance, strains of rats have been bred for high and low propensity to respond to (uncontrollable) aversive stimuli with so-called learned helplessness behaviour (Henn & Edwards, 1994). The effect of the same early life adversity on adult responsivity of the HPA axis was profoundly different in the two strains and also different from that in wild type rats (King & Edwards, 1999). A further example for the implication of genes is a recent study in 5-HT$_{1A}$ receptor knock-out mice. Disruption of the 5-HT$_{1A}$ receptor gene in early postnatal life produced a more anxious mouse, an effect not observed when mutagenesis was postponed until adulthood (Gross et al., 2002). The reverse effects of a 'caring environment' strengthens this conclusion.

In conclusion, then, in animals, rearing experiences may permanently alter behavioural and endocrine stress responses. Early adversity can lead to an anxious animal, more prone to develop depression-like behaviour if stressed, particularly so if the animal is genetically 'primed'. The mutual associations between early life stress, persistent overproduction of CRH, and anxiety-like behaviour speak in favour of a pathogenic role of CRH overdrive in disorders with disturbed anxiety and/or mood regulation.

Are these data obtained in animals valid in humans too? This question will be discussed in Section 8.4.5.

8.4.5 The behavioural effects of early life stress in humans

As was discussed in the previous section, animal studies indicate that disrupted parenting produces a persistent, deleterious biobehavioural impact on offspring (Newport et al., 2002). The same seems to be true for humans.

Table 8.8. Traumatizing events and situations that increase the risk of depression in adulthood.

Permanent parental separation (particularly in children < 9 years).
Child maltreatment
Poor parenting

Behavioural effects of childhood adversity

The possible relationship between childhood adversity and depression in later life has been studied for almost 100 years. A major impetus has been Freud's (1957) paper *Mourning and Melancholia* suggesting that early loss of a parent rendered an individual vulnerable to developing depression in later life, particularly after loss experiences. Later, attachment theorists hypothesized an innate pattern of attachment behaviours, the disruption of which would predispose someone to, amongst others, depression (Bowlby, 1961).

The older literature permits no firm conclusions, because of design problems (Agid *et al.*, 2000). Most studies were not well controlled; depression was ill-defined; type of loss (separation, divorce, death), duration of loss and age at loss varied greatly and the impact of quality of parenting pre-loss, and quality of parenting by foster parents post-loss, seldom taken into account. Agid *et al.* (1999) drew attention to the peculiar fact that two reviews both appearing in 1980 and both reviewing the literature on parental death and adult depression, reached opposite conclusions. Lloyd considered the data supportive of such an association; Crook and Eliot, on the other hand, concluded that the data were unconvincing.

More recent studies have avoided many of those pitfalls (Table 8.8). Type of parental loss and point of time whereupon it occurred were specified and DSM-based diagnostic criteria employed. Groups of depressed patients were compared as to rate of early parental loss with a control group matched with the patient group on as many variables as possible (Roy, 1985; Faravelli *et al.*, 1986; Harris *et al.*, 1986). Apart from clinical samples, i.e. samples drawn from a population of depressed patients in treatment, community (epidemiologic) samples have been studied in which the rate of early parental loss was determined in those qualifying for a diagnosis of depression and compared with those who did not, or vice versa in which the rate of depression was determined in those reporting early parental loss and compared with those who did not (Bifulco *et al.*, 1987; Hallstrom, 1987).

A relation between adult depression and early parental death is still somewhat controversial (Tennant, 1988; Kendler *et al.*, 1992); a relationship with (permanent) separation, however, is well established (Roy, 1985; Bifulco *et al.*, 1987; Kendler *et al.*, 1992). One of the best and largest studies on the subject (Agid *et al.*, 1999) studied 136 patients with major depression, 107 with bipolar disorder, 160 with schizophrenia and 170 normal controls. The patients were matched one to one to controls. The rates of early parental loss before the age of 17 in these groups were 29.1%, 17.7%, 22.4% and 7.6–7.9% respectively. The effect of loss through permanent separation was much more marked than that of early parental death, and the effect of early parental loss more pronounced in children under 9 years of age than in older ones and in adolescents. The nonspecificity of the early loss effects with regard to associated psychiatric disorder is remarkable, and has also been reported by other authors (Kendler et al., 1992).

It remains to be determined whether the impact of separation is a direct one, or mediated through pre-existing marital discord that so often precedes separation, or by poor parenting afterwards. Another possibility is proposed by Kendler et al. (1992), who suggested that the association of parental loss and depression may in part or entirely be determined by genetic factors that predispose to poor marital adjustment and/or poor health in the parental generation.

The impact of childhood adversity, other than parental loss, on the risk of adult depression has also been the subject of many studies. *Child maltreatment* has received most attention. Maltreatment is defined as intentional harm or a threat of harm to a child by someone acting in the role of caretaker, and is commonly divided into four categories, i.e. physical abuse, sexual abuse, emotional abuse and neglect (Wissow, 1995). Emotional abuse is defined as 'coercive, demeaning, or overly distant behaviour by a parent or other caretaker' and neglect as 'failure of a caretaker to provide shelter, supervision, medical care or support' (Wissow, 1995). More often than not various forms of child maltreatment occur combined and hand-in-hand with other manifestations of family disruption, such as alcoholism, spouse battering and violence between siblings (McKibben et al., 1989).

Of the many forms of child maltreatment *sexual abuse* received most attention. Both community studies and studies using subjects from clinical settings reported a relationship between sexual abuse in childhood and depression in later life (Weiss et al., 1999). This seems particularly true for atypical depression (Levitan et al., 1998) and the association is most pronounced in women. One has to take into account, however, that sexual abuse of boys is probably less common than that of girls and certainly less studied. The more severe the abuse is, the longer its duration and the greater its frequency, the more pronounced the relationship with adult depression is (Bifulco et al., 1991). Physically or sexually abused women also show increased rates of medical utilization for physical problems in adulthood (Newman et al., 2000). Childhood sexual abuse was shown to increase the risk of a variety of psychopathological states in later life, independent of unfavourable family background, which appeared to be a risk factor for later psychopathology in its own right (Nelson et al., 2002).

Just as in animals, positive relationships will buffer the adverse effects of early abuse in humans (Kaufman & Heinrich, 2000). Genetic factors, too, modify the impact of postnatal stress. For instance, individuals with high genetic risk for depression are at increased risk of developing depression following adverse events (Kendler *et al.*, 1995).

Though the relation between childhood maltreatment and the risk of depression later in life seems well established, several questions remain unanswered.

1 As was stated above, maltreatment of a child often occurs in several modes. Which is the decisive one in terms of adult depression? Is it physical or sexual abuse as such or poor parenting? Poor parenting, in its various manifestations, has been demonstrated to be a risk factor for later depression (Yama *et al.*, 1993) and other forms of psychopathology (Enns *et al.*, 2002). According to Dinwiddie *et al.* (2000) the association between childhood sexual abuse and psychopathology arises at least in part (Hill *et al.*, 2000) or even for the most part (Rind *et al.*, 1998), through the influence of shared familial factors, such as poor parental care increasing both risk of victimization and risk of psychopathology. Rightly, they remark that failure to take this into account may lead to an overly simplistic view on the aetiology of psychiatric illness as well as minimizing the role of less dramatic but highly significant environmental risk factors. On the other hand some evidence indicates that the relation between childhood sexual abuse and adult depression persists after controlling for other forms of maltreatment (Weiss *et al.*, 1999). Obviously the precise relation between poor parenting, child abuse and adult depression is yet to be established.

2 Most studies are retrospective in nature and thus liable to recall bias.

3 The manner in which data were collected varies from face-to-face interviews to questionnaires and telephone surveys, raising questions about the reliability of some of the data.

4 Many studies include both cases of actual physical contact and sexual experiences without bodily contact (such as watching sexual activity and exposure to exhibitionists), though the former seem to be much more damaging than the latter. Furthermore, the degree of coercion and force used by the perpetrator is often unclear and actually hard to judge reliably in retrospect. The youngster is often a priori considered to be the will-less victim. The possibility that the victim, particularly the adolescent one, may have been provocative or at least nonresistant is mostly ignored, though this variable might well impact on the ultimate damage inflicted. Fleming's (1997) observations that only 7% of victims of childhood sexual abuse report the use of physical force by the perpetrator while 64% reported verbal coercion, hints that this might be a relevant factor, worthy of study.

In general, studies on negative childhood experiences and adult psychopathology tend to disregard the notion that destructive parental behaviour might have been provoked by personality disturbances and behavioural problems on the part of the child.

5 The long-term effects of sexual abuse are nonspecific. Depression vulnerability may be increased, but likewise that of other forms of psychopathology, including anxiety disorders, somatization disorder, PTSD and substance abuse (McCauley et al., 1997). Moreover sexual abuse in childhood is correlated with increased probability of a variety of psychosocial problems later in life, such as instability of marital relationships, greater incidence of divorce, violent behaviours, greater risk of victimization (e.g. by rape), and greater risk of sexual dysfunction (Bifulco et al., 1991). This is true for girls, and, to the extent it has been studied, for boys as well (King et al., 2002).

In addition, childhood sexual abuse is correlated with the development of a variety of personality deviations, such as low self-esteem, interpersonal sensitivity, suicide-proneness, antisocial behaviour and borderline symptoms (Johnson et al., 1999). It remains unclear whether the impact of early sexual abuse on the risk of depression in adulthood is a direct one or one mediated via personality damage.

6 As has been stated above, early sexual abuse is by no means unique in its potential to increase the risk of psychopathology and interpersonal difficulties in adult life. Other forms of maltreatment in childhood and maladaptive parenting possess similar potential (Kessler et al., 1997; Johnson et al., 1999; Sadowski et al., 1999). Johnson et al. (2001) showed that maladaptive parental behaviour is associated with increased risk for the development of psychiatric disorders among the offspring of parents with and without psychiatric disorders. Suicide risk is considerably increased (Johnson et al., 2002). Little, if any specificity exists regarding the consequences of the various types of adverse experiences (Heim & Nemeroff, 1999).

7 A family history of depression, prior history of depression, certain personality traits, female gender, alcohol and drug abuse, likewise predispose to depression. Childhood adversity is one risk factor out of many.

Though many questions still remain open, one may conclude that maltreatment during childhood is a risk factor for depression. Does it also lead to (lasting) dysfunctions in the HPA axis, as it does in animals?

Childhood adversity and dysfunction of the HPA axis

Can childhood maltreatment lead to permanent dysfunction of the HPA axis? Pertinent data are scarce and not unequivocal. De Bellis et al. (1999a) studied prepubertal children 10 years of age on the average, who had experienced maltreatment, mostly sexual abuse at an average age of 4.7 ± 3 years, and with an average duration of 2.4 ± 1.8 years before disclosure. All of them suffered from PTSD and almost all showed additional psychopathology, such as various forms of depression and attention deficit disorder. The maltreated children were compared with nontraumatized children with over-anxious disorders and with healthy controls.

Renal excretion of both free cortisol and catecholamines in the traumatized group was increased as compared with the control groups and both excretion values were positively correlated with duration of the traumatizing situation and severity of the PTSD symptoms. Traumatized children without PTSD were not studied.

These data fit in well with the animal data indicating that early maltreatment may lead to hyper-responsiveness of the HPA axis. The few human data derived from adults traumatized in childhood, however, are puzzling. Both increased and decreased levels of plasma and urinary cortisol have been reported (Lemieux & Coe, 1995; Resnick *et al.*, 1995). Stein *et al.* (1997b) studied plasma cortisol responsivity to dexamethasone and lymphocyte GR density in adult survivors of childhood sexual abuse. The suppression of cortisol by dexamethasone was significantly enhanced as compared with that of women who reported no history of abuse. Significant GR density differences were not detected. A majority of the victimized women met criteria for PTSD and almost all suffered from additional psychiatric disorders as well, most commonly from various forms of depression and dissociative disorders. It is therefore hard to deduce from these data whether the enhanced cortisol suppression is related to childhood traumatization as such or more to PTSD or any of the other psychiatric disorders.

Nondepressed women abused in childhood exhibited a greater than usual ACTH-response to CRH, and blunted cortisol response to ACTH, as compared with abused and nonabused women suffering from major depression. Baseline plasma cortisol was also lowered (Heim *et al.*, 2001). According to the authors these data suggest sensitization of the anterior pituitary and counter-regulative adaptation of the adrenal cortex in the first mentioned group. Though the women in this group were not depressed, PTSD was a confounding factor. Adult women with a history of childhood abuse also showed sensitization of the stress response (plasma ACTH and cortisol) to a standardized psychosocial laboratory stressor. Sensitization was particularly robust in patients with symptoms of depression and PTSD (Heim *et al.*, 2000, 2001).

A recent study by Rinne *et al.* (2002, 2003) demonstrated that chronically abused borderline patients had a significantly enhanced ACTH and cortisol response to a DEX/CRH challenge as compared with nonabused subjects. This is probably due to the enhanced central drive towards pituitary ACTH release. Sustained childhood abuse rather than borderline pathology, major depression or PTSD seemed to account for this effect. Comorbid PTSD attenuated the ACTH response to the DEX/CRH test, probably due to an enhanced efficacy of dexamethasone in the suppression of pituitary ACTH release (Rinne *et al.*, 2002). A 6- and 12-week

Table 8.9. Neuroendocrine 'fingerprint' of patients with PTSD.

CRH overdrive	Hypocortisolism
↑ CSF CRH	↓ 24-hour urinary cortisol excretion
	↓ Morning plasma cortisol
	↑ Suppression of plasma cortisol by dexamethasone
	↑ Density of GRs on lymphocytes

treatment with fluvoxamine normalized the outcome of the DEX/CRH test in the borderline patients depending on a history of childhood abuse (Rinne *et al.*, 2003).

Though the available data suggest that early adversity may derange functioning of the HPA axis, one cannot conclude that hypersensitivity is the invariable outcome. PTSD is a possibly confounding variable.

Posttraumatic stress disorder

The possible role of the PTSD syndrome in the occurrence of CRH/HPA axis disturbances that might follow early traumatization is intriguing (National Research Council, 1993). PTSD is a stress-induced syndrome, that shows a peculiar neuroendocrine 'fingerprint', different from that found in certain types of depression and in states of unmanageable stress. The PTSD syndrome is characterized by sustained arousal and inability to put traumatic experiences to the past. Memories of traumatic events are repeatedly relived. The intrusive memories occur spontaneously or, more frequently, triggered by stimuli related to the orginal event. Patients are furthermore irritable, hypervigilant, complain of disturbed sleep, emotional numbing and inability to experience pleasure. Startle responses are abnormally strong and so are psychophysiological reactions to trauma-related stimuli (e.g. increases in heart rate and blood pressure). Challenged with mCPP, a $5\text{-}HT_{2c}$ receptor agonist or with yohimbine – a blocker of inhibitory presynaptic, $alpha_2$-adrenergic autoreceptors – many PTSD patients exhibit signs of physiological arousal, and they may also experience anxiety, panic attacks and activation of PTSD symptoms (Southwick & Yehuda, 1993; Van Praag, in press).

PTSD rarely appears alone, but most commonly in association with a host of other psychopathological syndromes and phenomena, such as depression, impulsivity, affective lability and aggression against oneself and others (Van der Kolk *et al.*, 1996).

The neuroendocrine 'fingerprint' of PTSD patients is a peculiar mixture of hypocortisolism and CRH overdrive (Table 8.9). CSF levels of CRH are increased. Yet the 24-hour urinary cortisol excretion is decreased, morning cortisol lowered and suppression of plasma cortisol levels in response to dexamethasone is greater than normal (Yehuda *et al.*, 1990, 1991, 1993, 1995b). Even if morning cortisol is normal, a negative correlation has been established between cortisol level and severity of PTSD symptoms (Yehuda *et al.*, 1996). The cortisol response in the immediate aftermath of the trauma also is low in those who will develop PTSD (Resnick *et al.*, 1995; Yehuda *et al.*, 1998), indicating that hypocortisolism is not a consequence of exhaustion of the HPA axis. It has been hypothesized that enhanced negative feedback regulation of cortisol is a characteristic feature of the pathophysiology of PTSD, and indeed the density of GRs on lymphocytes was found to be increased (Yehuda *et al.*, 1991). It is unknown whether this is a primary phenomenon or one secondary to low levels of circulatory cortisol. It is however hard to explain that CRH release, notwithstanding increased GR density, remains high, at least if GR upregulation would occur throughout the body.

Somatostatin (somatotrophin release-inhibiting factor) inhibits HPA axis activity. Its CSF concentration is elevated in PTSD and reduced in depression (Stout *et al.*, 1995), possibly explaining the HPA axis differences in both conditions.

Urinary NA excretion as well as plasma NA levels are generally elevated in patients with PTSD, and the alpha$_2$-adrenergic receptor density on platelets is decreased (Perry *et al.*, 1987), indicating activation of the NA ergic system. This is usually the case in states of increased arousal.

The data from De Bellis *et al.* (1999b) described above, indicate that CRH overdrive combined with signs of peripheral hypocortisolism, is not a universal sign of PTSD. The specificity of the endocrine 'fingerprint' of PTSD, moreover, has still to be analysed. Hypocortisolism, as such, is not not typical for PTSD. Lowered morning plasma levels of cortisol have also been reported in antisocial males with histories of repeated physical violence (Woodman *et al.*, 1978; Dolan *et al.*, 2001) and in boys and girls with antisocial behaviour (McBurnett *et al.*, 2000; Pajer *et al.*, 2001). Criminals referred to a maximum-security hospital showed little plasma cortisol elevations in response to experimental stressors (Woodman *et al.*, 1978). Low salivary cortisol was found to be associated with persistent aggression in boys referred for disruptive behaviour (McBurnett *et al.*, 2000). Lowered urinary free cortisol has also been reported in chronic fatigue syndrome and in depression with a chronic course (Cleare *et al.*, 2001; Oldehinkel *et al.*, 2001). In pregnant adolescents low plasma CRH was found to be related to greater number of depressive symptoms and more signs of conduct disorder (Susman *et al.*, 1999).

Besides that, it remains an open question why the psychopathology and biology of PTSD differ from that usually seen after traumatic experiences. Current opinion holds that severity of the stressor is responsible. PTSD is considered to be the result of 'an extreme traumatic stressor, involving actual or threatened death or serious injury, or other threat to one's physical integrity, or witnessing an event of that nature, leading to a subjective response of fear, helplessness or horror' (DSM–IV). Stressful events would be less severe and dramatic than traumata and, while the effects of trauma would be indelible, those of stressful events would often be alleviated after removal of the stressor (Yehuda, 2000).

The distinction between stressful event and trauma, seems more semantic/theoretical than practical/clinical in nature. The impact of injury on one's physical integrity is unduly accentuated. Psychological onslaughts can be at least as traumatic and damaging. Psychic devastation is no less unbearable than physical horror. Sudden death of a partner, sudden dismissal from a job, discriminatory experiences, for instance, can be upsetting, leading to as much despair and feelings of helplessness as threats in the bodily sphere may do. Removing a stressful event or its consequences (for instance by remarrying or finding a new job) may be feasible, but it would be light-hearted to assume that with that the impact of the blow would have been effaced. Memories may linger on for long if not for ever.

More cogent than to differentiate between trauma and stressful event, is to assume that the response to adversity – trauma or stressful event – apparently may vary substantially, dependent as it is on the ability of a personality to cope appropriately and on the robustness of the biological stress-absorbing systems. For instance the endocrine 'fingerprint' associated with PTSD may be related to high density of GRs in certain regions, in existence preceding trauma exposure. Individual differences in the number and functional activity of GRs have indeed been demonstrated (Yehuda *et al.*, 1993, 1995a,b).

Assuming a continuum between trauma and stressful life event, and taking heterogeneity of stress responses as a starting point, seems to be a more logical approach to the study of stress-conditioned disorders than introducing artificial cut-offs between 'stressful event' and 'trauma', and to delineate a variety of discrete, stress-related disorders each understood as a free-standing category. Data derived from animal studies support this viewpoint. In the same species different coping styles have been observed. A coping style is defined as 'a coherent set of behavioural and physiological stress responses which is consistent over time and characteristic to a certain group of individuals' (Koolhaas *et al.*, 1999). Different coping styles probably make the animals vulnerable to different types of disease (see also Section 8.2.5).

Childhood adversity and structural changes in the brain

In animals, stress and in particular inescapable stress, as well as exogenous administration of glucocorticoids, ultimately leads to functional and structural neuronal disturbances up to neuronal death (Sapolsky *et al.*, 1990; Woolley *et al.*, 1990; De Kloet *et al.*, 1997). The hippocampus is particularly vulnerable. Hippocampal dysfunction is thought to be responsible for the cognitive defects observed in conditions in which corticosteroid levels are increased, such as Cushing's disease and mood disorders (Wolkowitz *et al.*, 1990) (see Section 8.4.3).

In humans decreased hippocampal volume has been observed in combat-related PTSD (Bremner *et al.*, 1995; Gurvits *et al.*, 1996); in female survivors of sexual abuse with PTSD (Bremner *et al.*, 1997b; Stein *et al.*, 1997a); in women maltreated in childhood with borderline personality disorder, about half of the sample suffering also from PTSD (Driessen *et al.*, 2000); in patients with severe, drug-resistant major depression (Mervaala *et al.*, 2000); in women with major depression who had a history of severe and prolonged physical and/or sexual abuse in childhood (Vythilingam *et al.*, 2002); and in patients with a history of major depression but currently in remission (Sheline *et al.*, 1996). The degree of hippocampal volume reduction correlates negatively with total duration of major depression and number of hospitalizations (Axelson *et al.*, 1993; Sheline *et al.*, 1996). In maltreated children and adolescents with PTSD reduction of intracranial and cerebral volumes has been observed, but not the predicted decrease in hippocampal volume (De Bellis *et al.*, 1999b). It has been hypothesized, though not been proven, that the hippocampal damage is caused by hypercortisolaemia, due to long-lasting stress. If hypercortisolism is indeed in a major way involved in hippocampal atrophy, it is curious to find hippocampal damage also in PTSD, a condition for which hypocortisolism is considered to be typical.

A relation between hippocampal atrophy and depression has not been confirmed by all authors (Vakili *et al.*, 2000). A recent postmortem study by Lucassen *et al.* (2001) failed to find evidence for hippocampal atrophy in major depression, though in some other brain structures apoptosis was demonstrable. The status of the HPA axis before death, however, was not known nor was the possible use of antidepressants.

In summary, then, in humans early adversity may lead to increased vulnerability for a variety of psychiatric disorders later in life. Depression is one of them. Damage to certain brain structures, particularly in the hippocampus, has been demonstrated in people with early traumatization. It has not been excluded, however, that hippocampal abnormalities precede the traumatic experiences, constituting, possibly, vulnerability factors for stress-related disorders.

The role of PTSD is unclear. Is this the mediating syndrome between early adversity and adult psychic vulnerability, or do PTSD and later mental vulnerability share a common origin? HPA axis hyperactivity has not been unequivocably linked to early adversity. Also, in this case PTSD confounds matters, because this condition supposedly is characterized by CRH overactivity and hypocortisolaemia, though this seems not to be an obligatory finding. De Bellis *et al.* (1999b) showed that PTSD may also be accompanied by hypercortisolism, at least in children.

Clearly, the available data do not permit a definitive conclusion as to the possible effects of early adversity on the development of the biological stressor-processing systems in humans.

8.4.6 Cortisol and the functioning of monoaminergic systems

In Chapter 7 the extensive evidence was discussed indicating involvement of MA ergic systems in the pathophysiology (of certain components) of the depressive syndrome. In this chapter the question is discussed whether the overproduction of CRH demonstrable in a subgroup of depression, is a potential pathogenic factor, or rather a derivative phenomenon. The former possibility would gain in probability if CRH or cortisol were to interfere with MA ergic functioning in a way that would lead to disturbances as ascertained in (certain types of) depression.

HPA axis and serotonin

5-HT is among the neurotransmitters that act as excitatory mediators of CRH and AVP release, supposedly acting via 5-HT_{1A}, 5-HT_{2A} and 5-HT_{2C} receptors (Calogero et al., 1993). 5-HT ergic nerve terminals have been demonstrated on CRH-producing neurons in the PVN. ACTH release is enhanced by CRH as well as by several neurotransmitter systems, among which is the 5-HT ergic system (Owens et al., 1990). 5-HT seems to be involved in ACTH release induced by some (e.g. restraint stress) but not all (e.g. cold swim-stress) stressors. Apparently 5-HT responses are stressor-specific (Jorgensen et al., 1998).

In humans, more or less selective 5-HT_{1A} agonists, such as ipsapirone and bus-pirone and the 5-HT_{2C} agonist mCPP, bring about a rise in plasma cortisol (Kahn & Van Praag, 1988; Lesch et al., 1990). In animals, reduction of hippocampal 5-HT reduces the number of GRs and MRs and attenuates feedback inhibition of the HPA axis by cortisol (Seckl & Fink, 1991). Tryptophan administration for 1–2 weeks to depressed DST nonsuppressors diminishes the nonsuppression, indicating that increased 5-HT availability augments cortisol-induced feedback inhibition in humans too (Nuller & Ostroumova, 1980).

Conversely, increased plasma cortisol or increased stress influences the 5-HT system profoundly (Table 8.10). Initially, it leads to a rise in CNS 5-HT turnover by increasing tryptophan availability and stimulation of tryptophan hydroxylase activity (De Kloet et al., 1982, 1983; Chaouloff, 1993; Davis et al., 1995). Sustained stress or sustained increase of plasma cortisol, however, is accompanied by diminution of 5-HT turnover (Weiss et al., 1981) and reduced 5-HT release in all areas studied, possibly due in part to activation of liver tryptophan pyrrolase activity by cortisol and increased shunting of tryptophan into the kynurenine-nicotinamide pathway (Maes et al., 1990). Accordingly an inverse relation has been found between plasma corticosterone level and 5-HT turnover in the CNS (De Souza & van Loon, 1986),

Table 8.10. CRH /cortisol – 5-HT interactions.

5-HT overdrive	Sustained CRH/cortisol overdrive
↑ CRH release	↓ 5-HT turnover
↑ Cortisol release	↓ Activity of 5-HT ergic neurons
	↓ Expression of 5-HT$_{1A}$ receptors
	↓ 5-HT$_{1A}$ receptor binding
	↑ 5-HT$_2$ receptor binding

while in depressives hypercortisolaemia and prolactin response to l-tryptophan were found to be inversely correlated (Deakin *et al.*, 1990).

5-HT neurons in the dorsal raphe nuclei are innervated by CRH and express CRH receptors. CRH administered directly in the cerebral ventricles in low doses increase, and in higher doses decrease, 5-HT release. Neuronal activity in those neurons, however, was inhibited both at low and high CRH doses (Price *et al.*, 1998).

Just like the turnover of 5-HT, the 5-HT$_{1A}$ receptor responds biphasically to sustained stress and increased cortisol levels, initially with increased and later with decreased receptor response (Joëls & de Kloet, 1992; Watanabe *et al.*, 1993; Young *et al.*, 1994; Karten *et al.*, 1999) and diminished expression of 5-HT$_{1a}$ receptor mRNA (Meijer & De Kloet, 1994, 1998; Fernandes *et al.*, 1997) (Figure 8.16). Offspring of rats, who during lactation received drinking water with corticosterone, showed in adulthood decreased 5-HT$_{1A}$ receptor binding in the hippocampus (Meerlo *et al.*, 2001). Rats raised in overcrowded conditions were more anxious than controls, while numbers of 5-HT$_{1A}$ receptors in the hippocampus and binding capacity to the ligand were significantly decreased (Daniels *et al.*, 2000). Apparently, hippocampal 5-HT$_{1A}$ receptor function is, during conditions of chronic stress, under inhibitory control of cortisol. This effect is predominantly mediated by MRs (Meijer & De Kloet, 1995), to a lesser extent by GRs (Chaouloff, 1995) on the level of the 5HT$_{1A}$ receptor gene and the coupling to G proteins.

Acute stress leads to desensitization of 5-HT$_2$ receptors (Yamada *et al.*, 1995). Under conditions of chronic stress 5-HT$_2$ receptor binding is increased (Kuroda *et al.*, 1992; Fernandes *et al.*, 1997). In subordinate (i.e. chronically stressed) rats, 5-HT$_{1A}$ binding throughout the entire hippocampus was decreased, while 5-HT$_2$ binding in layer IV of the parietal cortex was increased (McKittrick *et al.*, 1995). It is unknown whether the effect of cortisol on 5-HT$_2$ receptors is a direct one or is mediated via downregulation of 5-HT$_{1A}$ receptors. The latter process generally leads to upregulation of 5-HT$_2$ receptors, particularly the 5-HT$_{2A}$ receptor (Takao *et al.*, 1997; Rënyi *et al.*, 2001). Additionally, decrease in hippocampal 5-HT binding

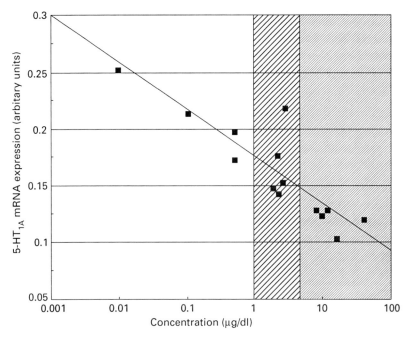

Figure 8.16. Adrenalectomized rats were treated with low, high, very high doses or no corticosterone replacement. The relationship between plasma corticosterone levels and 5-HT$_{1A}$ expression measured in the dentate gyrus is depicted. Hormone levels are on a logarithmic scale. $R^2 =$ 0.86 (after Meijer & De Kloet, 1994).
□: No corticosterone, ▨: low corticosterone, ▨: (very) high corticosterone.

to the 5-HT transporter has been reported under the influence of chronic stress (Maines et al., 1999).

Learned helplessness, a condition induced by exposure of an animal to inescapable stress, is associated with a decrease of 5-HT release in the frontal cortex (Petty et al., 1992). The level of presynaptic 5-HT$_{1B}$ receptor mRNA in the dorsal raphe nucleus is increased (Neumaier et al., 1997), with no 5-HT$_{1B}$ receptor changes in the postsynaptic membrane. The presynaptic 5-HT$_{1B}$ receptor is an autoreceptor, the stimulation of which leads to decrease in 5-HT release. Its over-expression will lead to a decrease in 5-HT ergic transmission.

Stimulation of 5-HT innervation from the median raphe to the hippocampus facilitates, via 5-HT$_{1A}$ receptors, the disconnection of previously learned associations between aversive stimuli and anxiety reactions. It would allow normal behaviours to gradually re-emerge, despite the persistence or repetition of noxious events. This mechanism would thus promote resilience through dissociation (Deakin, 1996). Downregulation of this system, too, would contribute to heightened anxiety and impaired adaptation to stressors and stress.

Dorsal raphe neurons projecting to the hippocampus and amygdala are believed to exert anxiogenic effects via 5-HT$_2$ receptors. Upregulation of the 5-HT$_2$ system would therefore contribute to heightened anxiety (McEwen, 1995).

Human data correspond with those found in animals. Several observations indicate that cortisol hypersecretion is associated with a decrease in tryptophan availability and thus possibly with reduced 5-HT synthesis. Depressed dexamethasone nonsuppressors, for instance, have lower plasma tryptophan levels and lower l-tryptophan/competing amino acid ratios than suppressors suffering from depression (Maes *et al.*, 1990). Moreover, patients with major depression in remission who showed depressive symptoms after tryptophan depletion had significantly higher plasma cortisol levels than subjects that did not respond to tryptophan depletion (Åberg-Wistedt *et al.*, 1998). In normal but stress-prone individuals a carbohydrate-rich, protein-poor diet prevents a deterioration of mood and performance under uncontrollable laboratory stress conditions. Such a diet raises insulin production and insulin sends the so-called competing amino acids into the skeletal muscles with the exception of tryptophan. The ratio tryptophan: competing amino acids increases, thereby augmenting tryptophan influx into the brain. This leads eventually to an increased synthesis of 5-HT (Markus *et al.*, 1998).

The cortisol and prolactin response to d-fenfluramine may be blunted in depression (see Chapter 7). After 1 week of treatment with ketoconazole, an inhibitor of cortisol synthesis, those responses normalized, irrespective of whether the patient did or did not improve (Thakore & Dinan, 1994). This suggests that subsensitivity of 5-HT receptors in depression is secondary to hypercortisolism.

As mentioned, the growth hormone response to l-tryptophan, a response probably mediated via 5-HT$_{1A}$ receptors (Smith *et al.*, 1991), is attenuated by hydrocortisone pretreatment (Porter *et al.*, 1998), confirming that in humans, just as in animals, corticosteroids decrease activity of the 5-HT$_{1A}$ receptor system. Remarkably, dexamethasone, a synthetic glucocorticosteroid, lacks this ability (Porter *et al.*, 1999).

Ketoconazole failed to enhance the neuroendocrine response to the partial and relative selective 5-HT$_{1A}$ receptor agonist ipsapirone (Price *et al.*, 1997). This, however, was a short-term experiment, in which ketoconazole was administered 1 day before the ipsapirone challenge. It is conceivable that more time is needed for 5-HT$_{1A}$ receptor downregulation to occur.

Recent data suggest a relationship between the functionality of the 5-HT transporter gene and strength of the stress response. Individuals with one or two copies of the short allele in the promoter region of this gene, seem to be more stressor-sensitive and more depression-prone than humans with one or two copies of the long allele (see Chapter 7, Section 7.2.5). These observations further demonstrate the inter-dependence of the 5-HT system and the stress response.

Table 8.11. CRH /cortisol – NA interactions.

NA overdrive	CRH overdrive	Hypercortisolaemia
↑ CRH release	↑ Firing rate NA ergic neurons (*initially*)	↓ Activity of CRH neurons in PVN (*regulating HPA axis*)
	↓ Firing rate NA ergic neurons (*eventually*)	↓ Activity of NA neurons in LC
		↑ Activity of hypothalamic CRH neurons projecting to LC and amygdala (*regulating anxiety*)

In conclusion, then, by chronic stress or sustained increase of plasma cortisol the 5-HT turnover as well as the responsivity of the 5-HT_{1A} receptor is reduced. Animal data indicate upregulation of the 5-HT_2 receptor system, but the results of human research are ambiguous. Similar 5-HT disturbances have been observed in depression, particularly in a new subtype of depression, named anxiety/aggression-driven depression, to be discussed in Chapter 9.

HPA axis and noradrenaline

The locus coeruleus (LC), located in the dorsal pons, is the main site of NA ergic cell bodies, of which the projections branch out throughout the entire brain. CRH pathways descend from the hypothalamus to the LC, whereas NA ergic fibres ascend to the paraventricular nuclei (PVN) in the hypothalamus (Cunningham *et al.*, 1990). Anatomical conditions, thus, allow for reciprocal relationships between the two systems, which indeed exist (Table 8.11).

CRH, for instance, applied to LC neurons increases their firing rate (Valentino *et al.*, 1983) and NA, in its turn, stimulates the release of CRH (Calogero *et al.*, 1988a,b). Centrally administered CRH antagonists, on the other hand, inhibit the response of the LC to a variety of stimuli, while β-blockers antagonize many of the behavioural effects of CRH applied directly into the brain (Dunn & Berridge, 1990). Both the CRH neurons in the PVN and the NA neurons in the LC are activated by 5-HT and inhibited by glucocorticoids (Calogero *et al.*, 1988a,b, 1989). Behaviourally, both activation of the LC and of the CRH circuitry leads to increased arousal, vigilance and ultimately to anxiety.

Close relationships between NA and corticosteroids have likewise been demonstrated in humans. Wong *et al.* (2000) reported that patients with major depression show elevated levels of CSF NA and plasma cortisol around the clock and that diurnal variations in CSF NA and plasma cortisol were virtually super-imposable. These data confirm the mutually reinforcing bidirectional links between a central hyper-NA ergic state and hyperfunction of particular CRH pathways. The levels of plasma ACTH and CSF CRH, though normal in absolute terms, were high if one takes into account the degree of hypercortisolism. Chrousos & Gold (1992) conclude: 'functionally, the CRH and LC-NE sympathetic systems seem to participate in a positive, reverberatory feedback loop so that activation of one system tends to activate the other as well'. Through stress both systems are activated, but it is hard to disentangle what comes first, but once one is activated, the other follows suit.

Glucocorticoids inhibit the CRH pathways orginating in the PVN, that regulate HPA axis activity. They stimulate, however, the hypothalamic CRH pathways to LC and amygdala (Makino *et al.*, 1994). Hence, the ultimate product of HPA axis activity, i.e. cortisol, contributes in its own right to overactivity of the LC. Moreover, acute stress or an acute rise in glucocorticoids leads to downregulation of presynaptic alpha-2-adrenergic receptors, and a rise in NA-release (Flügge, 1999).

All these data support the view that CRH, produced in excess, leads to hyperactivity of the NA ergic system. On the level of the hippocampus, however, cortisol suppressed NA-coupled adenylcyclase and the NA-induced increase in neuronal excitability (Joëls & De Kloet, 1989). Thus, cortisol has a permissive effect in that it promotes the activity of the PVN-LC system during stress but has a suppressive effect on NA-stimulated targets.

Ultimately, when a stressful situation is sustained, NA synthesis and NA utilization get out of step. Production cannot keep up with expenditure and NA stores get depleted (Anisman *et al.*, 1981; Lechin *et al.*, 1996). In addition, continued overproduction of NA will ultimately lead to downregulation of postsynaptic adrenergic receptor sites, another process detracting from the efficiency of NA ergic transmission. Finally, chronic stress or chronic overproduction of glucocorticoids induce upregulation of presynaptic α_2 adrenergic receptors, decreasing NA-release (Flügge, 1999).

In accordance with these observations it has been demonstrated that administration of l-tyrosine reduces or prevents several manifestations of chronic stress, both in animals (Lehnert *et al.*, 1984) and in humans (Deijen *et al.*, 1999). Tyrosine is the precursor of DA and NA, and enhances NA synthesis (Lehnert *et al.*, 1984).

α_2-Adrenergic receptors are also present at 5-HT ergic nerve endings, decreasing 5-HT release, once activated. Upregulation of these so-called heteroreceptors will diminish 5-HT release and contribute to reduction of 5-HT ergic transmission under conditions of sustained stress (Mongeau *et al.*, 1997).

Excessive activity of NA ergic systems generates feelings of anxiety. Reduced activity of that system leads in animals to behavioural changes such as decreased exploration in a novelty task, decreased appetite and deficits in previously well-learned tasks.

In depression both signs of reduced and increased NA ergic activity have been observed. The former phenomena have been hypothesized to contribute to such symptoms as motor retardation and emotional numbing, the latter to high levels of anxiety. Studies relating signs of NA ergic hypo- or hyperactivity to severity and duration of depression are not available.

In conclusion, sustained stress and hypercortisolaemia induce changes in the NA ergic system comparable with the ones that may be observed in depression.

HPA axis and dopamine

Stress has a major impact on the DA system. Several factors determine what the effects will be. The effects are to a degree *regionally specific*. For instance, in animals the rewarding value of stimulation of the mesocorticolimbic DA system is reduced, but self-stimulation from the nigrostriatal system is not influenced (Zacharko & Anisman, 1991). In the tubero-infundibular DA system stress exerts an inhibitory effect, leading amongst others to a rise in prolactin release. Apparently different DA systems in the brain show differential sensitivity to aversive experiences. *Severity* of the aversive stimulus is a further determinant of stress effects. Restraint stress, for example, enhances DA ergic impulse flow in the frontal cortex and nucleus accumbens, but not in the putamen. If, however, restraint stress is applied in a cold environment, DA ergic transmission in the putamen also gets involved (Imperato *et al.*, 1992).

Duration of stressor exposure is also an important determinant of the resultant changes in the DA system. Short exposure leads to increased DA release, prolonged exposure to decrease below the control level (Puglisi-Allegra *et al.*, 1991, Gambarana *et al.*, 1999). The latter effect is not a result of depletion of DA pools since rats, after the stress experience, are still able to respond to a stressor with increased DA release (Cabib & Puglisi-Allegra, 1996).

Another important factor controlling the DA response to stress, is the *(un)controllability* of the stressor. Mice, for instance, exposed to a series of foot shocks, show an increase in DA release if they have a possibility to interrupt shock delivery, but a decrease if they cannot exert any control (Weiss *et al.*, 1981; Zacharko & Anisman, 1991). Controllable and uncontrollable aversive experiences result in opposite effects, at least in the mesolimbic DA system. If coping is possible, increase in DA release continues as long as the stressful situation lasts. If, however, coping is impossible DA release is inhibited, and behaviourally a condition of motor inhibition, motivational blunting, impaired learning of active avoidance ('learned helplessness'), inhibition of escape attempts and disrupted responding to intra-cranial self-stimulation ensues (Weiss *et al.*, 1981; Garcia-Marquez & Armario, 1987; Cabib & Puglisi-Allegra, 1996).

Stress, thus, exerts a pronounced influence on DA ergic transmission. Much evidence indicates that this effect is in part mediated via increased release of cortisol.

Glucocorticoids stimulate DA ergic transmission. Corticosterone, for instance, activates tyrosine hydroxylase, the rate limiting step of catecholamine synthesis (Meyer, 1985). In rats dexamethasone as well as corticosterone enhances DA activity in the brain (Wolkowitz *et al.*, 1986), whereas in humans dexamethasone increases plasma levels of DA and its major degradation product homovanillic acid (Rothchild *et al.*, 1984; Wolkowitz *et al.*, 1985). Corticosterone, moreover, increases extracellular DA concentrations. Three mechanisms are presumably involved (Piazza *et al.*, 1996). First, increased firing of DA neurons; second, inhibition of DA degradation; third decrease of DA reuptake. Piazza *et al.* (1996) have characterized glucocorticoids as endogenous psychostimulants. Both types of substances, glucocorticoids and psychostimulants, increase extracellular DA concentrations, presumably by inhibiting monoamine oxidase and by reuptake inhibition. Both induce self-administration and enhance locomotor activity, whereas, finally, glucocorticoids facilitate self-administration of stimulants (Lindley *et al.*, 1999).

Several authors, however, have been unable to confirm a stimulating effect of glucocorticoids on mesotelencephalic DA neuronal firing (Imperato *et al.*, 1991; Lindley *et al.*, 1999). A possible explanation is that the stimulating effects of glucocorticoids seem to be contingent on behavioural activation and/or activation of DA neurons (Cabib & Puglisi-Allegra, 1996). They are, for instance, demonstrable in the dark phase, during eating and in high-responder rats, but absent in the light phase and in low-responder rats. Furthermore, glucocorticoids modify the membrane potential of hippocampal CA 1 cells in slice preparations when neurons are in a depolarized state, but they have no effects if the cells are in resting condition (Joëls & De Kloet, 1992). These findings could explain that some studies failed to find stimulatory effects of glucocorticoids on DA ergic transmission.

The factors responsible for the decrease of DA ergic activity after sustained stress are uncertain, but it is conceivable that, due to over-utilization of DA, DA synthesis rate fails to keep pace.

In depression reduction of DA metabolism may occur. Hypoactivity of the nigrostriatal and mesolimbic DA systems have been implicated in the pathophysiology of motor retardation and anhedonia respectively.

In conclusion, acute stress enhances, sustained (uncontrollable) stress ultimately attenuates DA ergic activity. Signs of DA ergic deficiency may also occur in depression.

Conclusions

The question discussed in this section was if (sustained) stress causes changes in the central MA ergic systems comparable with those that may be found in depression. The question can be answered in the affirmative. Decreased 5-HT metabolism, downregulated 5-HT$_{1A}$ receptor activity and upregulation of the 5-HT$_{2c}$ receptor system; findings that suggest both hyper- and hypoactivity of the NA ergic system and reduction of DA ergic activity are signs that are found both in the stressed condition and in some forms of depression (Chapter 7). This is a strong argument in favour of the hypothesis that stress may act as a pathogenetic (causative) factor in (subtypes of) depression.

8.4.7 Glucocorticoids and antidepressant action

If CRH overdrive and hypercortisolaemia would indeed play a role in the pathophysiology of depression or some of its components, one would expect suppression of CRH or cortisol activity to exert antidepressant effects. Indeed, antidepressants, at least some groups of antidepressants (see Section 8.4.2) as well as lithium and electroconvulsive treatment have the ability to increase GR mRNA, to enlarge in this manner the density of GRs on the pituitary and the hypothalamic PVN and thus to strengthen the cortisol-mediated negative feedback loop (Seckl & Fink, 1992; Reul *et al.*, 1993). MRs are likewise upregulated by tricyclic antidepressants (Seckl & Fink, 1992; Reul *et al.*, 1993). Activation of both GRs and MRs would result in downregulation of HPA axis activity. Recent research has focused on the development of compounds capable to decrease CRH and cortisol production or to block the receptors it acts on.

Inhibitors of steroid synthesis will lower raised cortisol levels. Ketoconazole has been used for this purpose, so far particularly in patients resistant to conventional antidepressants (Ravaris *et al.*, 1988; Wolkowitz *et al.*, 1999b), and in addition metyrapone and amino-glutethimide (Murphy *et al.*, 1991; Ghadirian *et al.*, 1995). Metyrapone inhibits the enzyme 11-hydroxylase resulting in decreased cortisol production and accumulation of 11-deoxycortisol; amino-glutethimide blocks the conversion of cholesterol to pregnenolone and ketoconazole inhibits steroid genesis in the same way (Price *et al.*, 1996) (Table 8.12).

Though the number of controlled observations is still small, most investigators report encouraging results, particularly in patients with hypercortisolaemia (Wolkowitz & Reus, 1999). Recently however Malison *et al.* (1999) published a negative study with ketoconazole in treatment-refractory patients with major depression. Diminution of cortisol production is, so it would seem, a double-edged sword. On the one hand it is expected to eliminate the noxious effects of excess cortisol, on the other hand it would weaken the cortisol-mediated brake on CRH production, a hormone supposed to play a key role in the pathogenesis of (certain types of) depression. However, Patchev *et al.* (1994) demonstrated that the latter probably does not occur, since steroid synthesis inhibitors do increase the pool of neuroactive steroids and some of those suppress CRH expression. Compensatory mechanisms, however, tend to return cortisol levels back to pretreatment levels in many patients (Price *et al.*, 1996), raising doubts on the usefulness of this treatment strategy.

Dehydroepiandrosterone (DHEA) and its sulphated metabolite (DHEA-S), are steroids secreted by the adrenal cortex, synchronously with cortisol. Both steroids

Table 8.12. Major pathways of adrenal steroidogenesis affected by cortisol synthesis inhibitors (Price *et al.*, 1996).

	Mineralocorticoid	Glucocorticoid	Androgen
Cholesterol → (1)	Pregnenolone → (2) ↓	17-OH-pregnenolone → (3) ↓	Dehydroepiandrosterone ↓
	Progesterone → (2) ↓	17-OH-progesterone → (3) ↓	Androstenedione ↓
	11-Deoxycorticosterone ↓	11-Deoxycortisol ↓ (4)	Testosterone
	Corticosterone ↓	Cortisol	
	18-OH-Corticosterone ↓		
	Aldosterone		

1 = cholesterol side chain cleavage; 2 = 17-hydroxylase; 3 = 17, 20-hydroxylase; 4 = 11-hydroxylase.

can also be synthesized de novo in the CNS. They possess *antiglucocorticoid properties*. Plasma levels of DHEA (S) as well as the ratio DHEA (S) to cortisol were found to be decreased in depression (Barrett-Connor *et al.*, 1999). Others failed to confirm these findings (Osran *et al.*, 1993) and increased plasma levels have also been reported (Heuser *et al.*, 1998). Some preliminary data suggest that DHEA might have antidepressant potential (Reus *et al.*, 1997; Wolkowitz *et al.*, 1999a). The available data base however is not sufficient for even an interim conclusion.

Another approach to normalize cortisol levels has been the application of *type 1 CRH receptor antagonists*. In animals such compounds reduce a repertoire of behaviours associated with anxiety (Basso *et al.*, 1999; Arborelius *et al.*, 2000; Habib *et al.*, 2000). A recently developed compound of this nature, R 121919, a pyrazolopyrimidine derivative, is now clinically tested and seems to exert anxiolytic and antidepressant effects (Holsboer, 2000; Zobel *et al.*, 2000). It does not suppress stress-induced HPA axis activity, possibly because it leaves type-2 CRH receptors, present at the pituitary, responsive. CRH-1 receptor deficiency, moreover, enhances hippocampal 5-HT ergic transmission (Penalva *et al.*, 2002). This might contribute to antidepressant activity. Several other lipophilic CRH antagonists, capable of penetrating the blood–brain barrier and possessing oral bio-availability are presently in development (Owens & Nemeroff, 1999).

Another strategy proposed to reduce circulating cortisol is *activation of GRs*, thus strengthening the cortisol-mediated negative feedback system. Dexamethasone is used for this purpose because this synthetic glucocorticoid suppressed HPA activity on the level of the pituitary (De Kloet *et al.*, 1975). As a consequence dexamethasone will lower plasma cortisol levels and deplete the brain from excess cortisol. Dexamethasone poorly penetrates the blood–brain barrier, and moreover occupies GR rather than MR. A few controlled, but small studies have been performed (Arana *et al.*, 1995; Bodani *et al.*, 1999; Scott *et al.*, 1999). All reported some antidepressant activity.

Activation of GRs can also be achieved by administering cortisol. In a study by DeBattista *et al.* (2000) a single intravenous administration of 15 mg cortisol produced a rapid improvement in patients with major depression.

Finally, *antagonists of GRs* appear to be a very promising therapy for patients suffering from psychotic depression (McQuade & Young, 2000; Belanoff *et al.*, 2001, 2002). Psychotic depression is a distinct syndrome in which hypercortiso-laemia and escape from the dexamethasone suppression are prominent (Schatzberg *et al.*, 1985). These patients are often resistant to the traditional treatment with antidepressants, but do respond to electroconvulsive therapy. In recent studies of Belanoff *et al.* (2001, 2002) patients were given either 600 or 1200 mg of the glu-cocorticoid antagonist mifespristone (RU 486) (Gaillard *et al.*, 1984) for 1 week in an open label, and in a double-blind, placebo-controlled crossover study. After this brief treatment the patients showed dramatic improvement in their Hamilton Rating Scale scores and the Brief Psychiatric Rating scales. Previously, Cushing's patients also experienced rapid disappearance of psychotic and depressive symptoms after RU 486 treatment (van der Lely, *et al.*, 1991; Sartor & Cutler, 1996).

The rationale of this approach is that the anti-glucocorticoid blocks the action of excess cortisol at GRs in afferent pathways, presumably in the frontal cortex, amygdala and hippocampus, to the PVN. It is intriguing that at the same time the anti-glucocorticoid disinhibits the HPA axis. The consequent rise in cortisol is likely to be counteracted by the extremely high dosage of the antagonist.

Spironolactone, a compound blocking the MRs, has an opposite effect and delays the recovery from depression after tricyclic antidepressants (Holsboer, 2001). Several GR antagonists are now in development (Karst *et al.*, 1997; Bachmann *et al.*, 1999).

In summary, compounds that diminish CRH and/or cortisol activity indeed seem to have therapeutic potential in mood disorders, at least in some mood disorders. Possibly, anxiety-aggression-driven depression (see Chapter 9) belongs in that

Table 8.13. Stress (CRH/HPA axis overactivity) might be a pathogenetic factor in a subtype of depression: supportive evidence.

CRH introduced directly into the brain of animals exerts anxiogenic effects and produces depression-like phenomena

In humans sustained hypercortisolaemia disrupts anxiety and aggression regulation and interferes with cognitive performance

Sustained hypercortisolaemia affects MA ergic systems in such a manner as the MA hypotheses presumes to underlie certain types of depression

Early life stress in animals causes lasting CRH overproduction, a persistent hyperactive HPA system and stressor hypersensitivity. Several observations suggest the same might happen in humans. Since early adversity is a risk factor for depression these data support the view that CRH/cortisol overdrive may play a causative role in depression

Many of the current antidepressants promote expression of MRs and GRs, thus enhancing feedback inhibition of CRH and cortisol production

CRH and cortisol antagonists seem to possess antidepressant potential

Conclusion: The CRH system is dually steered i.e. by CRH and urocortins, regulating the acutely activating and the late recovery responses to stress respectively. MRs and GRs participate in these stress modes by regulating the threshold or sensitivity and the termination or recovery of the stress responses. Imbalance of these stress responses leads possibly to enhanced depression vulnerability.

---

category. Biologically, hypercortisolaemia is possibly a predictor of good response. The risks of prolonged shortages of cortisol and/or CRH are not known.

These observations support the view that CRH overdrive might play a role in the pathophysiology of depression.

8.5 Conclusions

1 Stress is accompanied by CRH overdrive and cortisol overproduction. The same phenomena do occur in subtypes of depression.

2 CRH overdrive and cortisol overproduction generate MA ergic disturbances, similar to the ones that have been observed in subtypes of depression.

3 Several lines of evidence – behavioural and biological in nature – indicate that overactivity of stress hormones plays a role in the pathophysiology of depression, rather than being an epiphenomenon, associated with anxiety and tension, being prominent features of the depressive syndrome in some cases (Tables 8.13 and 8.14).

4 High CRH and cortisol are consequences of the stressed state, and at the same time produce stress phenomena, such as apprehension and anxiety. High CRH and cortisol operate in reverberating positive feedback loops on afferent pathways to the HPA axis. These afferents notably stem from circuits in amygdala,

Table 8.14. Stress (CRH /cortisol overproduction) might be a pathogenetic factor in a subtype of depression: cautionary notes.

Stress is not specifically linked to depression but precedes and accompanies many psychiatric disorders

CRH overproduction is not restricted to stress and stress-related disorders, but also occurs in disorders not typically linked to stress, e.g. anorexia nervosa

In some depressives plasma cortisol levels are decreased

These data indicate that:

In depression the CRH/HPA systems can be disordered in several ways.

These abnormalities are not linked to a particular category of mood disorder, but supposedly to certain psychopathological features, across diagnoses

hippocampus and frontal cortex that underlie cognitive and emotional aspects of the stress response. In this way those psychological features of the stress response are maintained, reinforced and may become independent of the stressor by which they were originally elicited.

5 Homeostatic regulations keeping the responses to stress at bay depend on the balance between two anti-parallel organized stress systems driven by CRH_1 and CRH_2 receptors. Corticosteroids operate in these stress systems via two receptor types: MR prevents disturbance of homeostasis, while GR promotes its recovery. MR/GR imbalance is induced by chronic stress and restored with antidepressant treatment.

   Once the balance in MR- and GR-mediated effects is disturbed, the individual loses the ability to maintain homeostasis, if challenged by an adverse event. This leads to a condition of neuroendocrine dysregulation and impaired behavioural adaptation, which may precipitate stress-related disorders such as depression in genetically predisposed individuals.

6 Antagonists of CRH and glucocorticoids, reducing CRH and cortisol overdrive and restoring MR/GR balance, can thus be expected to exert antidepressant activity (in subtypes of) depression. Preliminary clinical data confirm these expectations.

7 Theoretically CRH/cortisol overproduction could be a depressogenic condition in its own right, or exert depressogenic effects via MA ergic disturbances. Since states of CRH overdrive and cortisol overproduction may occur without depression, the latter possibility seems to be more likely than the former.

8 The data discussed in this chapter constitute strong evidence that stress indeed may be a causative factor in depression.

   The question arises whether the group of depression in which MA ergic and in particular 5-HT ergic disturbances have been ascertained, can be further specified. This is the subject of the next chapter.

REFERENCES

Åberg-Wistedt, A., Hasselmark, L., Stain-Malmgren, R., Apéria, B., Kjellman, B. F. & Mathé, A. A. (1998). Serotonergic 'vulnerability' in affective disorder: a study of the tryptophan depletion test and relationships between peripheral and central serotonin indexes in citalopram-responders. *Acta Psychiatr. Scand.*, **97**, 374–80.

Agid, O., Shapira, B., Zislin, J. *et al.* (1999). Environment and vulnerability to major psychiatric illness: a case control study of early parental loss in major depression, bipolar disorder and schizophrenia. *Mol. Psychiatry*, **4**, 163–72.

Agid, O., Kohn, Y. & Lerer, B. (2000). Environmental stress and psychiatric illness. *Biomed. Pharmacother.*, **54**, 135–41.

Amsterdam, J. D., Maislin, G., Droba, M. & Winokur, A. (1987). The ACTH stimulation test before and after clinical recovery from depression. *Psychiatry Res.*, **20**, 325–36.

Andrews, M. W. & Rosenblum, L. A. (1994). The development of affiliative and agonistic social patterns in differentially reared monkeys. *Child Dev.*, **65**, 1398–404.

Anisman, H., Ritch, M. & Sklar, L. S. (1981). Noradrenergic and dopaminergic interactions in escape behavior: analysis of uncontrollable stress effects. *Psychopharmacology*, **74**, 263–8.

Antoni, F. A. (1996). Calcium checks cyclic AMP-corticosteroid feedback in adenohypophyseal corticotrophs. *J. Neuroendocrinol.*, **9**, 659–72.

Arana, G. W., Santos, A. B., Laraia, M. T. *et al.* (1995). Dexamethasone for the treatment of depression: a randomized, placebo-controlled, double-blind trial. *Am. J. Psychiatry*, **152**, 265–7.

Arborelius, L., Owens, M. J., Plotsky, P. M. & Nemeroff, C. B. (1999). The role of corticotropin-releasing factor in depression and anxiety disorders. *J. Endocrinol.*, **160**, 1–12.

Arborelius, L., Skelton, K. H., Thrivikraman, K. V., Plotsky, P. M., Schulz, D. W. & Owens, M. J. (2000). Chronic administration of the selective corticotropin-releasing factor 1 receptor antagonist CP-154, 526: behavioral, endocrine and neurochemical effects in the rat. *J. Pharmacol. Exp. Ther.*, **294**, 588–97.

Austin, M. C., Rhodes, J. L. & Lewis, D. A. (1997). Differential distribution of corticotropin releasing hormone immunoreactive axons in monoaminergic nuclei of the human brainstem. *Neuropsychopharmacology*, **17**, 326–41.

Axelson, D. A., Doraiswamy, P. M., McDonald, W. M. *et al.* (1993). Hypercortisolemia and hippocampal changes in depression. *Psychiatry Res.*, **47**, 163–73.

Azmitia, E. (1999). Serotonin neurons, neuroplasticity and homeostasis of neural tissue. *Neuropsychopharmacology*, **21**, 33S–45S.

Bachmann, C. G., Linthorst, A. C. E. & Reul, J. M. H. M. (1999). Effect of chronic administration of the selective glucocorticoid receptor antagonists ORG 34850, ORG 34116, and ORG 34517 on the rat hypothalamic-pituitary-adrenocortical axis. *Eur. Neuropsychopharmacol.*, **9**, P.1.102.

Baker, D. G., West, S. A., Nicholson, W. E. *et al.* (1999). Serial CSF corticotropin-releasing hormone levels and adrenocortical activity in combat veterans with posttraumatic stress disorder. *Am. J. Psychiatry*, **156**, 585–8.

Bale, T. L., Contarino, A., Smith, G. W. *et al.* (2000). Mice deficient for corticotropin-releasing hormone receptor-2 display anxiety-like behaviour and are hypersensitive to stress. *Nat. Genet.*, **24**, 410–14.

Banki, C. M., Bissette, G., Arato, M., O'Connor, L. & Nemeroff, C. B. (1987). CSF corticotropin-releasing factor-like immunoreactivity in depression and schizophrenia, *Am. J. Psychiatry*, **144**, 873–7.

Banki, C. M., Karmacsi, L., Bissette, G. & Nemeroff, C. B. (1992). CSF corticotropin-releasing hormone and somatostatin in major depression: response to antidepressant treatment and relapse. *Eur. Neuropsychopharmacol.*, **2**, 107–13.

Barrett-Connor, E., von Mühlen, D., Laughlin, G. A. & Kripke, A. (1999). Endogenous levels of dehydroepiandrosterone sulfate, but not other sex hormones, are associated with depressed mood in older women: the Rancho Bernado study. *J. Am. Geriatr. Soc.*, **47**, 685–91.

Basso, A. M., Spina, M., Rivier, J., Vale, W. & Koob, G. F. (1999). Corticotropin-releasing factor antagonist attenuates the "anxiogenic-like" effect in the defensive burying paradigm but not in the elevated plus-maze following chronic cocaine in rats. *Psychopharmacology*, **145**, 21–30.

Belanoff, J. K., Flores, B. H., Kalezhan, M., Sund, B. & Schatzberg, A. F. (2001). Rapid reversal of psychotic deperssion using mifepristone. *J. Clin. Psychopharmacol.*, **21**, 516–21.

Belanoff, J. K., Rothschild, Cassidy, F. *et al.* (2002). An open label trial of C-1073 (Mifepristone) for psychotic major depression. *Biol. Psychiatry*, **52**, 386–92.

Benus, R. F., Bohus, B., Koolhaas, J. M. & Oortmerssen, G. A. (1991). Heritable variation in aggression as a reflection of individual coping strategies. *Experientia*, **47**, 1008–19.

Bifulco, A. T., Brown, G. W. & Harris, T. O. (1987). Childhood loss of parent, lack of adequate parental care and adult depression: a replication. *J. Affect. Disord.*, **12**, 115–28.

Bifulco, A., Brown, G. W. & Adler, Z. (1991). Early sexual abuse and clinical depression in adult life. *Br. J. Psychiatry*, **159**, 115–22.

Board, F., Persky, H. & Hamburg D. A. (1956). Psychological stress and endocrine functions. *Psychosom. Med.*, **18**, 324–33.

Bodani, M., Sheehan, B. & Philpot, M. (1999). The use of dexamethasone in elderly patients with antidepressant-resistant depressive illness. *J. Psychopharmacol.*, **13**, 196–7.

Boksa, P., Krishnamurthy, A. & Sharma, S. (1996). Hippocampal and hypothalamic type I corticosteroid receptor affinities are reduced in adult rats born by a Caesarean procedure with or without an added period of anoxia. *Neuroendocrinology*, **64**, 25–34.

Bowlby, J. (1961). Childhood mourning and its implications for psychiatry *Am. J. Psychiatry*, **118**, 481–98.

Bremner, J. D., Randall, P., Scott, T. M. *et al.* (1995). MRI-based measurement of hippocampal volume in patients with combat-related posttraumatic stress disorder. *Am. J. Psychiatry*, **152**, 973–81.

Bremner, J. D., Licinio, J., Darnell, A. *et al.* (1997a). Elevated CSF corticotropin-releasing factor concentrations in posttraumatic stress disorder. *Am. J. Psychiatry*, **154**, 624–9.

Bremner, J. D., Randall, P., Vermetten, E. *et al.* (1997b). Magnetic resonance imaging-based measurement of hippocampal volume in posttraumatic stress disorder related to childhood physical and sexual abuse: a preliminary report. *Biol. Psychiatry*, **41**, 23–32.

Bremner, J. D., Narayan, M., Anderson, E. R., Staib, L. H. & Miller, H. I. (2000). Hippocampal volume reduction in major depression. *Am. J. Psychiatry*, **157**, 115–18.

Britton, D. R., Varela, M., Garcia, A. & Rivier, J. (1986). Dexamethasone suppresses pituitary-adrenal but not behavioural effects of centrally administered CRF. *Life Sci.*, **38**, 211–16.

Brooke, S. M., de Haas-Johnson, A. M. & Kaplan, J. R. (1994). Dexamethasone resistance among nonhuman primates associated with a selective decrease of glucocorticoid receptors in the hippocampus and a history of social instability. *Neuroendocrinology*, **60**, 134–40.

Buijs, R. M., Wortel, J., Van Heerkhuize, J. J. *et al.* (1999). Anatomical and functional demonstration of a multisynaptic suprachiasmatic nucleus – adrenal (cortex) pathway. *Eur. J. Neurosci.*, **11**, 1535–44.

Cabib, S. & Puglisi-Allegra, S. (1996). Stress, depression and the mesolimbic dopamine system. *Psychopharmacology*, **128**, 331–42.

Caldji, C., Tannenbaum, B., Sharma, S., Francis, D., Plotsky, P. M. & Meaney, M. J. (1998). Maternal care during infancy regulates the development of neural systems mediating the expression of fearfulness in the rat. *Proc. Natl. Acad. Sci. USA*, **95**, 5335–40.

Calogero, A., Galluci, W. T., Gold, P. W. & Chrousos, G. P. (1988a). Multiple regulatory feedback loops on hypothalamic corticotropin releasing hormone secretion. *J. Clin. Invest.*, **82**, 767–74.

Calogero, A. E., Gallucci, W. T., Chrousos, G. P. & Gold, P. W. (1988b). Effect of the catecholamines upon rat hypothalamic corticotropin releasing hormone secretion in vitro: clinical implications. *J. Clin. Invest.*, **82**, 839–46.

Calogero, A. E., Bernardini, R., Magioris, A. N. *et al.* (1989). Serotonin stimulates rat hypothalamic corticotropin releasing hormone secretion in vitro. *Peptides*, **10**, 189–210.

Calogero, A. E., Bagdy, G., Moncada, M. L. & D'Agata, R. (1993). Effect of selective serotonin agonists on basal, corticotrophin-releasing hormone- and vasopressin-induced ACTH release in vitro from rat pituitary cells. *J. Endocrinol.*, **136**, 381–7.

Carroll, B. J. (1982). Use of the dexamethasone suppression test in depression. *J. Clin. Psychiatry*, **43**, 44–50.

Catalán, R., Gallart, J. M., Castellanos, J. M. & Galard, R. (1998). Plasma corticotropin-releasing factor in depressive disorders. *Biol. Psychiatry*, **44**, 15–20.

Chalmers, D. T., Lovenberg, T. W., Grigoriadis, D. E., Behan, D. P. & De Souza, E. B. (1996). Corticotrophin-releasing factor receptor: from molecular biology to drug design. *Trends Pharmacol. Sci.*, **17**, 166–72.

Chaouloff, F. (1993). Physiopharmacological interactions between stress hormones and central serotonergic systems. *Brain Res. Rev.*, **18**, 1–32.

(1995). Regulation of 5-HT receptors by corticosteroids: where do we stand? *Fundam. Clin. Pharmacol.*, **9**, 219–233.

Chrousos, G. P. (1998). Stressors, stress, and neuroendocrine integration of the adaptive response. *Annals N. Y. Acad. Sci.*, **750**, 311–35.

Chrousos, G. P. & Gold, P. W. (1992). The concepts of stress and stress system disorders. *J. Am. Med. Assoc.*, **267**, 1244–52.

Clarke, A. S., Wittwer, D. J., Abbott, D. H. & Schneider, M. L. (1994). Long-term effects of prenatal stress on HPA axis activity in juvenile rhesus monkeys. *Dev. Psychobiol.*, **27**, 257–69.

Cleare, A. J., Blair, D., Chambers, S. & Wessely, S. (2001). Urinary free cortisol in chronic fatigue syndrome. *Am. J. Psychiatry*, **158**, 641–3.

Cole, M. A., Kim, P. J., Kalman, B. A. & Spencer, R. L. (2000). Dexamethasone suppression of corticosteroid secretion: evaluation of the site of action by receptor measures and functional studies. *Psychoneuroendocrinol.*, **25**, 151–67.

Contarino, A., Dellu, F., Koob, G. F. *et al.* (1999). Reduced anxiety-like and cognitive performance in mice lacking the corticotropin-releasing factor receptor 1. *Brain Res.*, **835**, 1–9.

Cools, A. R., Brachten, R., Heeren, D., Willemsen, A. & Ellenbroek, B. (1990). Search after neurobiological profile of individual specific features of Wistar rats. *Brain Res. Bull.*, **24**, 49–69.

Cooney, J. M. & Dinan, T. G. (1996). Preservation of hypothalamic-pituitary-adrenal axis fast-feedback responses in depression. *Acta Psychiatr. Scand.*, **94**, 449–53.

  (2000). Hypothalamic-pituitary-adrenal axis early-feedback responses are preserved in melancholic depression: a study of sertraline treatment. *Hum. Psychopharm. Clin. Exp.*, **15**, 351–6.

Coplan, J. D., Andrews, M. W., Rosenblum, L. A. *et al.* (1996). Persistent elevations of cerebrospinal fluid concentrations of corticotropin-releasing factor in adult nonhuman primates exposed to early-life stressors: implications for the pathophysiology of mood and anxiety disorders. *Proc. Natl. Acad. Sci. USA*, **93**, 1619–23.

Coplan, J. D., Smith, E. L. P., Trost, R. C. *et al.* (2000). Growth hormone response to clonidine in adversely reared young adult primates: relationship to serial cerebrospinal fluid corticotropin-releasing factor. *Psychiatry Res.*, **95**, 93–102.

Crook, T. & Eliot, J. (1980). Parental death during childhood and adult depression: a critical review of the literature. *Psychol. Bull.*, **87**, 252–9.

Cullinan, W. E., Herman, J. P., Helmreich, D. L. & Watson, S. J. (1995). A neuroanatomy of stress. In *Neurobiological and Clinical Consequences of Stress: from Normal Adaptation to PTSD*, ed. M. J. Friedman, D. S. Charney & A. Y. Deutch. Philadelphia, PA: Lippincott-Raven Publishers.

Cunningham, E. T., Bohn, M. C. & Sawchenko, P. E. (1990). The organization of adrenergic inputs to the paraventricular and supraoptic nuclei of the rat hypothalamus. *J. Comp. Neurol.*, **292**, 651–67.

Czéh, B., Michaleis, T., Watanabe, T. *et al.* (2002). Stress-induced changes in cerebral metabolites, hippocampal volume, and cell proliferation are prevented by antidepressant treatment with tianeptine. *Proc. Natl. Acad. Sci. USA*, **98**, 12796–801.

Dallman, M. F., Viau, V. G., Bhatnagar, S., Gomez, F., Laugero, K. & Bell, M. E. (2002). Corticotropin-releasing factor, corticosteroids, stress, and sugar: energy balance, the brain and behavior. In *Hormones, Brain and Behavior Volume 3*, ed. D. W. Pfaff. Amsterdam: Elsevier.

Daniels, W. M. U., Pietersen, C. Y., Carstens, M. E., Daya, S. & Stein, D. (2000). Overcrowding induces anxiety and causes loss of serotonin 5-HT$_{1A}$ receptors in rats. *Metab. Brain Dis.*, **15**, 287–95.

Davis, S., Heal, D. J. & Stanfort, S. C. (1995). Long-lasting effects of and acute stress on the neurochemistry and function of 5-hydroxytryptaminergic neurones in the mouse brain. *Psychopharmacology*, **118**, 267–72.

Deakin, J. F. (1996). Does selectivity matter? *Int. Clin. Psychopharmacol.*, **11** (Suppl. 1), 13–17.

Deakin, J. F. W., Pennell, I., Upadhyaya, A. J. & Lofthouse, R. (1990). A neuroendocrine study of 5-HT function in depression: evidence for biological mechanisms of endogenous and psychosocial causation. *Psychopharmacology*, **101**, 85–92.

DeBattista, C., Posener, J. A., Kalehzan, B. M. & Schatzberg, A. F. (2000). Acute antidepressant effects of intravenous hydrocortisone and CRH in depressed patients: a double-blind, placebo-controlled study. *Am. J. Psychiatry*, **157**, 1334–7.

De Bellis, M. D., Gold, P. W., Geracioti, T. D. Jr., Listwak, S. J. & Kling, M. A. (1993). Association of fluoxetine treatment with reductions in CSF concentrations of corticotropin-releasing hormone and arginine vasopressin in patients with major depression. *Am. J. Psychiatry*, **150**, 656–7.

De Bellis, M. D., Baum, A. S., Birmaher, B. *et al.* (1999a). Developmental traumatology part I: Biological stress systems. *Biol. Psychiatry*, **45**, 1259–70.

De Bellis, M. D., Keshavan, M. S., Clark, D. B. *et al.* (1999b). Developmental traumatology part II: Brain development. *Biol. Psychiatry*, **45**, 1271–84.

De Kloet, E. R., Van der Vlies, J. & De wied, D. (1974). The site of the suppressive action of dexamethasone on pituitary-adrenal activity. *Endocrinology*, **94**, 61–73.

De Kloet, E. R., Wallach, G. & McEwen, B. S. (1975). Difference in binding of corticosterone and dexamethasone to rat brain and pituitary. *Endocrinology*, **96**, 598–611.

De Kloet, E. R., Kovacs, G. L., Szabo, G., Telegdy, G., Bohus, B. & Versteeg, D. H. G. (1982). Decreased serotonin turnover in the dorsal hippocampus of rat brain shortly after adrenalectomy: selective normalization after corticosterone substitution. *Brain. Res.*, **239**, 659–63.

De Kloet, E. R., Versteeg D. H. G. & Kovacs, G. L. (1983). Aldosterone blocks the response to corticosterone in the raphe-hippocampal serotonin system. *Brain. Res.*, **264**, 323–7.

De Kloet, E. R., Vreugdenhil, E., Oitzl, M. S. & Joëls, J. (1997). Glucocorticoid feedback resistance. *Trends Endocrinol. Metabol.*, **8**, 26–33.

De Kloet, E. R., Vreugdenhil, E., Oitzl, M. S. & Joëls, M. (1998). Brain corticosteroid receptor balance in health and disease. *Endocrinol. Rev.*, **19**, 269–301.

De Kloet, E. R., Oitzl, M. S. & Joëls, M. (1999). Stress and cognition: are corticosteroids good or bad guys? *Trends Neurosci.*, **22**, 422–6.

De Souza, E. B. (1995). Corticotropin-releasing factor receptors: physiology, pharmacology, biochemistry and role in central nervous system and immune disorders. *Psychoneuroendocrinology*, **20**, 789–819.

Deuschle, M., Schweiger, U., Standhardt, H., Weber, B. & Heuser, I. (1996). Corticosteroid-binding globulin is not decreased in depressed patients. *Psychoneuroendocrinology*, **21**, 645–9.

Deuschle, M., Schweiger, U., Weber, B. *et al.* (1997). Diurnal activity and pulsatility of the hypothalamus-pituitary-adrenal system in male depressed patients and healthy controls. *J. Clin. Endocrinol. Metab.*, **82**, 234–8.

Deijen, J. B., Wientjes, C. J. E., Vullinghs, H. F. M., Cloin, P. A. & Langefeld, J. J. (1999). Tyrosine improves cognitive performance and reduces blood pressure in cadets after one week of a combat training course. *Brain Res. Bull.*, **48**, 203–9.

Dinan, T. G. (1994). Glucocorticoids and the genesis of depressive illness. A psychobiological model. *Br. J. Psychiatry*, **164**, 365–71.

Dinan, T. G., Lavelle, E., Scott, L. V. *et al.* (1999). Desmopressin normalizes the blunted adrenocorticotropin response to corticotropin-releasing hormone in melancholic depression: evidence of enhanced vasopressinergic responsivity. *J. Clin. Endocrinol. Metab.*, **84**, 2238–40.

Dinwiddie, S., Heath, A. C., Dunne, M. P. *et al.* (2000). Early sexual abuse and lifetime psychopathology: a co-twin-control study. *Psychol. Med.*, **30**, 41–52.

Dolan, M., Anderson, I. M. & Deakin, J. F. (2001). Relationship between 5-HT function and impulsivity and aggression in male offenders with personality disorders. *Br. J. Psychiatry*, **178**, 352–9.

Drevets, W. C., Price, J. L., Simpson, J. R. Jr. *et al.* (1997). Subgenual prefrontal cortex abnormalities in mood disorders. *Nature*, **386**, 824–7.

Driessen, M., Herrmann, J., Stahl, K. *et al.* (2000). Magnetic resonance imaging volumes of the hippocampus and the amygdala in women with borderline personality disorder and early traumatization. *Arch. Gen. Psychiatry*, **57**, 1115–22.

Duman, R. S., Malberg, J., Nakgawa, S. & D'Sa, C. (2000). Neuronal plasticity in mood disorders. *Biol. Psychiatry*, **48**, 732–9.

Dunn, A. J. & Berridge, C. W. (1990). Physiological and behavioral responses to corticotropin-releasing factor administration: is CRF a mediator of anxiety or stress responses? *Brain Res. Rev.*, **15**, 71–100.

Eaves, M., Britton, K. T., Rivier, J., Vale, W. & Koob, G. F. (1985). Effects of corticotropin releasing factor on locomotor activity in hypophysectomized rats. *Peptides*, **6**, 923–6.

Enns, M. W., Cox, B. J. & Clara, I. (2002). Parental bonding and adult psychopathology: results from the US National Comorbidity Survey. *Psychol. Med.*, **32**, 997–1008.

Faravelli, C., Sacchetti, E., Ambonetti, A., Conte, G., Pallanti, S. & Vita, A. (1986). Early life events and affective disorder revisited. *Br. J. Psychiatry*, **148**, 288–95.

Feldker, D. E. M., Datson, N. A., Veenema, A. H., Meulmeester, E., De Kloet, E. R. & Vreugdenhil, E. (2003). Serial analysis of gene expression predicts structural differences in hippocampus of long and short attack latency mice. *Eur. J. Neurosci.*, **17**, 379–87.

Fernandes, C., McKittrick, C. R., File, S. E. & McEwen, B. S. (1997). Decreased 5-HT$_{1a}$ and increased 5-HT$_{2a}$ receptor binding after chronic corticosterone associated with a behavioural indication of depression but not anxiety. *Psychoneuroendocrinology*, **22**, 477–91.

Fleming, J. M. (1997). Prevalence of childhood sexual abuse in a community sample of Australian women. *Med. J. Australia*, **166**, 65–8

Flügge, G. (1999). Effects of cortisol on brain alpha$_2$-adrenoceptors: potential role in stress. *Neurosci. Biobehav. Rev.*, **23**, 949–56.

Fone, K. C. F., Shalders, K., Fox, Z. D., Arthur, R. & Marsden, C. A. (1996). Increased 5-HT$_{2c}$ receptor responsiveness occurs on rearing rats in social isolation. *Psychopharmacology*, **123**, 346–52.

Freud, S. (1957). Mourning and melancholia. In *The Complete Psychological Works of Sigmund Freud*, ed. L. Strachey. London: Hogarth Press and Institute of Psychoanalysis.

Fuchs, E. & Gould, E. (2000). Mini-review: in vivo neurogenesis in the adult brain: regulation and functional implications. *Eur. J. Neurosci.*, **12**, 2211–14.

Gaillard, R. C., Riondel, A., Muller, A. F., Herrmann, W. & Baulieu, E. E. (1984). RU 486: a steroid with antiglucocorticosteroid activity that only disinhibits the human pituitary-adrenal system at a specific time of day. *Proc. Natl. Acad. Sci. USA*, **81**, 3879–82.

Gambarana, C., Masi, F., Tagliamonte, A., Scheggi, S., Ghiglieri, O. & Graziella De Montis, M. (1999). A chronic stress that impairs reactivity in rats also decreases dopaminergic transmission in the nucleus accumbens: a microdialysis study. *J. Neurochem.*, **72**, 2039–46.

Garcia-Marquez, C. & Armario, A. (1987). Chronic stress depresses exploratory activity and behavioural performance in the forced swimming test without altering ACTH response to a novel acute stressor. *Physiol. Behav.*, **40**, 33–8.

Gass, P., Kretz, O. Wolfer, D. P. *et al.* (2000). Genetic disruption of mineralocorticoid receptor leads to impaired neurogenesis and granule cell degeneration in the hippocampus of adult mice. *EMBO Reports*, **1**, 447–51.

Geracioti, T. D., Loosen, P. T. & Orth, D. N. (1997). Low cerebrospinal fluid corticotropin-releasing hormone concentrations in eucortisolemic depression. *Biol. Psychiatry*, **42**, 165–74.

Gesing, A., Bilang-Bleuel, A., Droste, S. K., Linthorst, A. C. E., Holsboer, F. & Reul, J. M. H. M. (2001). Psychological stress increases hippocampal mineralocorticoid receptor levels: involvement of corticotropin releasing hormone. *J. Neurosci.*, **21**, 4822–9.

Ghadirian, A. M., Engelsmann, F., Dhar, V. *et al.* (1995). The psychotropic effects of inhibitors of steroid biosynthesis in depressed patients refractory to treatment. *J Biol. Psychiatry*, **37**, 369–75.

Gillies, G. E., Linton, E. A. & Lowry, P. J. (1982). Corticotropin releasing activity of the new CRF is potentiated several times by vasopressin. *Nature*, **299**, 355–7.

Gold, P. W., Loriaux, D. L., Roy, A. *et al.* (1986). Responses to corticotropin-releasing hormone in the hypercortisolism of depression and Cushing's disease: pathophysiologic and diagnostic implications. *New Engl. J. Med.*, **314**, 1329–35.

Gould, E. (1999). Serotonin and hippocampal neurogenesis. *Neuropsychopharmacology*, **21**, 46S–51S.

Gould, E., Beylin, A., Tanapat, P., Reeves, A. J. & Schors, T. J. (1999a). Hippocampal-dependent enhances adult neurogenesis in the hippocampal formation. *Nat. Neurosci.*, **2**, 260–5.

Gould, E., Reeves, A. J., Fallah, M., Tanapat, P., Gross, C. G. & Fuchs, E. (1999b). Hippocampal neurogenesis in adult old world primates. *Proc. Natl. Acad. Sci. USA*, **96**, 5263–7.

Gross, C., Zhuang, X., Stark, K. *et al.* (2002). Serotonin 1A receptor acts during development to establish normal anxiety-like behaviour in the adult. *Nature*, **416**, 396–400.

Gurvits, T. V., Shenton, M. E., Hokama, H. *et al.* (1996). Magnetic resonance imaging study of hippocampal volume in chronic, combat related posttraumatic stress disorder. *Biol. Psychiatry*, **40**, 1091–9.

Habib, K. E., Weld, K. P., Rice, K. C. *et al.* (2000). Oral administration of a corticotropin-releasing hormone receptor antagonist significantly attenuates behavioral, neuroendocrine, and autonomic responses to stress in primates. *Proc. Natl. Acad. Sci. USA*, **97**, 6079–84.

Haller, J., Millar, S., Van de Schraaf, J., De Kloet, E. R. & Kruk, M. R. (2000). The active phase-related increase in corticosterone and aggression are linked. *J. Neuroendocrinology*, **12**, 431–6.

Hallstrom, T. (1987). The relationships of childhood socio-demographic factors and early parental loss to major depression in adult life. *Acta Psychiatr. Scand.*, **75**, 212–16.

Harris, T., Brown, G. W. & Bufulco, A. (1986). Loss in parent in childhood and adult psychiatric disorder: the role of lack of adequate parental care. *Psychol. Med.*, **16**, 641–59.

Harris, T. O., Borsanyi, S., Messari, S. *et al.* (2000). Morning cortisol as a risk factor for subsequent major depressive disorder in adult women. *Br. J. Psychiatry*, **177**, 505–10.

Heim, C. & Nemeroff, Ch. B. (1999). The impact of early adverse experiences on brain systems involved in the pathophysiology of anxiety and affective disorders. *Biol. Psychiatry*, **46**, 1509–22.

Heim, C., Newport, D. J., Heit, S. *et al.* (2000). Pituitary-adrenal and autonomic responses to stress in women after sexual and physical abuse in childhood. *J. Am. Med. Assoc.*, **284**, 592–7.

Heim, C., Newport, J., Bonsall, R., Miller, A. H. & Nemeroff, Ch. B. (2001). Altered pituitary-adrenal axis responses to provocative challenge tests in adult survivors of childhood abuse. *Am. J. Psychiatry*, **158**, 575–81.

Heinrichs, S. C., Menzaghi, F., Merlo Pich E., Britton, K. T. & Koob, G. F. (1995). The role of CRF in behavioral aspects of stress. *Ann. N. Y. Acad. Sci.*, **771**, 92–104.

Heinrichs, S. C., Lapsansky, J., Lovenberg, T. W., De Souza, E. B. & Chalmers, D. T. (1997). Corticotropin-releasing factor CRF_1, but not CRF_2, receptors mediate anxiogenic-like behaviour. *Regul. Pept.*, **71**, 15–21.

Henn, F. A. & Edwards, E. (1994). Animal models in the study of genetic factors in human psychopathology. In *Genetics Studies in Affective Disorders*, ed. D. F. Papolos & H. M. Lachman. New York: Brunner Mazel.

Henry, J. P. & Stephens, P. N. (1977). *Stress, Health and the Social Environment. A Socio-biological Approach to Medicine.* New York: Springer.

Herman, J. P. & Cullinan, W. E. (1997). Neurocircuitry of stress: central control of the hypothalamo-pituitary-adrenocortical axis. *Trends Neurosci.*, **20**, 78–84.

Heuser, I., Deuschle, M., Luppa, P., Schweiger, U., Standhardt, H. & Weber, B. (1998). Increased diurnal plasma concentrations of dehydroepiandrosterone in depressed patients. *J. Clin. Endocrin. Metabol.*, **83**, 3130–3.

Hill, J., Davis, R., Byatt, M., Burnside, E., Rollinson, L. & Fear, S. (2000). Childhood sexual abuse and affective symptoms in women: a general population study. *Psychol. Med.*, **30**, 1283–91.

Hofer, M. (1983). On the relationship between attachment and separation processes in infancy. In *Early Development*, ed. R. Plutnik & B. Emtion. New York: Academic Press.

Holsboer, F. (1999). The rationale for corticotropin-releasing hormone receptor (CRH-R) antagonists to treat depression and anxiety. *J. Psychiatry Res.*, **33**, 181–214.

(2000). The corticosteroid receptor hypothesis of depression. *Neuropsychopharmacology*, **23**, 477–501.

(2001). Antidepressant drug discovery in the postgenomic era. *World J. Biol. Psychiatry*, **2**, 165–77.

Holsboer, F., von Bardeleben, U., Wiedemann, K., Muller, O. A. & Stalla, G. K. (1987). Serial assessment of corticotropin-releasing hormone response after dexamethasone in depression. Implications for pathophysiology of DST non-suppression. *Biol. Psychiatry*, **22**, 228–34.

Holsboer-Trachsler, E., Stohler, R. & Hatzinger, M. (1991). Repeated administration of the combined dexamethasone-human corticotropin releasing hormone stimulation test during treatment of depression. *Psychiatry Res.*, **38**, 163–71.

Hsu, S. Y. & Hsueh, A. J. W. (2001). Human stresscopin and stresscopin-related peptide are selective ligands for the type 2 corticotropin-releasing hormone receptor. *Nat. Med.*, **7**, 605–11.

Hucks, D., Lowther, S., Rufus Crompton, M., Katona, C. L. E. & Horton, R. W. (1997). Corticotropin-releasing factor binding sites in cortex of depressed suicides. *Psychopharmacology*, **134**, 174–8.

Imperato, A., Puglisi-Allegra, S., Casolini, P. & Angelucci, L. (1991). Changes in brain dopamine and acetylcholine release during and following stress are independent of the pituitary-adrenocortical axis. *Brain Res.*, **538**, 111–17.

Imperato, A., Angelucci, L., Casolini, P., Zocchi, A. & Puglisi-Allegra, S. (1992). Repeated stressful experiences differently affect limbic dopamine release during and following stress. *Brain Res.*, **577**, 194–9.

Joëls, M. & de Kloet, E. R. (1989). Effects of glucocorticoids and norepinephrine on the excitability in the hippocampus. *Science*, **245**, 1502–5.

(1992). Control of neuronal excitability by corticosteroid hormones. *Trends Neurosci.*, **15**, 25–30.

Johnson, J. G., Cohen, P., Brown, J., Smailes, E. M. & Bernstein, D. P. (1999). Childhood maltreatment increases risk for personality disorders during early adulthood. *Arch. Gen. Psychiatry*, **56**, 600–6.

Johnson, J. G., Cohen, P., Kasen, S., Smailes, E. & Brook, J. S. (2001). Association of maladaptive behavior with psychiatric disorder among parents and their offspring. *Arch. Gen. Psychiatry*, **58**, 453–60.

Johnson, J. G., Cohen, P., Gould, M. S., Kasen, S., Brown, J. & Brook, J. S. (2002). Childhood adversities, interpersonal difficulties and risk for suicide attempts during late adolescence and early adulthood. *Arch. Gen. Psychiatry*, **59**, 741–9.

Jorgensen, H., Knigge, K., Kjaer, A., Vadsholt, T. & Warberg, J. (1998). Sertonergic involvement in stress-induced ACTH release. *Brain Res.*, **811**, 10–20.

Joyce, P. R., Mulder, R. T. & Cloninger, C. R. (1994). Temperament and hypercortisolemia in depression. *Am. J. Psychiatry*, **151**, 195–8.

Kahn, R. S. & Van Praag, H. M. (1988). A serotonin hypothesis of panic disorder. *Hum. Psychopharmacol.*, **3**, 285–8.

Karssen, A. M., Meijer, O. C., Van der Sandt, I. C. J. et al. (2001). Multidrug resistance P-glycoprotein hampers the access of cortisol but not of corticosterone to mouse and human brain. *Endocrinology*, **142**, 2686–94.

Karst, H., De Kloet, E. R. & Joëls, M. (1997). Effect of ORG 34116, a corticosteroid receptor antagonist, on hippocampal Ca^{2+} currents. *Eur. J. Pharmacol.*, **339**, 17–26.

Karten, Y. J. G., Nair, S. M., van Essen, L., Sibug, R. & Joëls, M. (1999). Long-term exposure to high corticosterone levels attenuates serotonin responses in rat hippocampal CA1 neurons. *Proc. Natl. Acad. Sci USA*, **96**, 13456–61.

Kaufman, J. & Heinrich, C. (2000). Exposure to violence and early childhood trauma. In *Handbook of Infant Mental Health*, ed. C. Zeanah. New York: Guilford Press.

Kaufman, J., Plotsky, P. M., Nemeroff, C. B. & Charney, D. S. (2000). Effects of early adverse experiences on brain structure and function: clinical implications. *Biol. Psychiatry*, **48**, 778–90.

Keck, M. E., Welt, T., Wigger, A. *et al.* (2001). The anxiolytic effect of the CRH (1) receptor antagonist R121919 depends on innate emotionality in rats. *Eur. J. Neurosci.*, **13**, 373–80.

Kendler, K. S., Neale, M. C., Kessler, R. C., Heath, A. C. & Eaves L. J. (1992). Childhood parental loss and adult psychopathology in women. A twin study perspective. *Arch. Gen. Psychiatry*, **49**, 109–16.

Kendler, K. S., Kessler, R. C., Walters, E. E. *et al.* (1995). Stressful life events, genetic liability, and onset of an episode of major depression in women. *Am. J. Psychiatry*, **152**, 833–42.

Kessler, R. C., Davis, C. G. & Kendler, K. S. (1997). Childhood adversity and adult psychiatric disorder in the US National Comorbidity Survey. *Psychol. Med.*, **27**, 1101–19.

King, J. A. & Edwards, E. (1999). Early stress and genetic influences on hypothalamic-pituitary-adrenal axis functioning in adulthood. *Horm. Behav.*, **36**, 79–85.

King, M., Coxell, A. & Mezey, G. (2002). Sexual molestation of males: associations with psychological disturbance. *Br. J. Psychiatry*, **181**, 153–7.

Kishimoto, T., Radulovic, J., Radulovic, M. *et al.* (2000). Deletion of crhr2 reveals an anxiolytic role for corticotropin-releasing hormone receptor-2. *Nat. Genet.*, **24**, 415–19.

Koob, G. F., Heinrichs, S. C., Pich, E. M. *et al.* (1993). The role of corticotropin-releasing factor in behavioral responses to stress. In *Corticotropin-Releasing Factor: Basic and Clinical Studies of a Neuropeptide*, ed. E. B. De Souza & C. B. Nemeroff. Chichester: John Wiley & Sons.

Koolhaas, J. M., Korte, S. M., De Boer, S. F. *et al.* (1999). Coping styles in animals: current status in behavior and stress physiology. *Neurosci. Biobehav. Rev.*, **23**, 925–35.

Korte, S. M. (2001). Corticosteroids in relation to fear, anxiety and psychopathology. *Neurosci. Biobehav. Rev.*, **25**, 117–42.

Kovacs, K. J. & Sawchenko, P. (1993). Mediation of osmoregulation influences on neuroendocrine corticotropin releasing factor gene expression in the rat paraventricular. *Proc. Natl. Acad. Sci. USA*, **90**, 7981–5.

Krishnan, K. R. R., Doraiswamy, P. M., Lurie, S. N. *et al.* (1991). Pituitary size in depression. *J. Clin. Endocr. Metab.*, **72**, 256–9.

Krishnan, K. R., Miller, M. N., Helms, M. J. *et al.* (1993). Dose–response relationship between plasma ACTH and cortisol after the infusion of ACTH1-24. *Eur. Arch. Psychiat. Clin. Neurosci.*, **242**, 240–3.

Kuroda, Y., Mikuni, M., Ogawa, T. & Takahashi, K. (1992). Effect of ACTH, adrenalectomy and the combination treatment of the density of $5\text{-}HT_2$ receptor binding sites in neocortex of rat forebrain and $5\text{-}HT_2$ receptor-mediated wet-dog shake behaviours. *Psychopharmacology*, **108**, 27–32.

Ladd, C. O., Owens, M. J. & Nemeroff, C. B. (1996). Persistent changes in corticotropin-releasing factor neuronal systems induced by maternal deprivation. *Endocrinology*, **137**, 1212–18.

Lammers, C.-H., Garcia-Borreguero, D., Schmider, J. *et al.* (1995). Combined dexamethasone/corticotropin-releasing hormone test in patients with schizophrenia and in normal controls. *Biol. Psychiatry*, **38**, 803–7.

Lechin, F., van der Dijs, B. & Benaim, M. (1996). Stress versus depression. *Prog. Neuro-Psychopharmacol. Biol. Psychiatry*, **20**, 899–950.

Lehnert, H., Reinstein, D. K., Strowbridge, B. W. & Wurtman, R. J. (1984). Neurochemical and behavioral consequences of acute uncontrollable stress: effects of dietary tyrosine. *Brain Res.*, **303**, 215–23.

Lemieux, A. M. & Coe, C. L. (1995). Abuse-related posttraumatic stress disorder: evidence for chronic neuroendocrine activation in women. *Psychosom. Med.*, **57**, 105–15.

Lesch, K. P., Mayer, S., Disselkamp-Tietze, *et al.* (1990). 5-HT$_{1a}$ receptor responsivity in unipolar depression: evaluation of ipsapirone-induced ACTH and cortisol secretion in patients and controls. *Biol. Psychiatry*, **28**, 620–8.

Levine, S., Lyons, D. M. & Schatzberg, A. F. (1997). Psychobiological consequences of social relationships. *Ann N. Y. Acad. Sci.*, **807**, 210–18.

Levine, S., Dent, G. & De Kloet, E. R. (2000). Stress-hyporesponsive period. In *Encyclopedia of Stress, Volume 3*, ed. G. Fink. Academic Press.

Levitan, R. D., Parikh, S. V., Lesage, A. D. *et al.* (1998). Major depression in individuals with a history of childhood physical or sexual abuse: relationship to neurovegetative features, mania, and gender. *Am. J. Psychiatry*, **155**, 1746–52.

Lewis, K., Li, C. & Perrin, M. H. (2001). Identification of urocortin III, an additional member of the corticotropin releasing factor (CRF) family with high affinity for the CRH 2 receptor. *Proc. Natl. Acad. Sci. USA*, **98**, 7570–5.

Li, C., Vaughan, J., Sawchecko, P. E. & Vale, W. W. (2002). Urocortin III- immunoreactive projections in rat brain: partial overlap with sites of type 2 corticotropin releasing factor receptor expression. *J. Neurosci.*, **22**, 991–1001.

Liebsch, G., Landgraf, R., Engelmann, M., Lorscher, P. & Holsboer, F. (1999). Differential behavioural effects of chronic infusion of CRH 1 and CRH 2 receptor antisense oligonucleotides into the rat brain. *J. Psychiatry Res.*, **33**, 153–63.

Lindley, S. E., Bengoechea, T. G., Schatzberg, A. F. & Wong, D. L. (1999). Glucocortioid effects on mesotelencephalic dopamine neurotransmission. *Neuropsychopharmacology*, **21**, 399–407.

Liu D., Diorio J., Day, J. C., Francis, D. D. & Meaney, M. J. (2000). Maternal care, hippocampal synaptogenesis and cognitive development in rats. *Nat. Neurosci.*, **3**, 799–806.

Lopez, J. F., Akil, H. & Watson, S. J. (1999). Neural circuits mediating stress. *Biol. Psychiatry*, **46**, 1461–71.

Lucassen, P. J., Vollman-Holsdorf, G. K., Gleisberg, M., Czeh, B., De Kloet, E. R. & Fuchs, E. (2001). Chronic psychosocial stress differently affects apoptosis in hippocampal subregions and cortex. *Eur. J. Neurosci.*, **14**, 161–6.

Lupien, S. J. & McEwen, B. S. (1997). The acute effects of corticosteroids on cognition: integration of animal and human studies. *Brain Res. Rev.*, **24**, 1–27.

Lupien, S. J., Lecours, A., Lussier, I., Schwartz, G., Nair, N. & Meaney, M. (1994). Basal cortisol levels and cognitive deficits in human aging. *J. Neurosci.*, **14**, 2893–903.

Lyons, W. E., Mamounas, L. A., Ricaurte, G. A. *et al.* (1999). Brain-derived neurotrophic factor-deficient mice develop aggressiveness and hyperphagia in conjunction with brain serotonergic abnormalities. *Proc. Natl. Acad. Sci. USA*, **96**, 15239–44.

Lyons, D. M., Chou Yang, Sawyer-Glover, A. M., Moseley, M. E. & Schatzberg, A. F. (2001). Early life stress and inherited variation in monkey hippocampal volumes. *Arch. Gen. Psychiatry*, **58**, 1145–51.

Maccari, S., Piazza, P. V., Kabbaj, M., Barbazanges, A., Simon, H. & Le Moal, M. (1995). Adoption reverses the long-term impairment in glucocorticoid feedback induced by prenatal stress. *J. Neurosci.*, **15**, 110–16.

Maes, M., Vandewoude, M., Schotte, C. *et al.* (1990). The relationships between the cortisol responses to dexamethasone and to L-5-HTP, and the availability of L-tryptophan in
depressed females. *Biol. Psychiatry*, **27**, 601–8.

Magarinos, A. M., Verdugo, J. M. G. & McEwen, B. S. (1997). Chronic stress alters synaptic
terminal structure in hippocampus. *Proc. Natl. Acad. Sci. USA*, **94**, 14002–8.

Maines, L. W., Keck, B. J., Smith, J. E. & Lakoski, J. M. (1999). Corticosterone regulation of
serotonin transporter and 5-HT$_{1a}$ receptor expression in the aging brain. *Synapse*, **32**,
58–66.

Makino, S., Gold, P. W. & Schulkin, J. (1994). Corticosterone effects on corticotropin-releasing
hormone mRNA in the central nucleus of the amygdala and the parvocellular region of the
paraventricular nucleus of the hypothalamus. *Brain Res.*, **64**, 105–12.

Malison, R. T., Anand, A., Pelton, G. H. *et al.* (1999). Limited efficacy of ketoconazole in treatment-
refractory major depression. *J. Clin. Psychopharmacol.*, **19**, 466–70.

Markus, C. R., Panhuysen, G., Tuiten, A., Koppeschaar, H., Fekkes, D. & Peters, M. L. (1998).
Does carbohydrate-rich, protein-poor food prevent a deterioration of mood and cognitive performance of stress-prone subjects when subjected to a stressful task? *Appetite*, **31**,
49–65.

McBurnett, K., Lahey, B. B., Rathouz, P. J. & Loeber, R. (2000). Low salivary control and persistent
aggression in boys referred for disruptive behavior. *Arch. Gen. Psychiatry*, **57**, 38–43.

McCauley, J., Kern, D. E., Kolodner, K., Dill, L. & Schroeder, A. F. (1997). Clinical characteristics
of women with a history of childhood abuse. *J. Am. Med. Assoc.*, **277**, 1362–8.

McEwen, B. S. (1995). Adrenal steroid actions on brain. In *Neurobiological and Clinical Consequences of Stress: from Normal Adaptation to PTSD*, ed. M. J. Friedman, D. S. Charney & A. J.
Deutch. Philadelphia: Lippincott-Raven Publishers.

(1998). Protective and damaging effects of stress mediators. In *Seminars in Medicine of the Beth
Israel Deaconess Medical Center*, ed. J. S. Flier & L. H. Underhill. New York: Massachusetts
Medical Society.

McEwen, B. S. & Sapolsky, R. M. (1995). Stress and cognitive function. *Curr. Opin. Neurobiol.*,
5, 205–16.

McEwen, B. S. & Stellar, E. (1993). Stress and the individual: mechanisms leading to disease. *Arch.
Intern. Med.*, **153**, 2093–101.

McKibben, L., De Vos, E. & Newberger, E. H. (1989). Victimization of mothers of abused children:
a controlled study. *Pediatrics*, **84**, 531–5.

McKinney, W. T., Moran, A. & Kraemer, G. W. (1984). Separation in non-human primates
as a model for human depression: neurobiological implications. In *Neurobiology of Mood
Disorders*, ed. R. Post & J. Ballenger. Baltimore: Williams and Wilkins.

McKittrick, C. R., Blanchard, D. C., Blanchard, R. J., McEwen, B. S. & Sakai, R. R. (1995). Serotonin
receptor binding in a colony model of chronic social stress. *Biol. Psychiatry*, **37**, 383–93.

McQuade, R. & Young, A. H. (2000). Future therapeutic targets in mood disorders: the glucocorticoid receptor. *Br. J. Psychiatry*, **177**, 390–5.

Meaney, M. J., Aitken, D. H., Bhatnagar, S., Van Berkel, C. & Sapolsky, R. M. (1988). Postnatal
handling attenuates neuroendocrine, anatomical, and cognitive impairments related to the
aged hippocampus. *Science*, **283**, 766–8.

Meerlo, P., Horvath, K. M., Luiten, P. G. M., Angelucci, L., Catalani, A. & Koolhaas, J. M. (2001). Increased maternal corticosterone levels in rats: effects on brain 5-HT$_{1A}$ receptors and behavioral coping with stress in adult offspring. *Behav. Neurosci.*, **115**, 1111–17.

Mervaala, E., Föhr, J., Könönen, M. *et al.* (2000). Quantitative MRI of the hippocampus and amygdala in severe depression. *Psychol. Med.*, **30**, 117–25.

Meijer, O. C. & De Kloet, E. R. (1994). Corticosterone suppresses the expression of 5-HT$_{1a}$ receptor mRNA in rat dentate gyrus. *Eur. J. Pharmacol. Mol. Pharm. Sect.*, **266**, 255–61.

(1995). A role for the mineralocorticoid receptor in a rapid and transient suppression of hippocampal 5-HT$_{1a}$ receptor mRNA by corticosterone. *J. Neuroendocrinol.*, **7**, 653–7.

(1998). Corticosterone and serotonergic neurotransmission in the hippocampus: functional implications of central corticosteroid receptor diversity. *Critical Rev. Neurobiol.*, **12**, 1–20.

Meijer, O. C., De Lange, E. C. M., Breimer, D. D., De Boer, A. G., Workel, J. O. & De Kloet, E. R. (1998). Penetration of dexamethasone into brain glucocorticoid targets is enhanced in mdr1A P-glycoprotein knockout mice. *Endocrinology*, **139**, 1789–93.

Meyer, J. S. (1985). Biochemical effects of corticosteroids on neural tissues. *Physiol. Rev.*, **65**, 946–1020.

Mitchell, J. B., Rowe, W., Boksa, P. & Meaney, M. J. (1990). Serotonin regulates type II corticosteroid receptor binding in hippocampal cell cultures. *J. Neurosci.*, **10**, 1745–52.

Modell, S., Yassouridis, A., Huber, J. & Holsboer, F. (1997). Corticosteroid receptor function is decreased in depressed patients. *Neuroendocrinology*, **65**, 216–22.

Modell, S., Lauer, C. J., Schreiber, M., Huber, J., Krieg, J. C. & Holsboer, F. (1998). Hormonal response pattern in the combined DEX-CRH test is stable over time in subjects at high familial risk for affective disorders. *Neuropsychopharmacology*, **18**, 253–62.

Moghaddam, B. (1993). Related stress preferentially increases extraneuronal levels of excitatory amino acids in the prefrontal cortex: comparison to hippocampus and basal ganglia. *J. Neurochem.*, **60**, 1650–7.

Mongeau, R., Blier, P. & De Montigny, C. (1997). The serotonergic and noradrenergic systems of the hippocampus: their interactions and the effects of antidepressant treatment. *Brain Res. Rev.*, **23**, 145–95.

Montkowski, A., Barden, N., Wotjak, C. *et al.* (1995). Long-term antidepressant treatment reduces behavioural deficits in transgenic mice with impaired glucocorticoid receptor function. *J. Neuroendocrinol.*, **7**, 841–5.

Müller, M. B., Lucassen, P. J., Yassourides, A., Hoogendijk, W. J., Holsboer, F. & Swaab, D. F. (2001). Neither major depression not glucocorticoid treatment affects the cellular integrity of the human hippocampus *Eur. J. Neurosci.*, **14**, 1603–12.

Munck, A., Guyre, P. M. & Holbrook, N. J. (1984). Physiological functions of glucocorticoids in stress and their relation to pharmacological actions. *Endocr. Rev.*, **5**, 25–44.

Murphy, B. E. P., Dhar, V., Ghadirian, A. M., Chouinard, G. & Keller, R. (1991). Response to steroid suppression in major depression resistant to antidepressant therapy. *J. Clin. Psychopharmacol.*, **11**, 121–6.

Musselman, D. L., De Battista, Ch., Nathan, K. I., Kilts, C. D., Schatzberg, A. F. & Nemeroff, Ch. B. (1998). Biology of mood disorders. In *Textbook of Psychopharmacology*, ed. A. F. Schatzberg & Ch. B. Nemeroff. Washington, DC: American Psychiatric Press.

National Research Council (1993). *Understanding Child Abuse and Neglect.* Washington, DC: National Academy Press.

Nelson, E. C., Heath, A. C., Madden, P. A. F. *et al.* (2002). Association between self-reported childhood sexual abuse and adverse psychosocial outcomes. *Arch. Gen. Psychiatry*, **59**, 139–45.

Nemeroff, C. B. (1996). The corticotropin-releasing factor hypothesis of depression: new findings and directions. *Mol. Psychiatry*, **1**, 336–42.

Nemeroff, C. B., Widerlöv, E., Bissette, G. *et al.* (1984). Elevated concentrations of CSF corticotropin-releasing factor-like immunoreactivity in depressed patients. *Science*, **226**, 1342–4.

Nemeroff, C. B., Owens, M. J., Bissette, G., Andorn, A. C. & Stanley, M. (1988). Reduced corticotropin-releasing factor binding sites in the frontal cortex of suicide victims. *Arch. Gen. Psychiatry*, **45**, 577–9.

Nemeroff, C. B., Krishnan, K. R. R., Reed, D., Leder, D., Beam, C. & Dunnick, N. R. (1992). Adrenal gland enlargement in major depression: computed tomography study. *Arch. Gen. Psychiatry*, **49**, 196–202.

Neumaier, J. F., Petty, F., Kramer, G. L., Szot, P. & Hamblin, M. W. (1997). Learned helplessness increases 5-hydroxytryptamine$_{1b}$ receptor mRNA levels in the rat dorsal raphe nucleus. *Biol. Psychiatry*, **41**, 668–74.

Newman, M. G., Clayton, L., Zuellig, A. *et al.* (2000). The relationship of childhood sexual abuse and depression with somatic symptoms and medical utilization. *Psychol. Med.*, **30**, 1063–77.

Newport, D. J., Stowe, Z. N. & Nemeroff, Ch. B. (2002). Parental depression: animal models of an adverse life event. *Am. J. Psychiatry*, **159**, 1265–83.

Nuller, J. L. & Ostroumova, M. N. (1980). Resistance to inhibiting effect of dexamethasone in patients with endogenous depression. *Acta Psychiatr. Scand.*, **61**, 169–77.

Oitzl, M. S. & De Kloet, E. R. (1992). Selective corticosteroid antagonists modulate specific aspects of spatial orientation learning. *Behav. Neurosci.*, **106**, 62–71.

Oitzl, M. S., Fluttert, M., Sutanto, W. & De Kloet, E. R. (1998). Continuous blockade of brain glucocorticoid receptors facilitated spatial learning and memory in rats. *Eur. J. Neurosci.*, **10**, 3759–66.

Oitzl, M. S., Workel, J. O., Fluttert, M., Frösch, F. & De Kloet, E. R. (2000). Maternal deprivation affects behavior from youth to senescence: amplification of individual differences in spatial learning and memory in senescent brown Norway rats. *Eur. J. Neurosci.*, **34**, 372–8.

Oitzl, M. S., Reichardt, H. M., Joëls, M. & De Kloet, E. R. (2001). Point mutation in the mouse glucocorticoid receptor preventing DNA binding impairs spatial memory. *Proc. Natl. Acad. Sci. USA*, **98**, 12790–5.

Oldehinkel, A. J., Van den Berg, M. D., Flentge, F., Bouhuys, A. L., Ter Horst, G. J. & Ormel, J. (2001). Urinary free cortisol excretion in elderly persons with minor and major depression. *Psychiatry Res.*, **104**, 39–48.

Osran, H., Resit, C., Cheng-Chung, C., Lifrak, E. T., Aleksandra, C. & Lawrence, D. P. (1993). Adrenal androgens and cortisol in major depression. *Am. J. Psychiatry*, **150**, 806–9.

Owens, M. J. & Nemeroff, C. B. (1991). Physiology and pharmacology of corticotropin-releasing factor. *Pharmacol. Rev.*, **43**, 425–73.

(1999). Corticotropin-releasing factor antagonists. *CNS Drugs*, **12**, 85–92.

Owens, M. J., Edwards, E. & Nemeroff, C. B. (1990). Effects of 5-HT$_{1a}$ receptor agonists on hypothalamo-pituitary-adrenal axis activity and corticotropin-releasing factor containing neurons in the rat brain. *Eur. J. Pharmacol.*, **190**, 113–20.

Pajer, K., Gardner, W., Rubin, R. T., Perel, J. & Neal, S. (2001). Decreased cortisol levels in adolescent girls with conduct disorder. *Arch. Gen. Psychiatry*, **58**, 297–302.

Palkovits, M. (1999). Interconnections between the neuroendocrine hypothalamus and the central autonomic system. *Front. Neuroendocrinol.*, **20**, 270–95.

Pariante, C. M. & Miller, A. H. (2001). Glucocorticoid receptors in major depression: relevance to pathophysiology and treatment. *Biol. Psychiatry*, **49**, 391–404.

Patchev, V. K., Shoaib, M., Holsboer, F. & Almeida, O. F. (1994). The neurosteroid tetrahydroprogesterone counteracts corticotropin-releasing hormone-induced anxiety and alters the release and gene expression of corticotropin-releasing hormone in the rat hypothalamus. *Neuroscience*, **62**, 265–71.

Patten, S. B. (2000). Exogenous corticosteroids and major depression in the general population. *J. Psychosom. Res.*, **49**, 447–9.

Penalva, R. G., Flachskamm, C., Zimmermann, S. *et al.* (2002). Corticotropin-releasing hormone receptor type 1-deficiency enhances hippocampal serotonergic neurotransmission: an in vivo microdialysis study in mutant mice. *Neuroscience*, **109**, 253–66.

Perry, B. D., Giller, E. L. & Southwick, S. M. (1987). Altered platelet alpha-2- adrenergic binding sites in posttraumatic stress disorder. *Am. J. Psychiatry*, **144**, 1511–12.

Petrides, J. S., Gold, P. W., Mueller, G. P. *et al.* (1997). Marked differences in functioning of the hypothalamic-pituitary-adrenal axis between groups of men. *J. Appl. Physiol.*, **82**, 1979–88.

Petty, F., Kramer, G. & Wilson, L. (1992). Prevention of learned helplessness: In vivo correlation with cortical serotonin. *Pharmacol. Biochem. Behav.*, **43**, 3631–7.

Piazza, P. V. & Le Moal, M. (1997). Glucocorticoids as a biological substrate of reward: physiological and pathophysiological implications. *Brain Res. Rev.*, **25**, 359–72.

Piazza, P. V., Rougé-Pont, F., Derouche, V., Maccari, S., Simon, H. & Le Moal, M. (1996). Glucocorticoids have state-dependent stimulant effects on the mesencephalic dopaminergic transmission. *Proc. Natl. Acad. Sci. USA*, **93**, 8716–20.

Plotsky, P. & Meaney, M. (1993). Early postnatal experience alters hypothalamic corticotropin-releasing factor (CRF) mRNA, median eminence CRF content, and stress-induced release in adult rats. *Mol. Brain Res.*, **18**, 195–200.

Porter, R., McAllister-Williams, R. H., Lunn, B. & Young, A. (1998). 5- Hydroxytryptamine receptor function in man is reduced by acute administration of hydrocortisone. *Psychopharmacology*, **139**, 243–50.

Porter, R. J., McAllister-Williams, R. H., Jones, S. & Young, A. H. (1999). Effects of dexamethasone on neuroendocrine and psychological responses to L-tryptophan infusion. *Psychopharmacology*, **143**, 64–71.

Posener, J. A., DeBattista, C., Williams, G. H., Kraemer, H. C., Kalehzan, M. & Schatzberg, A. F. (2000). 24-hour monitoring of cortisol and corticotropin secretion in psychotic and nonpsychotic major depression. *Arch. Gen. Psychiatry*, **57**, 755–60.

Price, L. H., Malison, R. T., McDougle, C. J. & Pelton, G. H. (1996). Antiglucorticoids as treatments for depression. Rational use and therapeutic potential. *CNS Drugs*, **5**, 311–20.

Price, L. H., Cappiello, A., Malison, R. T. *et al.* (1997). Effects of antiglucocorticoid treatment on 5-HT$_{1a}$ function in depressed patients and healthy subjects. *Neuropsychopharmacology*, **17**, 246–57.

Price, M. L., Curtis, A. L., Kirby, L. G., Valentino, R. J. & Lucki, I. (1998). Effects of corticotropin-releasing factor on brain serotonergic activity. *Neuropsychopharmacology*, **18**, 492–502.

Pugh, C. R., Tremblay, D., Fleshner, M. & Rudy, J. W. (1997). Selective role for corticosterone in contextual-fear conditioning. *Behav. Neurosci.*, **111**, 503–11.

Puglisi-Allegra, S., Imperato, A., Angelucci, L. & Cabib, S. (1991). Acute stress induces time-dependent responses in dopamine mesolimbic system. *Brain Res.*, **554**, 217–22.

Purba, J. S., Hoogendijk, W. J. G., Hofman, M. A. & Swaab, D. F. (1996). Increased number of vaso-pressin neurons in the paraventricular nucleus of the human hypothalamus in depression. *Arch. Gen. Psychiatry*, **53**, 137–43.

Raadsheer, F. C., Hoogendijk, W. J. G., Hofman, M. A. & Swaab, D. F. (1994). Increased numbers of corticotropin-releasing hormone neurons in the hypothalamic-paraventricular nucleus of depressed patients. *Clin. Neuroendocrinology*, **60**, 436–44.

Raadsheer, F. C., Van Heerikhuize, J. J., Lucassen, P. J., Hoogendijk, W. J., Tilders, F. J. & Swaab, D. F. (1995). Corticotropin-releasing hormone mRNA levels in the paraventricular nucleus of patients with Alzheimer's disease and depression. *Am. J. Psychiatry*, **152**, 1372–6.

Rasmusson, A. M., Shi, L. & Duman, R. (2002). Downregulation of BDNF mRNA in the hippocampal dentate gyrus after re-exposure to cues previously associated with footshock. *Neuropsychopharmacology*, **27**, 133–42.

Ratka, A., Sutanto, W., Bloemers, M. & De Kloet, E. R. (1989). On the role of mineralocorticoid (type I) and glucocorticoid (type 2) receptors in neuroendocrine regulation. *Neuroendocrinology*, **50**, 117–23.

Ravaris, C. L., Sateia, M. J., Beroza, K. W., Noordsy, D. L. & Brinck-Johnsen, T. (1988). Effect of ketoconazole on a hypophysectomized hypercortisolemic, psychotically depressed woman. *Arch. Gen. Psychiatry*, **45**, 966–7.

Rënyi, L., Evenden, J. L., Fowler, C. J. *et al.* (2001). The pharmacological profile of (*R*)-3,4-Dihydro-*N*-isopropyl-3-(*N*-isopropyl-*N*-propylamino)-2*H*-1-benzopyran-5-carboxamide, a selective 5-hydroxytryptamine$_{1A}$ receptor agonist. *J. Pharmacol. Exper. Ther.*, **299**, 883–93.

Resnick, H. S., Yehuda, R., Foy, D. W. & Pitman, R. K. (1995). Effect of prior trauma on acute hormonal response to rape. *Am. J. Psychiatry*, **152**, 1675–7.

Reul, J. M. H. M. & Holsboer, F. (2002). Corticotropin-releasing factor receptors 1 and 2 in anxiety and depression. *Curr. Opin. Pharmacol.*, **2**, 23–33.

Reul, J. M., Stec, I., Soder, M. & Holsboer, F. (1993). Chronic treatment of rats with the antidepressant amitriptyline attenuates the activity of the hypothalamic-pituitary-adrenocortical system. *Endocrinology*, **133**, 312–20.

Reul, J. M., Labeur, M. S., Grigoriadis, D. E., De Souza, E. B. & Holsboer, F. (1994). Hypothalamic-pituitary-adrenocortical axis changes in the rat after long-term treatment with the reversible monoamine oxidase-A inhibitor moclobemide. *Neuroendocrinology*, **60**, 509–19.

Reus, V. I., Wolkowitz, O. M. & Frederick, S. (1997). Antiglucocorticoid treatments in psychiatry. *Psychoneuroendocrinology*, **22**, S121–4.

Reyes, T. M., Lewis, K. & Perrin, M. H. (2001). Urocortin II: a member of the corticotropin releasing factor (CRF) neuropeptide family that is selectively bound to type 2 CRF receptors. *Proc. Natl. Acad. Sci. USA*, **98**, 2843–8.

Ribeiro, S. C. M., Tandon, R., Grunhaus, L. & Greden, J. F. (1993). The DST as a predictor of outcome in depression: a meta-analysis. *Am. J. Psychiatry*, **150**, 1618–29.

Rind, B., Tromovitch, Ph. & Bauserman, R. (1998). A meta-analytic examination of assumed properties of child sexual abuse using college samples. *Psychol. Bull.*, **124**, 22–53.

Rinne, Th., De Kloet, E. R., Wouters, L., Goekoop, J. G., De Rijk, R. H. & Van den Brink, W. (2002). Hyperresponsiveness of hypothalamic-pituitary-adrenal axis to combined dexamethasone/corticotropin-releasing hormone challenge in female borderline personality disorder subjects with a history of sustained childhood abuse. *Biol. Psychiatry*, **52**, 1102–12.

(2003). Fluvoxamine reduces responsiveness of HPA axis in adult female BPD patients with a history of sustained childhood abuse. *Neuropsychopharmacology*, **28**, 126–32.

Rodgers, R. J., Haller, J., Holmes, A., Halasz, J., Walton, T. J. & Brain, P. F. (1999). Corticosterone response to the plus-maze: High correlation with risk assessment in rats and mice. *Physiol. Behavior*, **68**, 47–53.

Romero, L. M. & Sapolsky, R. M. (1996). Patterns of ACTH secretagog secretion in response to psychological stimuli. *J. Neuroendocrinol.*, **8**, 243–58.

Rosenblum, L. A. & Paully, G. S. (1984). The effects of varying environmental demands on maternal and infant behavior. *Child Dev.*, **55**, 305–14.

Rosenblum, L. A., Coplan, J. D., Friedman, S., Bassoff, T., Gorman, J. M. & Andrews, M. W. (1994). Adverse early experiences affect noradrenergic and serotonergic functioning in adult primates. *Biol. Psychiatry*, **35**, 221–7.

Rothchild, A. J., Langlais, P. J., Schatzberg, A. F., Walsh, F. X., Cole, J. O. & Bird, E. D. (1984). Dexamethasone increases plasma free dopamine in man. *J. Psychiatry Res.*, **18**, 217–23.

Roy, A. (1985). Early parental separation and adult depression. *Arch. Gen. Psychiatry*, **42**, 987–91.

Sachar, E., Hellman, L., Fukushima, D. K. & Gallagher, T. F. (1970). Cortisol production in depressive illness. *Arch. Gen. Psychiatry*, **23**, 289–98.

Sadowski, H., Ugarte, B., Kolvin, I., Kaplan, C. & Barnes, J. (1999). Early life family disadvantages and major depression in adulthood. *Br. J. Psychiatry*, **174**, 112–20.

Sapolsky, R. M. (1992). *Stress, the Aging Brain and the Mechanism of Neuron Death*. Cambridge, MA: MIT Press.

(1996). Why stress is bad for your brain. *Science*, **273**, 749–50.

Sapolsky, R. M., Uno, H., Rebert, C. S. & Finch, C. E. (1990). Hippocampal damage associated with prolonged glucocorticoid exposure in primates. *J. Neurosci.*, **10**, 2897–902.

Sapolsky, R. M., Romero, L. M. & Munck, A. U. (2000). How do glucocorticoids influence stress responses? Integrating permissive, suppressive, stimulatory and preparative actions. *Endocr. Rev.*, **21**, 55–89.

Sartor, O. & Cutler, G. B, Jr (1996). Mifepristone: treatment of Cushing's syndrome. *Clin. Obstet. Gynecol.*, **39**, 506–10.

Schaaf, M. J. M., Workel, J. O., Lesscher, M., Vreugdenhil, E., Oitzl, M. S. & De Kloet, E. R. (2001). Correlation between hippocampal BDNF mRNA expression and memory performance in senescent rats. *Brain Res.*, **915**, 227–33.

Schatzberg, A. F., Rothschild, A. J., Langlais, P. J., Bird, E. D. & Cole, J. O. (1985). A corticosteroid/dopamine hypothesis for psychotic depression and related states. *J. Psychiatry Res.*, **19**, 57–64.

Schmidt, M., Enthoven, L., Van der Maark, M., Levine, S., de Kloet, E. R. & Oitzl, M. S. (2003). The postnatal development of the hypothalamic-pituitary-adrenal axis in the mouse. *Int. J. Dev. Neurosci.*, **21**, 125–32.

Schreiber, W., Lauer, C. J., Krumrey, K., Holsboer, F. & Krieg, J. C. (1996). Dysregulation of the hypothalamic-pituitary-adrenocortical system in panic disorder. *Neuropsychopharmacology*, **15**, 7–15.

Schulkin, J., Gold, P. W. & McEwen, B. S. (1998). Induction of corticotropin- releasing hormone gene expression by glucocorticoids: implication for understanding the states of fear and anxiety and allostatic load. *Psychoneuroendocrinology*, **23**, 219–43.

Scott, L. V. & Dinan, T. G. (1998). Vasopressin and the regulation of hypothalamic-pituitary-adrenal axis function: implications for the pathophysiology of depression. *Life Sci.*, **62**, 1985–98.

Scott, L. V., Thakore, J., Burnett, F. & Dinan, T. G. (1999). A preliminary study of dexamethasone treatment on pituitary-adrenal responsivity in major depression. *Hum. Psychopharm. Clin. Exp.*, **14**, 587–91.

Seckl, J. & Fink, G. (1991). Use of in situ hybridization to investigate the regulation of hippocampal corticosteroid receptors by monoamines. *J. Steroid Biochem. Mol. Biol.*, **40**, 685–8.
  (1992). Antidepressants increase glucocorticoid and mineralocorticoid receptor mRNA expression in rat hippocampus in vivo. *Neuroendocrinology*, **55**, 621–6.

Selye, H. (1936). Syndrome produced by diverse nocuous agents. *Nature*, **138**, 32.

Sheline, Y. I., Wang, P. W., Gado, M. H., Csernansky, J. G & Vannier, M, W. (1996). Hippocampal atrophy in recurrent major depression. *Proc. Natl. Acad. Sci. USA*, **93**, 3908–13.

Sheline, Y. I., Sanghavi, M., Mintun, M. A. & Gado, M. H. (1999). Depression duration but not age predicts hippocampal volume loss in medically healthy women with recurrent major depression. *J. Neurosci.*, **19**, 5034–43.

Shively, C. A., Laber-Laird, K. & Anton, R. F. (1997). Behavior and physiology of social stress and depression in female cynomolgus monkeys. *Biol. Psychiatry*, **41**, 871–82.

Singh, A., Petrides, J. S., Gold, Ph. W., Chrousos, G. P. & Deuster, P. A. (1999). Differential hypothalamic-pituitary-adrenal axis reactivity to psychological and physical stress. *J. Clin. Endocrinol. Metab.*, **84**, 1944–8.

Skutella, T., Criswell, H., Moy, S. *et al.* (1994). Corticotropin-releasing hormone (CRH) antisense oligodeoxynucleotide induces anxiolytic effects in rat. *Neuroreport*, **2**, 2181–5.

Smith, C. E., Ware, C. J. & Cowen, P. J. (1991). Pindolol decreases prolactin and growth hormone responses to intravenous L-tryptophan. *Psychopharmacology*, **103**, 140–2.

Smith, M. A. (1996). Hippocampal vulnerability to stress and aging: possible role of neurotrophic factors. *Behav. Brain Res.*, **78**, 25–36.

Southwick, S. M. & Yehuda, R. (1993). The interaction between pharmacotherapy and psychotherapy in the treatment of posttraumatic stress disorder. *Am. J. Psychother.*, **47**, 404–10.

Souza, E. B. de & van Loon, G. R. (1986). Brain serotonin and catecholamine responses to repeated stress in rats. *Brain Res.*, **367**, 77–86.

Spencer, R. L., Miller, A. H., Moday, H. *et al.* (1996). Chronic social stress produces reductions in available splenic type II corticosteroid receptor binding and plasma corticosteroid binding globulin levels. *Psychoneuroendocrinology*, **21**, 95–109.

Starkman M. N., Gebarski, S. S., Berent, S. & Schteingart, D. E. (1992). Hippocampal formation volume, memory dysfunction, and cortisol levels in patients with Cushing syndrome. *Biol. Psychiatry*, **32**, 756–65.

Stein, M. B., Koverola, C., Hanna, C., Torchia, M. G. & McClarty, B. (1997a). Hippocampal volume in women victimized by childhood sexual abuse. *Psychol. Med.*, **27**, 951–9.

Stein, M. B., Yehuda, R., Koverola, C. & Hanna, C. (1997b). Enhanced dexamethasone suppression of plasma cortisol in adult women traumatized by childhood sexual abuse. *Biol. Psychiatry*, **42**, 680–6.

Sterling, P. & Eyer, J. (1981). Allostasis: a new paradigm to explain arousal pathology. In *Handbook of Life Stress, Cognition and Health*, ed. S. Fisher & J. Reason. New York: John Wiley & Sons.

Stout, S. C., Kilts, C. D. & Nemeroff, C. B. (1995). Neuropeptides and stress. Preclinical findings and implications for pathophysiology. In *Neurobiological and Clinical Consequences of Stress: from Normal Adaptation to PTSD*, ed. M. J. Friedman, D. S. Charney & A. Y. Deutch. Philadelphia: Lippincott-Raven Publishers.

Sullivan, E. V., Pfefferbaum, A., Swan, G. E. & Carmelli, D. (2001). Heritability of hippocampal size in elderly twin men: equivalent influence from genes and environment. *Hippocampus* **11**, 754–62.

Susman, E. J., Schmeelk, K. H., Worrall, B. K., Granger, D. A., Ponirakis, A. & Chrousos, G. P. (1999). Corticotropin-releasing hormone and cortisol: longitudinal associations with depression and antisocial behavior in adolescents. *J. Am. Acad. Child Adolesc. Psychiatry*, **38**, 460–7.

Takao, K., Nagatani, T., Kitamura, Y. & Yamawaki, S. (1997). Effects of corticosterone on 5-HT$_{1a}$ and 5-HT$_2$ receptor binding and on the receptor-mediated behavioral responses of rats. *Eur. J. Pharmacol.*, **333**, 123–8.

Tennant, C. (1988). Parental loss in childhood: its effect in adult life. *Arch. Gen. Psychiatry*, **45**, 1045–50.

Thakore, J. H. & Dinan, T. G. (1994). D-fenfluramine-induced prolactin release in depression: the acute effects of ketoconazole. *J. Seroton. Res.*, **3**, 207–13.

Timpl, P., Spanagel, R., Sillaber, I. *et al.* (1998). Impaired stress response and reduced anxiety in mice lacking a functional corticotropin-releasing hormone receptor 1. *Nat. Genet.*, **19**, 162–6.

Vakili, K., Pillay, S. S., Lafer, B. *et al.* (2000). Hippocampal volume in primary unipolar major depression: a magnetic resonance imaging study. *Biol. Psychiatry*, **47**, 1087–90.

Vale, W. J., Spies, J., Rivier, C. & Rivier, J. (1981). Characterization of a 41-residue ovine hypothalamic peptide that stimulates secretion of corticotropin and ß-endorphin. *Science*, **213**, 1394–6.

Valentino, R. J., Foote, S. L. & Aston-Jones, G. (1983). Corticotropin-releasing hormone activates noradrenergic neurons of the locus coeruleus. *Brain Res.*, **270**, 363–7.

Van den Berg, D. T. W. M., De Kloet, E. R., Van Dijken, H. H. & De Jong, W. (1990). Differential central effects of mineralocorticoid and glucocorticoid agonists and antagonists on blood pressure. *Endocrinology*, **126**, 118–24.

Van den Berg, D. T. W. M., De Jong, W. & De Kloet, E. R. (1994). Mineralocorticoid antagonist inhibits stress-induced blood pressure response after repeated daily warming. *Am. J. Physiol. (Endocrinol. Metab.)*, **267**(30), E921–6.

Van den Buuse M., Van Acker, S. A. B. E, Fluttert, M. J. & De Kloet, E. R. (2002). Involvement of corticosterone in cardiovascular responses to an open field novelty stressor in freely moving rats. *Physiol. Behav.*, **75**, 207–15.

Van der Kolk, B. A., Pelcovitz, D., Roth, S., Mandel, F. S., McFarlane, A. & Herman, J. L. (1996). Dissociation, somatization, and affect dysregulation: the complexity of adaptation to trauma. *Am. J. Psychiatry*, **153**, (suppl. 7) 83–93.

Van der Lely, A. J., Foeken, K., van der Mast, R. C. & Lamberts, S. W. J. (1991). Rapid reversal of acute psychosis in the Cushing syndrome with the cortisol receptor antagonist mifepristone (RU 486) *Ann. Int. Med.* **114**, 143–4.

Van der Pool, J., Rosenthal, N., Chrousos, G. P. *et al.* (1991). Evidence for hypothalamic CRH deficiency in patients with seasonal affective disorder. *J. Clin. Endocrinol. Metab.*, **72**, 1382–87.

Van Eck, M., Berkhof, H., Nicolson, N. & Sulon, J. (1996). The effects of perceived stress, traits, mood states, and stressful daily events on salivary cortisol. *Psychosom. Med.*, **58**, 447–58.

Van Haarst, A. D., Oitzl, M. S., Workel, J. O. & De Kloet, E. R. (1996). Chronic glucocorticoid receptor blockade enhances the rise in circadian and stress-induced pituitary-adrenal activity. *Endocrinology*, **137**, 4935–43.

Van Londen, L., Goekoop, J. G., van Kempen, G. M. *et al.* (1997). Plasma levels of arginine vasopressin elevated in patients with major depression. *Neuropsychopharmacology*, **17**, 284–92.

Van Oers, H. J. J., De Kloet, E. R., Whelan, T. & Levine, S. (1998). Maternal deprivation effect on the infants neural stress markers is reversed by tactile stimulation and feeding but not by suppressing corticosterone. *J. Neurosci.*, **18**, 10171–9.

Van Praag, H. M. (2002). Crossroads of corticotropin-releasing hormone, corticosteroids and monoamines: about a biological interface between stress and depression. *Neurotox. Res.*, **4**, 531–55.

Lest thou forget. About recollections one wants to erase but cannot. *Prog. Neuropsychopharm. Biol. Psychiatry*, in press.

Van Praag, H., Schinder, A. F., Christie, B. R., Toni, N., Palmer, T. D. & Gage, F. H. (2002). Functional neurogenesis in the adult hippocampus. *Nature*, **415**, 1030–4.

Virgin, C. E. Jr., Ha, T. P., Packan, D. R. *et al.* (1991). Glucocorticoids inhibit glucose transport and glutamate uptake in hippocampal astrocytes: implications for glucocorticoid neurotoxicity. *J. Neurochem.*, **57**, 1422–8.

Von Bardeleben, U., Holsboer, F., Stalla, G. K. & Muller, O. A. (1985). Combined administration of human corticotropin-releasing factor and lysine vasopressin induces cortisol escape from dexamethasone suppression in healthy subjects. *Life Sci.*, **37**, 1613–18.

Vythilingam, M., Heim, Ch., Newport, J. *et al.* (2002). Childhood trauma associated with smaller hippocampal volume in women with major depression. *Am. J. Psychiatry*, **159**, 2027–80.

Watanabe, Y., Gould, E. & McEwen, B. S. (1992). Stress induces atrophy of apical dendrites of hippocampal CA3 pyramidal neurons. *Brain Res.*, **588**, 341–5.

Watanabe, L. Y., Sakai, R. R., McEwen, B. S. & Mendelson, S. (1993). Stress and antidepressant effects on hippocampal and cortical 5-HT$_{1a}$ and 5-HT$_2$ receptors and transport sites for serotonin. *Brain Res.*, **615**, 87–94.

Watson, S., Gallagher, P., Del-Estal, D., Hearn, A., Ferrier, I. N. & Young, A. H. (2002). Hypothalamic-pituitary-adrenal axis function in patients with chronic depression. *Psychol. Med.*, **32**, 1021–8.

Webster, M. J., O'Grady, J. O., Orthmann, C. & Freed, W. J. (1999). Decreased glucocorticoid receptor mRNA levels in individuals with depression, bipolar disorder and schizophrenia. *Schizophr. Res.*, **41**, III.

Weinstock, M. (1997). Does prenatal stress impair coping and regulation of hypothalamic-pituitary-adrenal axis? *Neurosci. Biobehav. Rev.*, **21**, 1–10.

Weinstock, M. (2001). Alterations induced by gestational stress in brain morphology and behaviour of the offspring. *Progr. Neurobiol.*, **65**, 427–51.

Weinstock, M., Fride, E. & Hertzberg, R. (1988). Prenatal stress effects on functional development of the offspring. *Progr. Brain Res.*, **73**, 319–31.

Weiss, E. L., Longhurst, J. G. & Mazure, C. M. (1999). Childhood sexual abuse as a risk factor for depression in women: psychosocial and neurobiological correlates. *Am. J. Psychiatry*, **156**, 816–28.

Weiss, J. M., Goodman, P. A., Losito, B. G., Corrigan, S., Charry, J. M. & Bailey, W. H. (1981). Behavioral depression produced by an uncontrollable stressor: relationship to norepinephrine, dopamine, and serotonin levels in various regions of rat brain. *Brain Res. Rev.*, **3**, 167–205.

Weninger, S. C., Dunn, A. J., Muglia L. J. *et al.* (1999). Stress-induced behaviors require the corticotropin-releasing hormone (CRH) receptor, but not CRH. *Proc. Natl. Acad. Sci. USA*, **96**, 8283–8.

Whalley, L. J., Borthwick, N., Copolov, D., Dick, H., Christie, J. E. & Fink, G. (1986). Glucocorticoid receptors and depression. *Br. Med. J.*, **292**, 859–61.

Wissow, L. S. (1995). Child abuse and neglect. *New Engl. J. Med.*, **332**, 1425–31.

Wolkowitz, O. M. & Reus, V. I. (1999). Treatment of depression with antiglucocorticoid drugs. *Psychosom. Med.*, **61**, 698–711.

Wolkowitz, O. M., Sutton, M. E., Doran, A. R. *et al.* (1985). Dexamethasone increases plasma HVA but not MHPG in normal humans. *Psychiatry Res.*, **16**, 101–9.

Wolkowitz, O., Sutton, M., Koulu, M. *et al.* (1986). Chronic corticosterone administration in rats: behavioral and biochemical evidence of increased central dopaminergic activity. *Eur. J. Pharmacol.*, **122**, 329–38.

Wolkowitz, O. M., Reus, V. I., Weingartner, H. *et al.* (1990). Cognitive effects of corticosteroids. *Am. J. Psychiatry*, **147**, 1297–303.

Wolkowitz, O. M., Reus, V. I., Weingartner, H. *et al.* (1999a). Treatment of depression with antiglucocorticoid drugs. *Psychosom. Med.*, **61**, 698–711.

(1999b). Antiglucocorticoid treatment of depression: double-blind ketoconazole. *Biol. Psychiatry*, **45**, 1070–4.

Wong, M.-L., Kling, M. A., Munson, P. J. *et al.* (2000). Pronounced and sustained central hyper-noradrenergic function in major depression with melancholic features: relation to hyper-corticolism and corticotropin-releasing hormone. *Proc. Natl. Acad. Sci. USA*, **97**, 325–30.

Woodman, D. D., Hinton, J. W. & O'Neill, M. T. (1978). Cortisol secretion and stress in maximum security hospital patients. *J. Psychosom. Res.*, **22**, 133–6.

Woolley, C. S., Gould, E. & McEwen, B. S. (1990). Exposure to excess glucocorticoids alters dendritic morphology and adult hippocampal neurons. *Brain Res.*, **531**, 225–31.

Workel, J. O., Oitzl, M. S., Fluttert, M., Lesscher, H., Karssen, A. & De Kloet, E. R. (2001). Differential and age-dependent effects of maternal deprivation on the hypothalamic-pituitary-adrenal axis of brown Norway rats from youth to senescence. *J. Neuroendocrinol.*, **13**, 1–13.

Yama, M. F., Tovey, S. L. & Fogas, B. S. (1993). Childhood family environment and sexual abuse as predictors of anxiety and depression in adult women. *Am. J. Orthopsychiatry*, **63**, 136–41.

Yamada, S., Watanabe, A., Nankai, M. & Toru, M. (1995). Acute immobilization stress reduces ($\pm$)DOI-induced 5-HT_{2a} receptor-mediated head shakes in rats. *Psychopharmacology*, **119**, 9–14.

Yan, W., Wilson, C. C. & Haring, J. H. (1997). 5-HT_{1a} receptors mediate the neurotrophic effect of serotonin on developing dentate granule cells. *Dev. Brain Res.*, **98**, 185–90.

Yehuda, R. (2000). Biology of posttraumatic stress disorder. *J. Clin. Psychiatry*, **61**, (suppl. 7) 14–21.

Yehuda, R., Southwick, S. M., Nussbaum, G., Wahby, V., Giller, E. L., & Mason, J. (1990). Low urinary cortisol excretion in patients with posttraumatic stress disorder. *J. Nerv. Ment. Dis.*, **187**, 366–9.

Yehuda, R., Lowy, M. T., Southwick, S. M., Shaffer, D. & Giller, E. L. (1991). Lymphocyte glucocorticoid receptor number in posttraumatic stress disorder. *Am. J. Psychiatry*, **148**, 499–504.

Yehuda, R., Southwick, S. M., Krystal, J. H., Bremner, D. C. & Mason, J. W. (1993). Enhanced suppression of cortisol following dexamethasone administration in posttraumatic stress disorder. *Am. J. Psychiatry*, **150**, 83–6.

Yehuda, R., Boisoneau, D., Lowy, M. T. & Giller, E. L. (1995a). Dose-response changes in plasma cortisol and lymphocyte glucocorticoid receptors following dexamethasone administration in combat veterans with and without posttraumatic stress disorder. *Arch. Gen. Psychiatry*, **52**, 583–93.

Yehuda, R., Kahana, B., Binder-Brynes, K., Southwick, S. M., Mason, J. W. & Giller, E. L. (1995b). Low urinary cortisol excretion in Holocaust survivors with posttraumatic stress disorder. *Am. J. Psychiatry*, **152**, 982–6.

Yehuda, R., Teicher, M. H., Trestman, R. L., Levengood, R. A. & Siever, L. J. (1996). Cortisol regulation in posttraumatic stress disorder and major depression: a chronobiological analysis. *Biol. Psychiatry*, **40**, 79–88.

Yehuda, R., McFarlane, A. C. & Shalev, A. Y. (1998). Predicting the development of posttraumatic stress disorder from the acute response to a traumatic event. *Biol. Psychiatry*, **44**, 1305–13.

Young, A. H., Goodwin, G. M., Dick, H. & Fink, G. (1994). Effects of glucocorticoids on 5-HT$_{1a}$ presynaptic function in the mouse. *Psychopharmacology*, **114**, 360–4.

Young, E. A. & Vazquez, D. (1996). Hypercortisolemia, hippocampal glucocorticoid receptors, and fast feedback. *Mol. Psychiatry*, **1**, 149–59.

Young, E. A., Haskett, R. F., Murphy-Weinberg, V., Watson, S. J. & Akil, H. (1991). Loss of glucocorticoid fast feedback in depression. *Arch. Gen. Psychiatry*, **48**, 693–9.

Young, E. A., Lopez, J. F., Murphy-Weinberg, V., Watson, S. J. & Akil, H. (2000). Hormonal evidence for altered responsiveness to social stress in major depression. *Neuropsychopharmacology*, **23**, 411–18.

Young, E. A., Lopez, J. F., Murphy-Weinberg, V., Watson, S. J. & Akil, H. (2003). Mineralocorticoid receptor function in major depression. *Arch. Gen. Psychiatry*, **60**, 24–8.

Zacharko, R. M. & Anisman, H. (1991). Stressor-induced anhedonia and the mesocorticolimbic system. *Neurosci. Biobehav. Rev.*, **15**, 391–405.

Zobel, A. W., Yassourides, A., Frieboes R. M. & Holsboer, F. (1999). Prediction of medium term outcome by cortisol response to the combined dexamethasone-CRH test in patients with remitted depression. *Am. J. Psychiatry*, **156**, 949–51.

Zobel, A. W., Nickel, T., Künzel, H. E. *et al.* (2000). Effects of the high affinity corticotropin releasing hormone receptor 1 antagonist R 121919 in major depression: the first 20 patients treated. *J. Psychiatry Res.*, **34**, 171–81.

Zobel, A. W., Nickel, T., Sonntag, A., Uhr, M., Holsboer, F. & Ising, M. (2001). Cortisol response in the combined dexamethasone/CRH test as predictor of relapse in patients with remitted depression: a prospective study. *J. Psychiatry Res.*, **35**, 83–94.

Stress, the brain and depression

9.1 The stress syndrome and depression: psychopathological and biological overlap

Depression is often preceded by life events, i.e. traumatizing occurrences that the stricken individual was unable to process and assimilate adequately, and/or by difficulties and worries that linger on for some time or for a long time and for which no solution seems to come in sight (Chapter 4). Such events and circumstances generate states of psychic distress which vary phenomenologically inter-individually, and over time also intra-individually. Yet certain features are seldom missed. This holds in particular for anxiety and (manifest or suppressed) anger. The psychic manifestations of distress are accompanied by a host of hormonal, autonomic and immunological alterations (Chapter 8). Collectively the behavioural and bodily changes are named the stress response or the stress syndrome.

The trigger of the stress syndrome may be a severe disturbance of corporeal integrity, but more often it is experiential in nature. In that case it is the feeling of frustration or of being endangered, either in a physical or psychological sense that gets the stress reaction underway. Such experiences lead to activation of the corticotrophin releasing hormone (CRH) and noradrenaline (NA) systems (Chapter 8), two systems that are thought to be the driving forces behind the ensuing cascade of stress phenomena.

Behaviourally, enhanced NA ergic activity leads initially to a state of arousal and increased vigilance and, if pronounced or prolonged, to heightened anxiety. In the long run, however, the NA ergic system may become exhausted and the state of NA ergic hypoactivity that follows is associated with motor retardation, cognitive inhibition and defects in emotional memory (Chapter 8).

Activation of CRH-producing cells in the parvocellular part of the hypothalamic paraventricular nucleus (PVN), gives rise to increased release of CRH, subsequently of ACTH and ultimately of cortisol. Activation of the extrahypothalamic CRH nerve cells probably activates anxiety-related circuitry and provokes behaviours reminiscent of depression, at least in animals (Chapter 8).

Increased cortisol levels stimulate central NA ergic systems as well as extrahypothalamic CRH neurons and in this way will reinforce the anxious state. Usually a rise in cortisol level will be self-limiting. Via stimulation of glucocorticoid receptors (GRs), cortisol inhibits the release of CRH and ACTH. This negative feedback system, however, may fail. In that case sustained stress will be accompanied by sustained hypercortisolism. Add to all this that extra-hypothalamic CRH pathways and NA ergic pathways interact in a reverberative stimulatory fashion, and it follows that ongoing hypercortisolism will be associated with a persistent state of increased tension and anxiety.

Persistent hypercortisolism, moreover, has a pronounced impact on the 5-HT ergic system. Initially cortisol stimulates 5-hydroxytryptamine (5-HT, serotonin) metabolism. Sustained increase of cortisol levels, however, lead to a decline of 5-HT synthesis. Furthermore 5-HT receptor function is influenced by persisting hypercortisolaemia. The expression of 5-HT_{1A} receptors is decreased, while 5-HT_{2c} and 5-HT_{2A} receptors are upregulated either as a primary cortisol effect or secondary to 5-HT_{1A} downregulation.

The 5-HT system comprises both anxiolytic and anxiogenic components (Chapter 7). The 5-HT innervation of the amygdala and hippocampus, originating from the dorsal raphe nuclei, exerts anxiogenic effects, mediated most likely via 5-HT_2 receptors. Pathways from the median raphe nuclei to the hippocampus, acting via 5-HT_{1A} receptors, exert anxiolytic effects. Therefore, upregulation of 5-HT_2 receptors and downregulation of 5-HT_{1A} receptors will both contribute to the anxious state.

Generally speaking, enhancing 5-HT ergic activity reduces aggressive behaviours, while inhibiting 5-HT ergic activity has opposite effects. This has been demonstrated in animals, at least for particular forms of aggression, most notably for offensive aggression (Chapter 7). 5-HT_{1A} and $5\text{-HT}_{1B/D}$ receptors are involved in aggression-modulation, most likely those with postsynaptic localization (Olivier *et al.*, 1999). Activation of these receptor types by selective agonists leads to pronounced reduction in, for instance, the resident-intruder paradigm, whereby intrusion of an unfamiliar male into the home territory of a congener provokes aggression in the resident. The effect is specific in that disruptive effects on exploration and motor activity do not appear (Saudou *et al.*, 1994; Olivier *et al.*, 1995; De Boer *et al.*, 1999). Downregulation of 5-HT_{1A} receptors, then, can be expected to facilitate (particular forms of) aggressive behaviours.

Several biological sequelae of the stressed state are also found in certain forms of depression: increased activity of the HPA axis, signs of hyper- or hypoactivity of the CA ergic system, lowering of 5-HT metabolism, and decreased density of

Table 9.1. Biological sequelae of the stressed state also found in (certain forms of) depression.

Stress	Depression
↑ CRH	↑ CRH
↑ cortisol	↑ cortisol
↑ MA ergic activity (initially)	↑ NA ergic activity
	↓ DA ergic activity
↓ MA ergic activity (subsequently)	↓ 5-HT metabolism
	↓ responsivity 5-HT$_{1A}$ receptor

5-HT receptors, among which is the 5-HT$_{1A}$ receptor (Table 9.1; Chapter 7). The two conditions overlap psychopathologically, too. In a subgroup of depressed patients, for instance, anxiety and/or signs of increased aggression directed to oneself or towards others, are prominent features just as they often are in stress syndromes.

Taking the psychopathological and biological data summarized above together, the following questions arise.

1 Are states of increased anxiety/aggression and states of depression causally related? In other words, might anxiety/aggression dysregulation trigger a depressed state?

2 Are the 5-HT disturbances demonstrable in subgroups of patients with recurrent depression associated with disturbances in anxiety and aggression regulation, taking into account that such disturbances are prominent in some depressed patients?

3 Are patients with recurrent depression and signs of 5-HT ergic disturbances stress-prone, in that they respond more easily and vehemently with anxiety and anger to adversities and frustrations than control populations?

In other words, is there any evidence for the existence of a subtype of depression in which defective coping abilities, destabilization of 5-HT ergic circuits, defective anxiety and aggression regulation and ultimately mood lowering coalesce?

Before addressing these questions a brief and general account will be given of the interconnections of anxiety, aggression and depression and subsequently on the ways the resulting diagnostic problems have been handled.

9.2 Depression, anxiety and aggression: the concept of comorbidity

Very frequently mood and anxiety disorders appear hand in hand (Kessler, 1998). Depression and disturbed aggression regulation, too, are strongly intertwined. Depression is a major suicide precursor (van Heeringen, 2001) and manifestations of increased outward directed aggression, too, frequently form part of depressive syndromes (see next section). The two prevailing taxonomies – DSM and ICD – however, do not recognize a category of aggression disorders. Hence no data are available on mood pathology and anxiety in conditions in which aggression dysregulation is a major feature. Yet, it seems likely that mood, anxiety and aggression (disorders) show a high degree of comorbidity.

The concept of comorbidity is a typical product of the nosological disease model, according to which mental pathology is subdividable in discrete and separable entities, called disorders. In the absence of clear data on causation, a disorder is defined in terms of symptoms, course, outcome, and if possible treatment response. The alleged discreteness of mental disorders allows several disorders to be diagnosed in the same patient, at the same time. In diagnosing comorbid conditions an allusion as to their possible mutual interrelation is generally lacking. Has one disorder index-status, to which the others are subsequent, or do they occur independently, and in the former case does it seem likely that the index disorder is causally related to the later ones? The term comorbidity is used in a purely descriptive sense and without relational suppositions. As such it seems a handy term to avoid the diagnostic problems referred to and the questions raised by the intertwinement of anxiety and mood disturbances (Van Praag, 1996a). Yet, the concept of comorbidity is less practically useful than it seems. A major confounder is that anxiety and mood disorders share a number of symptoms – not only feelings of tension and restlessness, anxiety and sadness, but in addition sleep disturbances, fatigue, difficulties with concentration, various somatic symptoms, lack of self-esteem and feelings of uncertainty. This can make it difficult to decide whether we deal with comorbid anxiety and mood disorders, or with a depression with pronounced anxiety, or with an anxiety disorder with marked signs of mood dysregulation.

Furthermore, the introduction of diagnoses such as subsyndromal mood and anxiety disorders has complicated matters (Chapter 1). These constructs refer to syndromes that do not meet DSM-formulated criteria (Judd et al., 1997). Those syndromes, however, are ill-defined. It is often unclear whether severity has been the critical diagnostic factor or number of symptoms. In fact many different definitions are in circulation. Moreover the border between subsyndromal psychopathology and still-normal states of dreariness and restlessness is ill-defined. It is also undecided if one symptom is enough for a subsyndromal diagnosis, or if more symptoms are required, and which symptoms are decisive, if any. Listing a number of comorbid syndromal conditions in what is supposed to be a comprehensive diagnosis is often equivalent to setting up a smoke screen to conceal diagnostic impotence.

Finally, states of disordered mood and anxiety regulation are not stable over time. Symptoms wax or wane, and vary in intensity. Sometimes they reach case level with respect to number and intensity; at other times they sink beneath threshold levels. Comorbidity statements, thus depend on time of evaluation.

The concept of comorbidity, then, leaves plenty of room for diagnostic uncertainty.

9.3 Comorbidity of depression, anxiety and aggression: some numbers

9.3.1 Intercorrelation of the symptoms of mood lowering, anxiety and aggressivity

Mood lowering and feelings of anxiety and tension frequently go hand in hand. This holds for normal individuals in trouble and for patients with mental disorders. Patients with depression very often report feeling anxious, without qualifying for a DSM 'certified' anxiety disorder, and vice versa patients with an anxiety disorder regularly feel depressed, without suffering from a regular depression (Pini *et al.*, 1997). Patients with depression, for instance, score high on depression as well as on anxiety scales (Wetzler *et al.*, 1990). Patients with major depression or dysthymia had even higher scores on anxiety scales than patients with anxiety disorders (Di Nardo & Barlow, 1990).

Disturbances of aggression regulation are a frequent component of mood disorders. The aggression can be turned inward, manifesting itself as self-denigration or suicidality, or can be directed outward with symptoms such as irritability, short-temperedness, impatience and anger attacks. Sudden spells of anger have been observed in approximately 30–40% of depressed patients, both in major depression and dysthymia (Fava *et al.*, 1990). In panic disorder increased suicidality has been reported (Weissman *et al.*, 1989) – though there are also negative reports (Arnold *et al.*, 1995) – as well as anger outbursts (Korn *et al.*, 1992, 1997). Lifetime outward directed aggression is increased in suicide attempters and vice versa (Mann, 1998), while suicide attempts are frequently preceded by intense anxiety, sometimes assuming panic proportions (Van Praag *et al.*, 1986). As said, aggression disorders are not a recognized category in present-day psychiatric taxonomies and thus no data are available on the symptoms of mood lowering and anxiety in the (hypothetical, but by no means imaginary) group of aggression disorders.

In other psychiatric disorders, too, feelings of anxiety, tenseness and downheartedness are often found, alone or in combination.

It comes as no surprise, then, that strong intercorrelations exist between the symptoms of anxiety, aggression, impulsivity and mood lowering across diagnoses, i.e. independent of the diagnostic categories within which those phenomena occur (Apter *et al.*, 1990) (Table 9.2).

9.3.2 Comorbidity of mood disorders and anxiety disorders

The comorbidity rates of anxiety and mood disorders are quite impressive, but published data vary considerably (Kessler, 1998).

Table 9.2. Correlation between anxiety, impulsivity and aggression in acute psychiatric patients from various diagnostic categories (Apter *et al.*, 1990).

	Suicide risk	Violence risk	Impulsivity	State anxiety	Trait anxiety
Suicide risk		0.53*	0.50*	0.47*	0.67*
Violence risk			0.39**	0.33**	0.48*
Impulsivity				0.33**	0.48*

* $P < 0.001$; ** $P < 0.01$.

Pini *et al.* (1997) diagnosed panic disorder in 36.8% of patients with bipolar depression, in 31.4% with unipolar depression, and in 13% of those with dysthymia, while generalized anxiety disorder was found in 31.6% of patients with bipolar disorder, in 37.1% with unipolar depression, and in 65.2% with dysthymia.

If a history of depression is used as a criterion of comorbidity, the number of patients with panic disorder and comorbid depression increases substantially, to over 60% according to some authors (Breier *et al.*, 1984; Sanderson *et al.*, 1990; Stein *et al.*, 1990). A history of panic disorder in patients with depression is less frequent (Sanderson *et al.*, 1990).

From a meta-analysis of comorbidity literature, Dobson & Cheung (1990) concluded that 42–100% (mean 67%) of patients with depression also suffered from an anxiety disorder concurrently or in their life time, and in 17–65% (mean 40%) of patients with anxiety disorders depression is also present. In family studies, moreover, a high rate of cotransmission of mood and anxiety disorders has been reported (Rende *et al.*, 1997).

The overlap between social phobia and both major depression and dysthymia also varies greatly in different studies but is considerable, irrespective of whether the index case is social phobia or depression. Figures up to 70% have been reported (Merikangas & Angst, 1995).

The overlap of PTSD and mood/anxiety disorders is likewise substantial. Fifty per cent of war veterans suffering from PTSD report singular panic attacks (Davidson *et al.*, 1990). More than 40% of patients with PTSD suffer from panic disorder as well (Davidson *et al.*, 1990; McFarlane & Papay, 1992). Overall the comorbidity of depression and PTSD is estimated to be up to 56% concurrent, and up to 95% life time (Bleich *et al.*, 1997).

9.3.3 Comorbidity of depression and personality disorder

The co-occurrence of depression and personality disorder is very high (Wetzler *et al.*, 1990) (Table 9.3). This holds equally true for major depression and dysthymia, and for major depression melancholic type (synonymous with endogenous

Table 9.3. Comorbidity of depression and personality disorder (Flick *et al.*, 1993).

	Personality disorder	
	Present (%)	Not present (%)
Major depression	61	39
Dysthymia	71	29
Bipolar/cyclothymia	70	30

depression and, in symptomatological terms, with vital depression) as well, albeit to a somewhat lesser extent. Initially this latter depression type was thought to appear 'out of the blue' and in stable personalities. This point of view appeared to be wrong. In a substantial proportion of patients precipitants are demonstrable and neurotic personality features are by no means rare, though not virtually ubiquitous as is the case in the other subtypes of depression (Pilkonis & Frank, 1988; Van Praag, 1989; Sanderson *et al.*, 1992; Mulder *et al.*, 1994).

In particular those dysfunctional personalities, characterized by high degrees of dependency, insecurity, affiliative disabilities and discomfort with life are frequent in depressive disorders (Chapter 4). These personality features lead to a state of existential anxiety, a fear to live.

The conclusion seems justified that disturbances in the regulation of mood, anxiety and aggression frequently appear together.

9.4 Comorbidity of anxiety and depression: ways the problem has been approached

Diagnostically, the issue of symptomatological, syndromal and nosological overlap between disorders of mood regulation and anxiety regulation has been addressed in different ways: via hierarchical exclusion rules and via combination diagnoses.

9.4.1 Hierarchical exclusion rules

The third edition of the DSM applied the hierarchical principle, according to which psychiatric disorders are ranked according to severity (Foulds, 1976). Schizophrenia is considered to be more serious than depression, and depression more serious than an anxiety disorder. Only one Axis I diagnosis is allowed, and the higher-ranked diagnosis takes priority over a lower-ranked one. In a patient suffering from depression and panic disorder, the latter is simply ignored. The hierarchical principle, however, is hard to reconcile with accurate diagnosing. Firstly, because the concept of severity remains unspecified and is so hard to specify. Is social disability decisive, or should the degree of personal suffering or the measure of psychological disorganization be taken into account? Actually, it is impossible to argue that paranoid schizophrenia is a more serious condition than major depression, or that melancholia and dysthymia are more serious than panic disorder. Moreover, it remains unproven that subordinate diagnoses are the consequence of higher-positioned ones; for instance, that anxiety disorders are secondary to depression (Sanderson *et al.*, 1990). Finally, psychiatric research is corrupted by the hierarchical approach. One studies a depressed patient and correlates the findings with depression, being 'officially' allowed to disregard coexisting diagnoses. Burying one's head in the sand does not make the problem of comorbidity disappear.

In the DSM–III–R and DSM–IV, the hierarchical principle has been mitigated, but not abandoned. Several diagnoses are permitted, but one has to be designated as the 'principal' diagnosis, i.e. the one that is considered as the main reason for admission or referral to a clinic. But what is, for instance, the principal diagnosis in a patient addicted to alcohol, who feels chronically low, has panic attacks, and qualifies for two or three personality disorders? For the purpose of treatment, an answer has to be given, but in most cases it will be arbitrary. The temptation to solve the comorbidity problem by concealing it has not disappeared.

A more relevant question to be answered in cases of comorbidity is that of 'primary diagnosis' (Sanderson *et al.*, 1990), i.e. the (Axis I) diagnosis that appeared first chronologically. It seems logical to hypothesize that this is the basic disturbance to which the other Axis I diagnoses are indeed subordinate. Evidence in support of this contention would provide a scientific basis to the hierarchical principle. Retrospectively, the question of primary diagnosis is difficult to answer. It is an issue requiring prospective studies, but few such studies have been carried out.

9.4.2 Combination diagnoses

Atypical depression

The concept of atypical depression combining pronounced anxiety and mood dysregulation, was introduced in 1959 by West and Dally and modified shortly after by Sargant (1960), Pollitt (1965) and Hordern (1965). It was based on observations in a group of patients who had responded poorly to tricyclic antidepressants (TCAs) and electroconvulsive therapy (ECT), but did improve upon treatment with the monoamine oxidase inhibitor (MAOI) iproniazid. Symptomatologically, these patients were depressed, but also showed a variety of anxiety disorders, such as generalized anxiety disorder, panic attacks and phobias. Compared with the classic syndrome of vital (endogenous) depression, vegetative symptoms were often 'reversed', i.e. hyperphagia instead of anorexia, hypersomnia instead of insomnia, increased rather than decreased libido, and symptom intensity culminating in the evening rather than in the morning. Mood disturbances were described as fluctuating, and mood reactivity (the ability to be lifted out of a sorrowful low) was preserved. Hysterical personality features were prominent.

Atypical depression thus defined was a loose and confusing concept. It did not, for instance, specify how this condition related to what was, at the time, a current diagnostic construct: neurotic depression. The possibility that depression in these cases was secondary to an anxiety disorder, and that the latter responded positively to MAOIs was left undiscussed. Finally, the hypothetical specific action of MAOIs in this type of depression had not been verified in double-blind studies. Once such studies were carried out, West and Dally's claim was not confirmed. Both amitriptyline and the MAOI phenelzine, for instance, surpassed the placebo effect in atypical depression (Ravaris et al., 1980; Nies & Robinson, 1981; Rowan et al., 1981).

Pitt (1968) contended that the group of atypical depression was heterogeneous and encompassed 'anxious depressions' and forms of depression with reversed, i.e. so-called atypical vegetative, symptoms. Davidson et al. (1982) referred to these as group A and V depression, respectively. Klein et al. (1980) divided the group of atypical depression in yet another way, i.e. a group with reversed vegetative symptoms and a group dubbed 'hysteroid dysphoria', characterized by hysterical personality features, a high activity level when in remission, and rejection sensitivity. Finally, when Ravaris et al. (1980) reported that depressed patients who could still be cheered up by pleasant events responded better to phenelzine than amitriptyline, the concept of mood reactivity was 'officially' added to the definition of atypical depression.

The concept of atypical depression, poorly operationalized as it was, barely distinguishable from bordering diagnoses, and ever expanding, thus represented a true diagnostic monstrosity. Meanwhile, a few studies were published that concluded that certain atypical symptoms responded better to MAOIs than to TCAs (eg. hyperphagia and hypersomnia) (Davidson et al., 1982). Based on these data, the Columbia group, led by Donald Klein, (Liebowitz et al., 1984; Quitkin et al., 1988, 1989; Rabkin et al., 1996) suggested an operational definition of the concept of atypical depression, with the following criteria: depression according to the RDC- (Research Diagnostic Criteria) or DSM-defined criteria; mood reactivity, one of the following symptoms: increased appetite/overeating/increase in body weight; hypersomnia; intense fatigue; and rejection sensitivity. Symptoms of anxiety are no longer required for the diagnosis, though they are frequently reported in this type of depression. Clear, this definition of atypical depression is; balanced, it is not. Reversed vegetative symptoms indeed seem to constitute a cluster (though even this contention has been challenged by Levitan et al., 1997). The hypothesis that depression with those symptoms differs fundamentally from depression with 'typical' vegetative symptoms stands to reason. Mood reactivity, however, is a symptom of a different order and, moreover, difficult to establish. It is not reasonable to combine this phenomenon with 'reversed' vegetative symptoms. Recently, Posternak & Zimmerman (2002) demonstrated that the two sets of phenomena are actually unconnected.

Based on the above definition, the Columbia group demonstrated that phenelzine was more efficacious in atypical depression than imipramine (Liebowitz *et al.*, 1984; Quitkin *et al.*, 1988, 1989; Rabkin *et al.*, 1996). However, no difference was found between phenelzine and fluoxetine (Pande *et al.*, 1996). An additional argument that atypical depression, according to the above definition, is possibly a valid concept was provided by the experiments of Asnis and coworkers (Asnis *et al.*, 1995; McGinn *et al.*, 1996), who demonstrated that the cortisol response to the noradrenaline reuptake inhibitor desipramine was greater in this type of depression than in 'typical' depression.

All in all, it can be concluded that attempts to define atypical depression as a combination of anxiety and depression have failed. In contrast, there are pharmacotherapeutic and biological data suggesting that depressions with 'reversed' vegetative symptoms constitute a specific type of depression.

Mixed anxiety–depression disorder

If the overlap between DSM-defined anxiety and mood disorders may be called substantial, the coexistence of symptoms of mood-lowering and anxiety is even more frequent. This mixture of complaints is more often seen in general practice than by psychiatrists. Eight per cent of the patients treated in five general practices in different parts of the USA showed a mixture of depressive and anxiety symptoms that did not qualify as a 'true' anxiety or mood disorder, but which handicapped the patients occupationally as well as socially (Zinbarg *et al.*, 1994). Nonspecific affective disturbances, which Dohrenwerd (1990) termed demoralization phenomena, occur with a high frequency in the general population. Murphy (1990) for instance, found that, in a random sample of the general population, 12.5% complained of bouts of depression and anxiety severe enough to interfere with occupational and social functioning, and which lasted for more than 1 month.

This type of data prompted the proposal of a new type of depression, i.e. 'mixed anxiety–depression disorder' (Dohrenwerd, 1990; Murphy, 1990; Katon & Roy-Byrne, 1991; Zinbarg *et al.*, 1994; McGinn *et al.*, 1996) which was incorporated in the DSM–IV (as a category to be studied) and the ICD–10.

The (semi-)acceptance of this diagnosis can be qualified as unfortunate, for various reasons. First of all, it is ill-defined. According to DSM–IV, the main symptom is dysphoria, but, curiously, the symptom of anxiety is not required. Moreover, 4 symptoms out of a series of 10 have to be present, but most of those are also part of the definition of major depression and dysthymia. Finally, the patient must not qualify for any other mood or anxiety disorder. These concepts, however, overlap so strongly that the criterion of severity becomes decisive. The proposed diagnostic category thus represents a miscellany of mild forms of mood and anxiety disorders. This, however, is not explicitly stated, and the criterion of severity is never defined.

The concept under discussion, moreover, has not been differentiated from the affective state called worrying. This entails the risk that taxing, but not pathological periods in a person's life are drawn into the realm of psychiatry. Psychiatry, then, flows beyond its designated limits and this will not serve mental health goals well. Public authorities, moreover, misled by inflationary figures about the prevalence of depression, might take the wrong policy decisions.

Another failing is that the concept of mixed anxiety–depression disorder is not in any way linked to the dominion of personality disorders. Feelings of discomfort, including dejection and anxious tension, are frequently related to intrapersonal or interpersonal conflicts, which, in turn, originate in deviant or dysfunctional personality traits.

A further question is whether mixed anxiety–depression disorder could be a mild form or a precursor of a 'true' (DSM-defined) anxiety or mood disorder, rather than an independent diagnostic entity. DSM criteria for 'true' anxiety or mood disorders (such as duration, severity and course) are, after all, largely arbitrary.

Unknown is whether the proposed depression type might be a reaction to a physical disease. This question is relevant because most studies on this type of depression have been conducted in the general population and in general practice. Little is known, moreover, about specific treatments for this category of depression, its course and the psychiatric history and the family history of afflicted patients.

Finally, it is unclear whether mixed anxiety–depression disorder should be differentiated from subsyndromal mood and anxiety disorders, and if so, what the differentiating criteria are.

In short, the concept of mixed anxiety–depression disorder is poorly defined and badly validated. The introduction of such a shaky concept into clinical practice carries the risk of sloppy diagnosis. The patient reports vague complaints, including anxious tension and downheartedness. A (pseudo)diagnosis is at hand, distracting a diagnostician from making a precise analysis of the condition and leading him to abusive prescription of antidepressant and/or anxiolytic drugs.

Clearly the current category of mixed anxiety–depression disorder lacks the qualifications to serve as a diagnostic framework to those psychiatric conditions in which disorders of mood and anxiety regulation go hand in hand.

In short, then, hierarchical exclusion rules seem unacceptable, both from a clinical and research point of view. The available combination diagnoses have not clarified the relationship between anxiety and mood disorders either, nor have they contributed to their differential diagnosis.

9.5 Relationship between anxiety and mood disorders

The relationship between anxiety disorders and mood disorders is unclear. One can conceive of three possibilities. Firstly, the anxiety disorder is caused by the mood disorder or vice versa. This possibility will be discussed in the next section. Secondly, both disorders could rest on the same predisposition, that is: anxiety and mood disorders are different phenotypic expressions of a common genotype. Studies in females lend some support to this possibility (Kendler *et al.*, 1992). Conflicting data however also exist. In the case of a common susceptibility factor, one would expect relatives of patients with depression to show an increased rate of anxiety disorders, and relatives of patients with anxiety disorders an increased risk of depression. Though reported (Rende *et al.*, 1997), the issue is still controversial (Coryell *et al.*, 1992).

Finally, it is conceivable that the notion of discreteness of anxiety and mood disorders as such is flawed, in that disturbances in affect regulation manifest themselves, unpredictably, in mixed clusters of symptoms caused by disturbances in anxiety and mood regulation. In this case attempts to draw borders would be of no avail (Van Praag *et al.*, 1987, 1990; Van Praag, 1992a, 1993, 1997a,b).

9.6 Anxiety and aggression as pacemakers of depression

9.6.1 Anxiety, aggression and mood

In Section 9.5 it was proposed that the high rate of comorbidity of mood and anxiety disorders might be attributable to a causal relationship between those groups of disorders. The following discussion is restricted to the question whether disordered anxiety regulation might kindle depression. We raise the same question with reference to disturbances in aggression regulation, based on the following considerations:

1 Disorders of aggression regulation are a major psychopathological feature in some depressed patients.
2 Mood lowering, anxiety and aggression dysregulation are highly intercorrelated, irrespective of the categorical context in which these phenomena occur (Table 9.2) (Apter *et al.*, 1990).
3 Disturbances in the 5-HT system, as observed in some depressed patients, were demonstrated to correlate with both anxiety and disturbed inward and outward directed aggression (see Chapter 7).

9.6.2 Anxiety/aggression and depression: psychopathological aspects

Tentative evidence suggests that disorders in anxiety and aggression regulation may cause disturbances in mood regulation, inducing in this way a fully fledged depressive syndrome. That evidence is first of all psychopathological in nature.

Table 9.4. Precursor symptoms of a depressive episode in 100 patients with major depression (per cent) (Van Praag, 1996a).

Precursor symptoms	Percentage of patients
Anxiety/aggression	39
Anxiety/aggression and mood lowering	14
Mood lowering and/or other symptoms, save anxiety/aggression	47

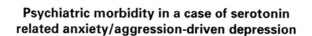

Psychiatric morbidity in a case of serotonin related anxiety/aggression-driven depression

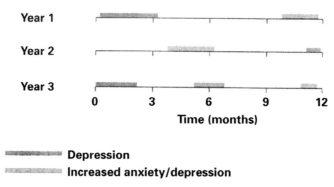

Figure 9.1. Psychiatric morbidity in a case of anxiety/aggression-driven depression.

In some patients a depressive episode is heralded by growing anxiety and tension and by manifestations of outward directed aggression, such as irritability, impatience, short-temperedness and outbursts of anger after only slight provocations (Table 9.4). Obviously, regulation of aggressive impulses gets disturbed (Van Praag, 1992b). One patient's wife expressed this sequence in the following way: 'When he becomes impossible again, I know another episode is near'. Mood lowering in those cases is a relatively late phenomenon. Moreover it does not necessarily develop. At times there are episodes with increased anxiety and aggressiveness, in which mood regulation remains undisturbed and a full depressive syndrome fails to turn up (Figure 9.1).

Based on these findings, it was hypothesized that this type of depression is characterized primarily by disturbances in anxiety and aggression regulation, that *might* lead to disturbances in mood regulation in which case a depressive syndrome will develop (Van Praag, 1994a,b). The name proposed for this type of depression was: anxiety/aggression-driven depression. Moreover the concept of '*pacemaker symptoms*' was introduced, defined as disturbances in psychological control systems – in this case those involved in anxiety and aggression regulation – that have the power to disrupt others, in this case mood regulation (Van Praag, 2001). Anxiety/aggression-driven depression, then, was hypothesized not to be a primary mood disorder.

9.6.3 Anxiety/aggression and depression: biological aspects

Serotonin

The biological findings in a subgroup of depressed patients, discussed in Chapter 7, lend support to the posited construct of anxiety/aggression-driven depression. They hinted at diminished metabolism of 5-HT and disturbed 5-HT receptor function. In challenge tests with relative selective, partial 5-HT_{1A} receptor agonists this subtype of 5-HT receptors was found to be hyporesponsive. PET scanning indicated a diminution of 5-HT_{1A} receptors, both pre- and postsynaptically in some depressed patients. Data on 5-HT_2 receptors are controversial. Both increased, decreased and unchanged densities have been reported (Yatham *et al.*, 2000). Due to lack of sufficiently selective agonists, data on the state of other 5-HT receptors are lacking.

The disturbances in 5-HT metabolism and 5-HT receptor function turned out not to be specific for a particular subtype of depression as presently distinguished, but seem to be associated with components of the depressive syndrome, particularly with disturbed anxiety and aggression regulation (Van Praag *et al.*, 1987, 1990). Animal research has demonstrated that the 5-HT_{1A} receptor system plays a role in the regulation of both anxiety and (offensive) aggression (Olivier *et al.*, 1995, 1999).

The 5-HT disturbances are trait-related, i.e. not bound to the depressive syndrome as such, but persisting in times of remission. They were assumed to be vulnerability factors increasing the risk of disturbances in anxiety and aggression regulation in times of mounting stress (Van Praag & De Haan, 1980a,b).

These observations raised the question whether the 5-HT disturbances under discussion are over-represented in depression in which anxiety and aggression are hypothesized to be key features, i.e. in anxiety/aggression-driven depression. This has indeed been reported, at least with regard to the metabolic disturbances. Low levels of 5-HIAA in CSF were significantly more frequent in depression heralded by anxiety and aggression than in depression with other precursor symptoms (Van Praag, 1996a,b) (Table 9.5). No data are as yet available on possible associations between 5-HT receptor dysfunctions and anxiety/aggression-driven depression.

Stress (CRH/cortisol) – serotonin interactions

As has been extensively discussed in Chapter 8, stress is generally accompanied by CRH overdrive and cortisol overproduction. Sustained hypercortisolaemia will

Table 9.5. Percentage of depressed patients with increased anxiety and/or aggressiveness as early symptoms, in the groups with low and normal CSF 5-HIAA (Van Praag, 1996b).

	Early symptoms	
	Anxiety and/or aggression	Others
Low CSF 5-HIAA	62	38
Normal CSF 5-HIAA	30	70

reduce 5-HT turnover and 5-HT$_{1A}$ receptor gene expression. In this way a 5-HT system marginally operating due to acquired or genetic influences, might be pushed into deficit functioning.

Another risk factor for anxiety/aggression-driven depression might be a (again: acquired or genetic) defect in corticosteroid gene expression. Such an impairment would lead to marginal glucocorticoid feedback inhibition of CRH and ACTH release under normal conditions and early failure of this mechanism under stressful conditions. Depressed patients in whom the dexamethasone/CRH test is disturbed, show after remission still abnormal values: lower than in the depressed phase, but higher than in normal controls. This suggests a trait-related defect in glucocorticosteroid receptor-mediated feedback inhibition.

Psychopharmacological observations

If indeed anxiety and increased aggression were to be key features in some forms of depression it would be a logical expectation that in those disorders successful treatment with antidepressants would follow a certain sequence, in that manifestations of anxiety and aggression would be the first to abate, followed by mood elevation and amelioration of other components of the depressive syndrome.

Some preliminary data hint that this indeed might be the case (Table 9.6). In a subgroup of depression, anxiety and hostility were the first symptoms to improve on treatment with tricyclic antidepressants, only to be followed one or more weeks later by mood elevation (Katz et al., 1987). Patients with an early response of anxiety and aggression to antidepressants were significantly more likely to be found in the group of anxiety/aggression-driven depression than in patients with other precursor symptoms (Van Praag, 1996b).

9.6.4 Anxiety/aggression-driven depression: aspects of personality structure

Anxiety and (manifest or suppressed) anger are key features of the stress syndrome. If indeed in some individuals suffering from depression the regulation of anxiety and aggression is vulnerable, possibly due to trait-related 5-HT ergic disturbances, one would expect them to be stress-prone, i.e. to react to (certain?) untoward experiences

Table 9.6. Responder vs. nonresponder patient groups: comparison of affective factors at 1 and 2 weeks of treatment (mean ± SD) (Katz *et al.*, 1987).

State constructs	Responders			Nonresponders			Significant differences changes from baseline responders vs. nonresponders	
	Baseline	1 Week	2 Weeks	Baseline	1 Week	2 Weeks	1 Week	2 Weeks
Depressed	4.31	3.75	3.08	5.84	5.73	5.39	–	$P < 0.01$
mood	(1.56)	(1.58)	(1.42)	(1.63)	(2.34)	(1.92)		
Anxiety	3.92	3.29	2.88	4.35	4.64	4.72	$P < 0.01$	$P < 0.001$
	(1.75)	(1.39)	(1.19)	(1.29)	(1.37)	(1.54)		
Hostility	1.56	1.16	0.76	2.05	2.00	2.19	$P < 0.01$	$P < 0.001$
	(1.28)	(0.93)	(0.070)	(1.36)	(1.15)	(1.24)		

more readily or more vehemently than individuals in whom those regulatory systems function normally. Phrased differently, patients with anxiety/aggression-driven depression can be expected to show neurotic traits. Preliminary and tentative evidence supports this expectation (Van Praag, 1996c).

Low CSF 5-HIAA depressives in remission were contrasted with remitted depressives with normal CSF 5-HIAA levels, in terms of character-neurotic traits. As discussed, anxiety/aggression-driven depression is over-represented in the group of low CSF 5-HIAA depressives. The Freudian concept of character neurosis is defined as a personality disorder, the features of which the patient experiences as ego-syntonic ('it is just the way I am, doctor') rather than as pathological, though the quality of life of the patient and/or those near to him can be seriously compromised. Examples are feelings of insecurity, dependence, and isolation; difficulties in accepting authority; excessive desire to assert; inability to admit to having been wrong, and many others. This type of personality disorder is frequent, but neglected in the DSM system. Character neurotic personality disorders weaken mental resilience and thus will increase vulnerability to (certain) stressors.

To trace symptoms of ego-syntonic personality disorder we did not rely on available questionnaires because they are largely geared towards the ego-dystonic counterparts. Instead we used structured interview techniques focusing on phenomenological phenomena in the sense of Jaspers (1948). That is, we concentrated on the individual's own experiences (Van Praag, 1989, 1992a). In this case we tried to explore whether the patient experienced his or her personality make-up as being neurotic, i.e. as a source of dissatisfaction and displeasure. We qualified a personality as (character-) neurotically disturbed if, in a semi-structured interview, the following experiential qualities were thought to be present by at least two independently scoring clinicians:

1 Basic feelings of discontent with one's life situation and one's own psychological make-up. Feelings that life has treated one unfairly, in that it had blessed most others with more pleasure and satisfaction than oneself.

2 Unhappiness with one's personal relations, ranging from parental relations and school and work experiences, to marital relations and relations with one's children. The other is felt to be not forthcoming, distant, threatening, cold, abrasive or in any other way not meeting the individual's expectations and needs. As a consequence, a chronic feeling of loneliness and solitude has developed.

3 Emotional instability, in that the basic discontent ignites a range of emotions varying from mood-lowering to guilt, anger, despair and anxiety. These emotions are generally intense, vary abruptly and frequently, sometimes ignited by traceable events in the life situation, sometimes not clearly so.

Each of the three factors we scored on a 5-point scale ranging from 4 to 0, so that a maximum score of 12 and a minimum score of 0 could be obtained. Interviews were done when the patients were in remission.

The average score on the three items was 9.8 in the group of 25 patients with the lowest CSF 5-HIAA concentration, extracted from a cohort of 203 depressed patients, and 6.1 in the 25 patients of that cohort with the highest 5-HIAA levels in CSF. The former group thus held a larger proportion of (ostensibly) 'asymptomatic' or 'minor' personality disorders than the group of high 5-HIAA depressives.

In order to get an impression of the stress level prior to the onset of depression the life event scale developed by Paykel *et al.* (1971) was employed. Based on data obtained from 213 psychiatric patients and 160 relatives of psychiatric patients, these authors rank-ordered 61 life events according to their psychotraumatic weight. We extended the 'top' five events a score of 12, the subsequent five a score of 11, and so on, so that the last six events received a score of 1. If a patient mentioned more than one event the scores were averaged.

From the above-mentioned cohort of 203 patients with depression, of whom CSF 5-HIAA had been measured, we contrasted those 25 with the lowest CSF 5-HIAA concentrations with those with the highest CSF 5-HIAA values in terms of the seriousness, i.e. the 'weight' of the life events that had occurred in the 3 months prior to the onset of the depression (Figure 9.2).

The average weight of life events that had occurred in that period was significantly less in the low-CSF 5-HIAA group than in the high-CSF 5-HIAA group. This observation permits two explanations. First, 5-HT-related depression arises in large measure autonomously, i.e. independent of psychotraumatic events. Second, in 5-HT-related depression the susceptibility for (certain) psychotraumatic events

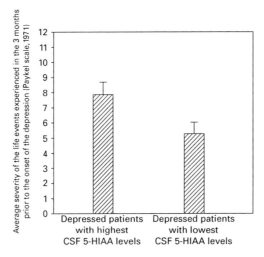

Figure 9.2.   Average weight of the stressor(s) in 25 depressive patients with the lowest CSF 5-HIAA concentration and the 25 depressed patients with the highest CSF 5-HIAA values, sampled from a group of 203 patients suffering from various types of depression, in whom CSF 5-HIAA was measured.

is increased, which is why ostensibly insignificant events still exercise a powerful decompensating effect. The latter hypothesis seems more likely than the former. In detailed free interviews life events that had occurred in the 3 months prior to onset of the depression were explored as to 'objective' (i.e. Paykel Scale) severity and in terms of emotional impact they had had on a particular subject. In the low 5-HIAA group the majority of events ranked rather low on the Paykel scale. Rating them on a global impact scale ranging from 0 (unimportant) to 4 (severely disruptive) the patients themselves, however, considered them to be severe (mean rating 3.1), i.e. as serious blows to an already meagre sense of independence and self-appreciation. Examples are a derogatory remark by one's employer, a disappointing date, an expected invitation that had not been forthcoming. Due to personality imperfections these individuals were vulnerable for ostensibly rather innocent psychotraumatic events, particularly those that reinforced feelings of insecurity, loneliness, nonacceptance and dependence.

In sum, some – admittedly tentative – evidence suggests that in low-CSF 5-HIAA depressives, contrasted with their high-CSF 5-HIAA counterparts, neurotic personality traits are prevalent and the threshold for (certain) stressors seems to be lowered. 5-HT disturbances, thus, seem to be associated with neurotic personality traits, labile anxiety and aggression regulation, stress sensitivity and consequently the propensity to develop anxiety/aggression-driven depression.

9.6.5 Anxiety/aggression-driven depression: a psycho-bio-psychopathological bridge hypothesis

As discussed in the previous section, in a subgroup of depressed subjects the following observations were made.

1 Psychopathological observations: i.e. signs of disturbed anxiety and aggression regulation heralding and possibly eliciting a depressive syndrome.

2 Biological observations: i.e. signs of particular metabolic and receptor disturbances of the 5-HT system that are trait-related and accumulate in depressives in whom increased aggression and anxiety dysregulation is pronounced. Responsivity of the 5-HT_{1A} system has been demonstrated to be reduced.

3 Psychopharmacological observations: i.e. early therapeutic response of anxiety and aggression to TCAs in depressions heralded by anxiety and aggression.

4 Personality-related observations: i.e. high prevalence of character neurotic traits, responsible for enhanced vulnerability for the destabilizing effects of (certain?) psychotraumatic events.

These observations were hypothesized to hang together in the following manner (Van Praag, 1994a,b, 1996d, 2001).

In a subgroup of depression 5-HT metabolism in the brain is reduced, being a trait-related phenomenon. Moreover the density of 5-HT_{1A} receptors is diminished, both pre- and postsynaptically, likewise in a trait-related fashion. The functioning of the 5-HT_{1A} receptor circuitry will thus be compromised, leading to instability of anxiety and aggression regulation. Hypofunction of 5-HT_{1A} receptor circuitry is considered to be a key disturbance in these patients. Theoretically it could be due to genetic defects, or to acquired damage, either biological in nature (e.g. perinatal brain damage) or of psychological character (e.g. traumatic childhood experiences).

Under normal circumstances the 5-HT_{1A} system can just manage; under conditions of sustained stress the system fails due to the resulting overproduction of cortisol. Cortisol will further reduce 5-HT turnover and the expression of 5-HT_{1A} receptors. Hypoactivity of the 5-HT_{1A} system will disrupt anxiety and aggression regulation and this might subsequently lead to disturbances in mood regulation. If so, depression ensues. Activation of the HPA axis will occur the more readily if, constitutionally, its setpoint is raised to begin with. Cortisol also downregulates 5-HT_6 and 5-HT_7 receptors but the clinical significance of these effects is unknown.

Because of anxiety/aggression-proneness, subjects with the above-mentioned imperfections in the 5-HT and/or CRH-HPA system can be expected to be hypersensitive to the stress-inducing effects of negative life events, since anxiety and (manifest or suppressed) anger are key features of the stress syndrome. Anxiety and aggression proneness is due to two factors. Firstly, a marginally functioning 5-HT_{1A} system, and secondly, because of debilitating personality traits thwarting successful

Table 9.7. Vulnerability factors for
anxiety/aggression-driven depression.

Marginally functioning 5-HT(1A) system.
Raised setpoint HPA axis activity.
Personality frailties/deficient coping skills.

Table 9.8. Anxiety/aggression-driven depression: its development.

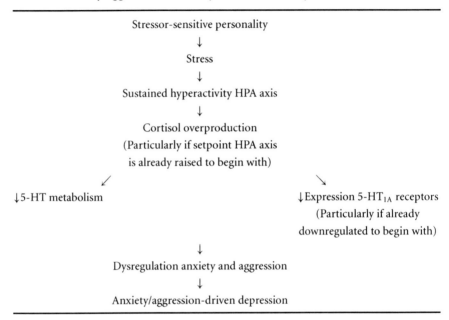

Stressor-sensitive personality
↓
Stress
↓
Sustained hyperactivity HPA axis
↓
Cortisol overproduction
(Particularly if setpoint HPA axis
is already raised to begin with)

↓5-HT metabolism   ↓Expression 5-HT$_{1A}$ receptors
                                     (Particularly if already
                                     downregulated to begin with)

↓
Dysregulation anxiety and aggression
↓
Anxiety/aggression-driven depression

coping. A raised setpoint of the CRH/HPA system will be an additional risk factor (Table 9.7).

In short, in a subgroup of depression, biological combined with psychological stressor vulnerability is the starting point of a cascade that via psychotraumatic experiences as a starting point leads to disturbances in affect regulation, with defective 5-HT/cortisol interactions as the biological interface (Table 9.8).

The phenomena discussed above, seem to show enough mutual coherence to justify the hypothesis of a new depression type, that was named stressor-precipitated, cortisol-induced, 5-HT related, anxiety/aggression-driven depression; in short, anxiety/aggression-driven depression (Van Praag, 1994a,b, 1996b,c) (Table 9.9). Rihmer & Pestality (1998) reported that this type of depression is predominantly seen in males.

Table 9.9. Evidence that anxiety and aggression dysregulation may be key symptoms in a subgroup of depression.

In a subgroup of depression:
    Anxiety/aggression are precursor symptoms
    Anxiety/aggression are pacemaker symptoms
    Anxiolysis and 'mellowing', herald full antidepressive response
    Accumulation of 5-HT disturbances
    5-HT disturbances associated with disturbed anxiety and aggression regulation

Table 9.10. Preferential treatment of anxiety/aggression-driven depression.

Selective, postsynaptic 5-HT_{1A} agonist
Selective, postsynaptic 5-HT_{2c} antagonist
CRH or cortisol antagonist
To be administered in the anxiety/aggression phase of the disorder
    Psychological interventions
       ↓ stressor vulnerability
       ↑ coping skills

9.6.6 Anxiety/aggression-driven depression: therapeutic expectations

If indeed a subgroup of depression exists, in which 5-HT related disruption of anxiety and aggression regulation are the driving forces, one would expect those depressions to respond preferentially to compounds that normalize the regulation of anxiety and aggression via normalization of the 5-HT ergic and/or CRH-HPA systems. It has been hypothesized that optimal treatment of this depression type would include the following components (Van Praag, 1996b) (Table 9.10).

1 Administration, not of one of the usual antidepressants, but of a selective, postsynaptic, full 5-HT_{1A} agonist. Such a compound would normalize 5-HT_{1A} receptor-mediated transmission, harmonize anxiety and aggression regulation, and ultimately – in second instance – lead to mood normalization. Preferably this treatment should start at the stage in which only anxiety and aggression are dysregulated. In the depressive phase this intervention might be too late.

Such compounds are now on their way, so this hypothesis can shortly be put to the test (Borsini & Cesana, 2001). Partial, and not very selective 5-HT_{1A} receptor agonists of the azapirone group (e.g. buspirone and ipsapirone) have been shown to exert anxiolytic and antidepressive actions in humans (Stahl, 1992; Deakin, 1993).

2 An antagonist or inverse agonist of $5\text{-}HT_{2A}$ and/or $5\text{-}HT_{2C}$ receptors might be considered. In humans, hyper-responsivity of this receptor system has not been convincingly demonstrated (see Chapter 7), but animal experiments indicate that this type of compound might exert anxiolytic and antidepressant effects (Sibille *et al.*, 1997; Wood *et al.*, 2001; Yamada & Sugimoto, 2001).

3 A $5\text{-}HT_{1A}$ agonist should be combined with a cortisol or CRH antagonist to remove the break on $5\text{-}HT_{1A}$ receptor functioning.

   Compounds of that nature are presently being studied, and thus it will be possible to evaluate this hypothesis too, in due course.

4 Psychological intervention methods should be employed to boost ego strength, improve coping abilities and reverse inadequate adaptive reaction patterns.

5 Prophylactically a combination of pharmacotherapy, with a $5\text{-}HT_{1A}$ agonist and/or cortisol or CRH antagonist, in combination with continued psychological treatment should be employed.

9.7 Anxiety/aggression-driven depression: diagnostic implications

9.7.1 Diagnostic acuity: a condition sine qua non for biological stress research

Study of the biological interface between stress and psychopathology could start from either side. From the stress side; in which case well-defined stress phenomena are the starting point, and the central question will be whether stress phenomena can induce brain disturbances found to be associated with a particular stress-related psychopathological condition, such as a mood or anxiety disorder, syndromal or subsyndromal in format.

Alternatively, stress-related psychopathological conditions, for instance a syndromal or subsyndromal mood or anxiety disorder can be the starting point. In that case the question is raised whether that condition is associated with neurobiological disturbances known to be stress-inducible. Following the second route, careful multi-level characterization of the psychopathological condition to be studied is as crucial as it is on the former track. It seems unlikely that heterogeneous, and coarsely outlined psychopathological constructs, like major depression or dysthymia, are associated with well-defined and definable faults in cerebral circuitry.

The research that ultimately led to the construct anxiety/aggression-driven depression had followed the second route. In order to achieve the necessary diagnostic acuity two new diagnostic approaches were applied, called functionalization and verticalization. They will be briefly discussed in the next sections (for a more extensive discussion see Van Praag, 1989, 1990, 1992a, 1993, 1997a, 2001).

Table 9.11. Functionalization of psychiatric diagnosing

Diagnosing should comprise four steps:
   Categorical diagnosis
   Syndrome characterization
   Symptom characterization
   Assessment of the psychological dysfunctions underlying psychopathological symptoms

9.7.2 Functionalization of psychiatric diagnosing

The term functionalization stands for a way of diagnosing a current psychiatric disorder that proceeds according to four steps (Table 9.11) (see also Chapter 1).

1 Establishment of the categorical diagnosis.

Since the disease entities we presently distinguish are symptomatologically greatly variable and also heterogeneous in terms of course, outcome, treatment response and concomitant biological variables, the categorical diagnosis provides no more than a first and crude diagnostic clue. A diagnosis like schizophrenia or major depression has little more acuity than a medical diagnosis like cardiac disorder or pulmonary disorder.

2 Precise definition of the (predominant) syndrome.

In the current diagnostic system x out of a series of y symptoms suffice to establish a diagnosis. Each diagnostic category thus covers a variety of syndromes. Hence a categorical diagnosis provides little information about the syndrome one is dealing with.

3 Analysis of the symptoms the psychiatric syndrome(s) consists of.

Most psychiatric patients suffer simultaneously from several psychiatric syndromes, or, more frequently, parts of those syndromes. Hence indicating one predominant syndrome or several syndromes of equal 'weight', does not provide sufficient diagnostic accuracy. To acquire that, a precise analysis of the psychopathological phenomena the mental condition consists of is needed.

4 Determination of the psychic dysfunctions underlying the psychopathological phenomena.

Psychopathological phenomena and psychic dysfunctions are not identical. A psychopathological symptom is the expression of a psychic dysfunction. The symptom is the way the dysfunction is experienced by the patient and perceived by the observer. The psychic dysfunction is its generator. For instance: hearing voices is a symptom, certain perceptual disturbances the underlying psychological dysfunction; anhedonia is a symptom, inability to link a particular perception to a particular emotion the generating psychological dysfunction.

Table 9.12. Why is functionalization of psychiatric diagnosing important?

Present-day diagnostic constructs	Functionalized diagnoses
Symptomatologically heterogeneous	Symptomatological finesse
Hard to measure	Measurable
'Diffuse'	Detailed map of psychic 'apparatus'
Hardly correlate with biological variables	Correlate much better with biological variables

Psychometric instruments to carry out such functional analysis are only in part available, and have to be further developed and refined, jointly by research psychiatrists and experimental clinical psychologists.

9.7.3 Importance of functionalization for the diagnostic process in psychiatry

For several reasons, functionalization of the diagnostic process seems to be an essential exercise to optimize psychiatric diagnosing (Table 9.12).

1 Present-day diagnostic constructs are symptomatologically utterly heterogeneous. For research, and particularly for brain and behaviour research, it is essential that the object of study is precisely defined. Functionalization of diagnosis provides that finesse.

2 Psychological dysfunctions are measurable; in several instances even quantitatively. Syndromes and categorical entities permit at best a qualitative estimate about their presence or absence.

3 A functionalized diagnosis provides a detailed map of those components of the mental 'apparatus' that function deficiently and those that still function within normal limits. This is important, because it enables us to focus therapeutic interventions and (biological) research efforts more sharply than the nosological approach current today permits.

4 Biological disturbances established in psychiatric disorders do not correlate well with categorical entities such as schizophrenia, major depression, dysthymia or any one of the personality disorders. Hence biology's role in diagnosing psychiatric disorders has so far been next to nothing. This is hardly surprising, because the way psychiatric disease categories have been defined is to a large extent arbitrary and not based on systematically collected empirical data. On the other hand, significant correlations have been established with psychic dysfunctions. Examples are the associations between 5-HT ergic dysfunctions and disturbances in anxiety and aggression regulation and impulse control and between dopaminergic dysfunctions and disturbances in motoricity (Van Praag *et al.*, 1990; Coccaro, 1992). As long as psychiatry does not have a taxonomy consisting of well-delineated and validated diagnostic constructs at its disposal,

Table 9.13. Procedures to determine 'diagnostic valence' of psychopathological phenomena.

Temporal sequence of occurrence
Relationship of precursor symptoms to biological disturbances (if any)
Therapeutic effect of interventions aimed at normalizing the biological abnormalities

biological psychiatry's main target should be the psychic dysfunction rather than the present-day disease categories.

Functionalization of psychiatric diagnosing provides the diagnostic framework for functionalization of biological research in psychiatry.

9.7.4 Functionalization of diagnosis and the construct of anxiety/aggression-driven depression

Applying the principles of functionalized diagnosing, depression was studied as a conglomerate of interacting dysfunctions within the psychic 'apparatus': dysfunctions in the provinces of affectivity, cognition and motor regulation.

In that way, we were able to trace disturbed anxiety and aggression regulation as precursor dysfunctions and possibly key (i.e. pacemaker) components of a certain type of depression.

9.7.5 Verticalization of psychiatric diagnosing

Verticalization is the term Van Praag (1992a, 1997a) used for the process of prioritizing psychopathological symptoms/psychic dysfunctions that together constitute a mental disorder. Prioritizing means that their relationship towards the neurobiological substratum underlying a particular psychiatric condition is established. Are they a direct consequence of the neurobiological substratum underlying a particular psychiatric disorder, or associated in a derivative manner? The former symptoms/dysfunctions are called primary, the latter secondary. It is very well conceivable that primary symptoms possess 'pacemaker qualities', that is the ability of eliciting disturbances in other psychic regulatory systems (see also Section 9.6.2).

9.7.6 Approaches towards verticalization of psychiatric diagnoses

Acknowledging that as yet we know little about biological determinants of abnormal behaviour, what means do we presently have to verticalize the psychopathology constituting a psychiatric disorder, i.e. to determine its relationship towards the underlying pathophysiology (Table 9.13)?

The first step is sequential analysis, i.e. determination of the sequence of appearance of the psychopathological phenomena, preferably in a prospective manner.

Table 9.14. Why is verticalization of psychiatric diagnosing important?

Present-day diagnosing	Verticalized diagnosing
Psychopathological phenomena ordered horizontally	Psychopathological phenomena weighted as to their 'diagnostic valence'.
Biological and psychopharmacological research unfocused	Biological and psychopharmacological research focused on primary psychopathological phenomena/psychic dysfunctions

The hypothesis that the frontrunners carry a primary character seems to make sense.

Next the question is studied whether neurobiological disturbances that might have been revealed in a given case – such as dysfunctions in monoaminergic or other transmitter circuits or in stress-regulating systems such as the HPA axis – are associated with any of the phenomena hypothesized to be primary.

If indeed such associations are demonstrable, pharmacological interventions will be applied or developed aimed at normalizing the neurobiological abnormalities. If the associated psychopathological (primary) phenomena are responsive, the hypothesis about their primary nature is strengthened. If those psychopathological phenomena would have served as pacemakers of the psychiatric disorder, one would expect the remaining (secondary) symptoms to ameliorate subsequently.

It was in applying the verticalization principle that it was possible to (1) conceptualize the construct of anxiety/aggression-driven depression, (2) to establish its relationship with 5-HT ergic dysfunctions and (3) to formulate a hypothesis on its preferential treatment and prophylaxis.

9.7.7 Importance of verticalization for the diagnostic process in psychiatry

Presently psychiatrists diagnose in a horizontal manner. The symptoms observed in a given psychopathological condition are counted and placed in a horizontal plane as if they all had the same diagnostic weight. This however is quite improbable. It is much more likely, that some are the direct consequences of the underlying cerebral dysfunctions while others are of a subsidiary nature. The former (primary) phenomena are diagnostically the most important. They should be the focus of biological studies, and they should be the main target of psychopharmacological interventions (Table 9.14).

It goes without saying, that verticalization is not a diagnostic strategy ready for practical use. It is a research domain the development of which will require long-term collaboration of psychiatrists and experimental (clinical) psychologists. It

Table 9.15. Changes in biological psychiatric research brought about by functionalization/verticalization of diagnoses.

Categorically defined entities → Dysfunctioning psychological domains
↓
Psychiatric physiology

Table 9.16. Changes in psychopharmacological research brought about by functionalization/verticalization of diagnoses.

Categorically defined entities → Dysfunctioning psychological domains
↓
Functional psychopharmacology

seems to be, however, a quintessential domain to gain insight into the relationships between abnormal behaviour and abnormal brain functions.

9.8 Consequences of diagnostic renewal for biological psychiatric and psychopharmacological research

General application of the principles of functionalization and verticalization of psychiatric diagnosing would have profound consequences for biological psychiatric and psychopharmacological research.

Firstly, it would lead to a change of focus of biological psychiatric research. To unravel the biology of dysfunctioning psychic domains would be its ultimate goal, rather than elucidation of the cause of categorically defined entities like major depression or schizophrenia. The latter are considered to be too heterogeneous to make a uniform pathophysiology a likely supposition. Functionalization of diagnosis will ultimately lead to a *psychiatric physiology* (Table 9.15) (Van Praag, 1997a).

Secondly, drug research would also shift from categorical entities to dysfunctioning psychic domains, such as disturbed regulation of anxiety, aggression, mood and motoricity, disturbances in perception, in hedonic functions, in information processing and others. Psychopharmacological treatment would be geared toward dysfunctioning psychic domains – particularly those of a primary nature – rather than toward disease entities as such. This approach was called by Van Praag (1997a,b) *functional psychopharmacology* (Table 9.16).

Consequently systematic development of a functionalized and verticalized system of diagnosing in psychiatry would bring an era of psychiatric thinking gradually to a close. An era in which a static disease concept prevailed and mental disorders were categorically understood, while ushering in a new era of dynamic and functionally oriented psychiatry.

Conceptually as well as practically, such a change in orientation could be conceived as progress.

9.9 Conclusions

1 Quite frequently psychotraumatic life events, leading to a state of apprehension and powerlessness, precede depression. Tentative evidence suggests a causal relationship. Definite proof awaits demonstration that stress may induce changes in neuronal circuits that supposedly are associated with (certain types of) depression or certain components of depression.

2 States of severe apprehension (called stress) will lead to activation of the hypothalamic and extra-hypothalamic CRH system and to cortisol overproduction. Normally excess cortisol will shut off CRH and ACTH production, via activation of GRs, thus normalizing HPA axis activity and ending the state of hypercortisolaemia.

Sustained stress, however, might lead to sustained overproduction of cortisol; particularly so if the GR-mediated negative feedback system functions deficiently.

Acute stress also activates MA ergic systems, whereas under conditions of sustained stress or sustained cortisol overproduction DA ergic, NA ergic and 5-HT ergic activity will be reduced. Expression of the 5-HT_{1A}, 5-HT_7 and 5-HT_8 receptor genes goes down, while 5-HT_{2c} receptors are upregulated.

3 In some depressed patients the following biological disturbances have been established: CRH overproduction, HPA axis overactivity accompanied by hypercortisolaemia; signs indicative of both hyper- and hypoactivity of NA ergic systems, and of diminished DA ergic activity; reduced 5-HT metabolism; reduced numbers of 5-HT_{1A} receptors and (possibly) upregulation of 5-HT_{2c} receptors. Stress-induced changes in the CRH and MA systems and changes found in those systems in some depressed subjects thus show remarkable similarities.

4 In animals it has been demonstrated that the stress-induced changes in the CRH and MA systems have behavioural consequences, particularly in the domains of anxiety and aggression regulation.

Extra-hypothalamic CRH overdrive, NA ergic hyperactivity, downregulation of 5-HT_{1A} receptors and upregulation of 5-HT_{2c} receptors have all been associated with heightened anxiety, whereas downregulation of 5-HT_{1A} receptors will facilitate particular forms of aggressive behaviour.

5 Anxiety and (manifest or suppressed) anger are key constituents of the stress-syndrome. They are likewise prominent features in certain types of depression. Thus the question can be raised whether stress-induced disturbances in the CRH and MA systems, leading to disturbances in anxiety and aggression regulation,

might trigger a depression. If so, this would represent the first direct evidence that life events, inducing unmanageable stress, may indeed cause depression. So far, this relation was presumed to exist based on indirect evidence.

6 Tentative evidence exists that depression might indeed be stressor-precipitated and anxiety/aggression-driven. This type of depression can be characterized on various levels:

Personality-wise by a high prevalence of character-neurotic traits, thwarting successful coping.

Psychopathologically, the depression is preceded by anxiety and manifestations of increased outward direct aggression. In some episodes, however, mood lowering fails to occur. Psychopathology remains restricted to the domains of anxiety and aggression regulation. Disturbances in anxiety and aggression regulation thus probably have the potential to act as pacemakers of the depression.

Biologically these patients show an excess of 5-HT disturbances, most notably a reduction of 5-HT metabolism and supposedly downregulation of 5-HT receptors, in which the 5-HT_{1A} system is involved. Those 5-HT disturbances are not characteristic for a particular subtype of depression as presently distinguished, but were shown to correlate with disturbances in anxiety- and aggression regulation, irrespective of diagnosis.

The 5-HT disturbances persist in times of remission. This suggests that regulation of anxiety and aggression remains vulnerable, causing stressor-sensitivity and increased risk of pronounced stress reactions in response to adversity. A raised setpoint of the CRH/HPA systems would have similar behavioural consequences. This might indeed be the case in depression (Holsboer-Trachsler *et al.*, 1991).

These data seem to show sufficient coherence to hypothesize a new group of depression, named anxiety/aggression-driven depression or, in full: stressor-precipitated, cortisol-induced, 5-HT related, anxiety/aggression-driven depression. It constitutes the first direct evidence that stress may *cause* depression, assuming of course that the evidence validating this construct will be confirmed.

7 Therapeutically a combination of drugs (a selective, full, postsynaptic 5-HT_{1A} agonist, in combination with a cortisol or CRH antagonist) and psychological interventions aimed at augmenting ego strength are considered to be the treatment of choice in anxiety/aggression-driven depression.

The drugs mentioned should be administered in the anxiety/aggression-only stage, i.e. before the full depressive syndrome has developed.

Prophylactically the same drugs as recommended for treatment are indicated.

8 Downregulation of the 5-HT_{1A} receptor system and/or raised excitability of the HPA system (acquired or genetically determined), should lead to increased susceptibility for anxiety-aggression/driven depression.

Conceivably, certain polymorphisms of the 5-HT transporter gene could have similar consequences. Individuals with one or two copies of the short allele on the promoter region of that gene show signs of increased stressor-proneness and raised depression vulnerability, compared with humans with one or two long alleles. Short-allele monkeys, moreover, show signs of decreased 5-HT turnover (see Chapter 7, Section 7.2.5).

9 Studies of stress/brain/behaviour relationships should rest on detailed definition of the behavioural condition following stressor exposure. Psychiatric diagnosing as it is presently being practiced, based on a predominantly categorical disease model, does not provide this finesse. Biological-oriented stress research, to be fruitful, is in need of new diagnostic guidelines.

In conceptualizing the construct of anxiety/aggression-depression two new diagnostic approaches were applied, named functionalization and verticalization. Functionalization implies focusing on psychic dysfunction rather than on disease entities. Verticalization implies weighing of symptoms, i.e. attempting to distinguish symptoms directly related to the neurobiological substratum underlying a particular mental condition, from those that seem to be derivatives. Systematic application of these strategies will lead to a retreat of the categorical disease model in psychiatry, in favour of a dynamic, functionally oriented disease concept. This change in orientation is conceived as progress.

10 The strength of the – emphatically – still hypothetical construct anxiety/aggression-driven depression in diagnostic terms, lies in the fact that it is not merely a combination diagnosis, bringing anxiety (and aggression) and depression together in a purely descriptive and horizontal way. It postulates a causal (or vertical) relationship between dysfunctioning psychic domains (in other words, places them in a vertical connection). It relates those dysfunctions to unassimilated psychotraumatic events, and proposes a biological interface between precipitating psychological factors and ensuing psychopathological consequences. The proposed vertical arrangement of psychopathological phenomena, moreover, has clear therapeutic consequences.

This type of hypothesis 'cascade' – hypotheses, so to say – is clearly needed to advance human brain and behaviour research.

REFERENCES

Apter, A., Van Praag, H. M., Plutchik, R., Sevy, S., Korn, M. & Brown, S. L. (1990). Interrelationships among anxiety, aggression, impulsivity, and mood: A serotonergically linked cluster. *Psychiatry Res.*, **32**, 191–9.

Arnold, D. H., Sanderson, W. C. & Beck, A. T. (1995). Panic disorders and suicidal behavior. In *Panic Disorder. Clinical, Biological and Treatment Aspects*, ed. G. M. Asnis & H. M. van Praag. New York: John Wiley & Sons.

Asnis, G. M., McGinn, L. K. & Sanderson, W. C. (1995). Atypical depression: clinical aspects and noradrenergic function. *Am. J. Psychiatry*, **152**, 31–6.

Bleich, A., Kosolowsky, M., Dolev, A. & Lerer, B. (1997). Posttraumatic stress disorders and depression. *Br. J. Psychiatry*, **170**, 479–82.

Borsini, F. & Cesana, R. (2001). Further characterisation of potential antidepressant action of flibanserin. *Psychopharmacology*, **159**, 64–9.

Breier, A., Charney, D. S. & Heninger, G. R. (1984). Major depression in patients with agoraphobia and panic disorder. *Arch. Gen. Psychiatry*, **41**, 1129–35.

Coccaro, E. F. (1992). Impulsive aggression and central serotonergic system function in humans: an example of a dimensional brain – behavior relationship. *Int. Clin. Psychopharmacol*, **7**, 3–12.

Coryell, W., Endicott, J. & Winokur, G. (1992). Anxiety syndromes as epiphenomena of primary major depression: outcome and familial psychopathology. *Am. J. Psychiatry*, **149**, 100–7.

Davidson, J. R. T., Miller, R. D., Turnbull, C. D. & Sullivan, J. L. (1982). Atypical depression. *Arch. Gen. Psychiatry*, **39**, 527–34.

Davidson, J., Kudler, H. S., Saunders, W. B. & Smith, R. D. (1990). Symptoms and comorbidity patterns in world war II and Vietnam veterans with posttraumatic stress disorder. *Compr. Psychiatry*, **31**, 162–70.

Deakin, J. F. (1993). A review of clinical efficacy of 5-HT$_{1A}$ agonists in anxiety and depression. *J. Psychopharmacol.*, **7**, 283–9.

De Boer, S. F., Lesourd, M., Mocaer, E. & Koolhaas, J. M. (1999). Selective antiaggressive effects of alnespirone in resident-intruder test are mediated via 5-hydroxytryptamine$_{1a}$ receptors: a comparative pharmacological study with 8-hydroxy-2-dipropylaminotetralin, ipsapirone, buspirone, eltoprazine, and WAY-100635. *J. Pharmacol. Exp. Ther.*, **288**, 1125–33.

Di Nardo, P. A. & Barlow, R. D. (1990). Syndrome and symptom co-morbidity in the anxiety disorders. In *Comorbidity in Anxiety and Mood Disorders*, ed. J. D. Maser & C. R. Cloninger. Washington, DC: American Psychiatric Press.

Dobson, K. S. & Cheung, E. (1990). Relationship between anxiety and depression: conceptual and methodological issues. In *Comorbidity of Mood and Anxiety Disorders*, ed. J. D. Maser & C. R. Cloninger. Washington, DC: American Psychiatric Press.

Dohrenwerd, B. P. (1990). Notes on some epidemiologic studies of comorbidity. In *Comorbidity of Mood and Anxiety Disorders*, ed. J. D. Maser & C. R. Cloninger. Washington, DC: American Psychiatric Press.

Fava, M., Anderson, K. & Rosenbaum, J. F. (1990). "Anger attacks": possible variants of panic and major depressive disorders. *Am. J. Psychiatry*, **147**, 867–70.

Flick, S. N., Roy-Byrne, P. P., Cowley, D. S., Shores, M. M. & Dunner, D. L. (1993). DSM–II–R personality disorders in a mood and anxiety disorders clinic: prevalence, comorbidity, and clinical correlates. *J. Affect. Disord.*, **27**, 71–9.

Foulds, J. A. (1976). *The Hierarchical Nature of Personal Illness*. London: Academic Press.

Holsboer-Trachsler, E., Stohler, R. & Hatzinger, M. (1991). Repeated administration of the combined dexamethasone/CRH stimulation test during treatment of depression. *Psychiatry*, **38**, 163–71.

Hordern, A. (1965). The antidepressant drugs. *New Engl. J. Med.*, **272**, 1159–69.

Jaspers, K. (1948). *Allgemeine Psychopathologie*. Berlin: Springer.

Judd, L. L., Akiskal, H. S. & Paulus, M. P. (1997). The role and clinical significance of subsyndromal depressive symptoms (SSD) in unipolar, major depressive disorder. *J. Affect. Disord.*, **45**, 5–18.

Katon, W. & Roy-Byrne, P. P. (1991). Mixed anxiety and depression. *J. Abnorm. Psychol.*, **100**, 337–45.

Katz, M. M., Koslov, S., Maas, J. W. *et al.* (1987). The timing and specificity and clinical prediction of tricyclic drug effects in depression. *Psychol. Med.*, **17**, 297–309.

Kendler, K. S., Neale, M. C., Kessler, R. C., Heath, A. C. & Eaves, L. J. (1992). Major depression and generalized anxiety disorder. Same genes, (partly) different environments? *Arch. Gen. Psychiatry*, **49**, 716–22

Kessler, R. C. (1998). Comorbidity of depression and anxiety disorders. In *SSRIs in Depression and Anxiety*, ed. S. A. Montgomery & J. A. den Boer. Chichester: John Wiley & Sons.

Klein, D. F., Gittelman, R., Quitkin, F., Terzani, S. & Gastpar, M. (1980). *Diagnosis and Drug Treatment of Psychiatric Disorders in Adults and Children*. Baltimore: Williams & Wilkins.

Korn, M. L., Kotler, M., Molcho, A. *et al.* (1992). Suicide and violence associated with panic attacks. *Biol. Psychiatry*, **31**, 607–12.

Korn, M. L., Plutchik, R. & van Praag, H. M. (1997). Panic-associated suicidal and aggressive ideation and behavior. *J. Psychiatry Res.*, **31**, 481–7.

Levitan, R. D., Lesage, A., Parikh, S. V., Goering, P. & Kennedy, S. H. (1997). Reversed neurovegetative symptoms of depression: a community study of Ontario. *Am. J. Psychiatry*, **154**, 934–40.

Liebowitz, M. R., Quitkin, F. M., Stewart, J. W. *et al.* (1984). Phenelzine vs imipramine in atypical depression. *Arch. Gen. Psychiatry*, **41**, 669–77.

Mann, J. J. (1998). The neurobiology of suicide. *Nat. Med.*, **4**, 25–30.

McFarlane, A. C. & Papay, P. (1992). Multiple diagnoses in posttraumatic stress disorder in the victims of a natural disaster. *J. Nerv. Ment. Disord.*, **180**, 498–504.

McGinn, L. K., Asnis, G. M. & Rubinson, E. (1996). Biological and clinical validation of atypical depression. *Psychiatry Res.*, **60**, 191–8.

Merikangas, K. R. & Angst, J. (1995). Comorbidity and social phobia: evidence from clinical, epidemiologic, and genetic studies. *Eur. Arch. Psychiatry Clin. Neurosci.*, **244**, 297–303.

Mulder, R. T., Joyce, P. R. & Cloninger, C. R. (1994). Temperament and early environment influence comorbidity and personality disorders in major depression. *Compr. Psychiatry*, **35**, 225–33.

Murphy, J. (1990). Diagnostic comorbidity and symptom co-occurrence: The stirling county study. In *Comorbidity of Mood and Anxiety Disorders*, ed. J. D. Maser & C. R. Cloninger. Washington, DC: American Psychiatric Press.

Nies, A. & Robinson, D. S. (1981). Comparison of clinical effects of amitriptyline and phenelzine treatment. In *Monoamine Oxidase Inhibitors – The State of the Art*, ed. B. H. Youdim & E. Paykel. New York: John Wiley & Sons.

Olivier, B., Mos, J., van Oorschot, R. & Hen, R. (1995). Serotonin receptors and animal models of aggressive behavior. *Pharmacopsychiatry*, **28**, 80–90.

Olivier, B., Soudijn, W. & Van Wijngaarden, I. (1999). The 5-HT$_{1a}$ receptor and its ligands: structure and function. *Progr. Drug Res.*, **52**, 103–65.

Pande, A. C., Birkett, M., Fechner-Bates, S., Haskett, R. F. & Greden, J. F. (1996). Fluoxetine versus phenelzine in atypical depression. *Biol. Psychiatry*, **40**, 1017–20.

Paykel, E. G., Prusoff, B. & Ulenhuth, E. H. (1971). Scaling of life events. *Arch. Gen. Psychiatry*, **24**, 340–7.

Pilkonis, P. & Frank, E. (1988). Personality pathology in recurrent depression: Nature, prevalence and relationship to treatment response. *Am. J. Psychiatry*, **145**, 435–41.

Pini, S., Cassano, G. B., Simonini, E., Savino, M., Russo, A. & Montgomery, S. A. (1997). Prevalence of anxiety disorders comorbidity in bipolar depression, unipolar depression, and dysthymia. *J. Affect. Disord.*, **42**, 145–53.

Pitt, B. (1968). Atypical facial pain and depression. *Br. J. Psychiatry*, **114**, 1325–35.

Pollitt, J. (1965). Suggestions for a physiological classification of depression. *Br. J. Psychiatry*, **111**, 489–95.

Posternak, M. A. & Zimmerman, M. (2002). Partial validation of the atypical features subtype of major depressive disorder. *Arch. Gen. Psychiatry*, **59**, 70–6.

Quitkin, F. M., Stewart, J. W. & McGrath, P. J. (1988). Phenelzine versus imipramine in the treatment of probable atypical depression: defining syndrome boundaries of selective MAOI responders. *Am. J. Psychiatry*, **145**, 306–11.

Quitkin, F. M., McGrath, P. J., Stewart, J. W. *et al.* (1989). Phenelzine and imipramine in mood reactive depressives. Further delineation of the syndrome of atypical depression. *Arch. Gen. Psychiatry*, **46**, 787–93.

Rabkin, J. G., Stewart, J. W., Quitkin, F. M. & Klein, D. F. (1996). Should atypical depression be included in DSM–IV? In *DSM–IV Sourcebook*, ed. T. A. Widiger, A. J. Frances & H. A. Pincus. Washington, DC: American Psychiatry Press.

Ravaris, C. L., Robinson, D. S., Ives, J. O., Nies, A. & Bartlett, D. (1980). Phenelzine and amitriptyline in the treatment of depression. A comparison of present and past studies. *Arch. Gen. Psychiatry*, **37**, 1075–80.

Rende, R., Weissman, M. & Rutter, M. (1997). Psychiatric disorders in the relatives of depressed probands II. Familial loading for comorbid non-depressive disorders based upon proband age of onset. *J. Affect. Disord.*, **42**, 23–8.

Rihmer, Z. & Pestality, P. (1998). 'Anxiety/aggression-driven depression' and 'male depressive syndrome': are they the same? *Psychiatry Res.*, **77**, 209–10.

Rowan, P. R., Paykel, E. S., Parker, R. R. & Barber, H. E. (1981). Tricyclic antidepressant and MAO inhibitor: are there differential effects? In *Monoamine Oxidase Inhibitors – the State of the Art*, ed. B. H. Youdim & E. S. Paykel. New York: John Wiley & Sons.

Sanderson, W. C., Beck, A. T. & Beck, J. (1990). Syndrome comorbidity in patients with major depression or dysthymia: prevalence and temporal relationships. *Am. J. Psychiatry*, **147**, 1025–8.

Sanderson, W. C., Wetzler, S., Beck, A. T. & Betz, F. (1992). Prevalence of personality disorders in patients with major depression and dysthymia. *Psychiatry Res.*, **42**, 93–9.

Sargant, W. (1960). Drugs in the treatment of depression. *Br. Med. J.*, **1**, 225–7.

Saudou, F., Amara, D. A., Dierich, A. *et al.* (1994). Enhanced aggressive behavior in mice lacking 5-HT1B receptor. *Science*, **265**, 1875–8.

Sibille, E., Sarnyai, Z., Benjamin, D., Gal, J., Baker, H. & Toth, M. (1997). Antisense inhibition of 5-hydroxytryptamine$_{2A}$ receptor induces an antidepressant-like effect in mice. *Mol. Pharmacol.*, **52**, 1056–63.

Stahl, S. M. (1992). Serotonin neuroscience discoveries usher in a new era of novel drug therapies for psychiatry. *Psychopharmacol. Bull.*, **28**, 3–9.

Stein, M. B., Tancer, M. E. & Uhde, T. W. (1990). Major depression in patients with panic disorder: factors associated with course and recurrence. *J. Affect. Disord.*, **19**, 287–96.

Van Heeringen, K. (Ed.) (2001). *Understanding Suicidal Behavior. The Suicidal Process, Approach to Research, Treatment and Prevention.* Chichester: John Wiley & Sons.

Van Praag, H. M. (1989). Diagnosing depression. Looking backward into the future. *Psychiatr. Dev.*, **7**, 375–94.

(1990). Two-tier diagnosing in psychiatry. *Psychiatry Res.*, **34**, 1–11.

(1992a). *Make Believes in Psychiatry or the Perils of Progress.* New York: Brunner Mazel.

(1992b). About the centrality of mood lowering in mood disorders. *Eur. Neuropsychopharm.*, **2**, 393–402.

(1993). Diagnosis, the rate-limiting factor of biological depression research. *Neuropsychobiology*, **28**, 197–206.

(1994a). 5-HT related, anxiety- and/or aggression driven depression. *Intern. Clin. Psychopharmacol.* **9**, 5–6.

(1994b). Anxiety and aggression as pacemakers of depression: dimensional variation of the serotonin hypothesis of depression. In *Current Therapeutic Approaches to Panic and other Anxiety Disorders*, ed. G. Darcourt, J. Mendlewicz, G. Racagni & N. Brunello. *Int. Acad. Biomed. Drug Res.*, Vol. 8. Basel: Karger.

(1996a). Comorbidity (psycho-)analysed. *Br. J. Psychiatry*, **168**, 129–34.

(1996b). Serotonin-related, anxiety/aggression-driven, stressor-precipitated depression. A psychobiological hypothesis. *Eur. Psychiatry*, **11**, 57–67.

(1996c). Faulty cortisol/serotonin interplay. Psychopathological and biological characterisation of a new hypothetical depression subtype (SeCA depression). *Psychiatry Res.*, **65**, 143–57.

(1996d). Serotonin-related, anxiety and/or aggression induced stress-precipitated depressions. A psycho-biological hypothesis. In *Advances in the Neurobiology of Anxiety Disorders*, ed. H. G. M. Westenberg, D. L. Murphy & J. A. den Boer. Chichester: John Wiley & Sons.

(1997a). Over the mainstream: diagnostic requirements for biological psychiatric research. *Psychiatry Res.*, **72**, 201–12.

(1997b). Demoralisation and melancholy. Concerning the biological interface between traumatic life experiences and depression. In *Depression: Neurobiological, Psychopathological and Therapeutic Advances*, ed. A. Honig & H. M. van Praag. Chichester: John Wiley & Sons.

(2001). Anxiety/aggression-driven depression. A paradigm of functionalization and verticalization of psychiatric diagnosis. *Progr. Neuro-Psychopharm. Biol. Psychiatry*, **25**, 893–924.

Van Praag, H. M. & De Haan, S. (1980a). Depression vulnerability and 5-hydroxytryptophan prophylaxis. *Psychiatry Res.*, **3**, 75–83.

(1980b). Central serotonin deficiency. A factor which increases depression vulnerability? *Acta Psychiatr. Scand.*, **61**, 89–95.

Van Praag, H. M., Plutchik, R. & Conte, H. (1986). The serotonin-hypothesis of (auto)aggression. Critical appraisal of the evidence. *Ann. N.Y. Acad. Sci.*, **487**, 150–67.

Van Praag, H. M., Kahn, R., Asnis, G. M. *et al.* (1987). Denosologization of biological psychiatry or the specificity of 5-HT disturbances in psychiatric disorders. *J. Affect. Disord.*, **13**, 1–8.

Van Praag, H. M., Asnis, G. M., Kahn, R. S. *et al.* (1990). Monoamines and abormal behavior. A multi-aminergic perspective. *Br. J. Psychiatry*, **157**, 723–34.

Weissman, M. M., Klerman, G. L., Markowitz, J. S. & Onelette, R. (1989). Suicidal ideation and suicide attempts in panic disorder and attacks. *New Engl. J. Med.*, **321**, 1209–14.

Wetzler, S., Kahn, R. S., Cahn, W., Van Praag, H. M. & Asnis, G. M. (1990). Psychological test characteristics of depressed and panic patients. *Psychiatry Res.*, **31**, 179–92.

Wood, M. D., Reavill, C., Trail, B. *et al.* (2001). SB-243213; a selective 5-HT2C receptor inverse agonist with improved anxiolytic profile: lack of tolerance and withdrawal anxiety. *Neuropsychopharmacology*, **41**, 186–99.

Yamada, J. & Sugimoto, Y. (2001). Effects of 5-HT$_2$ receptor antagonists on the anti-immobility effects of imipramine in the forced swimming test with mice. *Eur. J. Pharmacol.*, **427**, 221–5.

Yatham, L. N., Liddle, P. F., Shiah, I.-S. *et al.* (2000). Brain serotonin$_2$ receptors in major depression. *Arch. Gen. Psychiatry.*, **57**, 850–8.

Zinbarg, R. E., Barlow, D. H., Liebowitz, M. *et al.* (1994). The DSM–IV field trial for mixed anxiety-depression. *Am. J. Psychiatry*, **151**, 1153–62.

Epilogue

Stress-induced depression

Can stress cause depression? This was the key question posed in this discourse. An affirmative answer, it was stated, cannot rest on clinical and epidemiological grounds alone but requires data indicating that stress may inflict neuronal disturbances similar to those that have been observed in (subtypes of) depression and presumably play a role in their pathophysiology. The answer to that key question is cautiously and tentatively confirmatory. The argument is as follows.

MA ergic disturbances may occur in depression (Chapter 7). They seem not to be linked to a particular diagnostic category or to a particular syndrome, but rather to some syndromal components. Lowering of 5-HT metabolism and downregulation of the 5-HT$_{1A}$ receptor system seem to be associated with disruption of regulation of anxiety and aggression. Anxiety may be further enhanced by hyperfunction of the 5-HT$_2$ receptor system, either directly or indirectly as a consequence of downregulation of the 5-HT$_{1A}$ receptor system. The NA-system can be likewise out of balance. Both signs of hypo- and hyperfunction have been reported, possibly stage-related: hyperfunction linked to anxiety and hyperarousal in the early phases, and NA ergic deficits developing later on accompanied, on a behavioural level, by fatigue and inertia.

DA metabolism has been found to be lowered in some depressed patients. Motor retardation and anhedonia are the likely behavioural correlates.

Many findings suggest the MA ergic disturbances to be causative, rather than being a consequence of depression. 5-HT depletion, for instance, induced by a tryptophan deficit, may induce depressive symptoms, particularly in individuals with a history of depression, while increasing 5-HT ergic activity generates antidepressant effects. Catecholamine (CA) agonists, too, possess antidepressant properties, while CA antagonists may generate depressive phenomena.

In a subgroup of *depression* the CRH/HPA axis is hyperactive and the balance between GRs and MRs disturbed (Chapter 8). Ample animal data indicate hyperactivity of extra-hypothalamic CRH tracts to be associated with anxiety-like and depression-like behaviour. Those behaviours are potentiated by excess cortisol release. Via hippocampal damage hypercortisolaemia is probably also involved in the pathophysiology of memory defects as they might occur in depression. Sustained overdrive of CRH systems and of the HPA axis in humans is accompanied by behavioural disturbances comparable with those found in test animals. Since preliminary data indicate that various compounds antagonizing the effects of CRH and cortisol behave as antidepressants, overproduction of these stress hormones probably represents a depressogenic condition.

All in all, the evidence that both the MA and the stress hormones CRH and cortisol may be implicated in the pathophysiology of depression is quite strong. Both systems, moreover, are intertwined. Sustained increase of cortisol release, for instance, leads to 5-HT_{1A} receptor downregulation and initially to stimulation and later to attenuation of 5-HT, NA and DA turnover.

Stress leads to CRH overdrive, hyperactivity of the HPA axis and imbalance of the GR/MR systems (Chapter 8). CRH is activated both extra-hypothalamically and within the hypothalamus, the latter leading to activiation of the HPA axis and ultimately to increased release of cortisol. As has been mentioned above, sustained CRH/cortisol overdrive affects MA functioning and both will produce anxiogenic and depressogenic effects.

Thus the biological effects of longlasting stress mirror quite closely those ascertained in (certain types of) depression. Behaviourally, excess CRH and cortisol generate phenomena familiar from depression and the same is true for the resulting MA ergic changes.

Taken together these data constitute strong evidence that stress indeed may cause depression.

Vulnerabilities

Emotionally, cognitively and behaviourally stress is a heterogeneous construct. Hence an obvious question is whether all forms of stress possess equal depressogenic power. The question permits no answer; since in most clinical studies stress is dealt with as a more or less homogeneous construct. Its phenomenological heterogeneity is not reckoned with. Stress research in psychiatry urgently needs diagnostic upgrading of the stress concept.

Reversing the question, one may ask whether everybody is equally susceptible for the depressogenic effects of stress. Obviously not. Some withstand stress without pathological consequences, others succumb. Who, from a biological point of view, might be particularly vulnerable? First of all, and theoretically speaking, those with a marginally functioning 5-HT_{1A} receptor system. Under normal conditions it functions just within normal limits; under taxing circumstances, when cortisol levels tend to be chronically elevated it will be further downregulated and fail. Consequently anxiety ensues or is intensified and signs of disturbed aggression regulation – such as irritability, spite and anger outbursts without (much) reason – will become manifest. Anxiety and/or increased aggression (the latter manifesting itself in overt or suppressed anger) are key features of all stress syndromes. If in 5-HT$_{1A}$ receptor compromised individuals the stress level rises, CRH and cortisol release will increase, leading to further downregulation of the 5-HT$_{1A}$ receptor system and disruption of the CA system. Thus a vicious circle is established with depression as the possible ultimate outcome.

This supposition is not without foundation. The group of patients suffering from major depression does indeed encompass patients in whom 5-HT metabolism is low and pre- and postsynaptic 5-HT$_{1A}$ receptor density is decreased, both during depression and in remission (Chapter 7).

A second group of patients that can be expected to be susceptible for stress-induced depression would be those in whom CRH production and/or the setpoint of the HPA axis are permanently increased. Slight mishaps, then, would give rise to a disproportionate increase in CRH drive and/or cortisol release. If taxing conditions endure, the 5-HT$_{1A}$ system will be downregulated and MA metabolism gradually decrease. Anxiety and aggression phenomena intensify, a full blown stress syndrome develops and eventually depression may ensue.

Also this supposition does not lack foundation. In nondepressed relatives of patients with major depression the results of the dexamethasone/CRH test – a sensitive indicator of HPA axis activity – are slightly abnormal and fall in between normal values and those recorded in major depression. Apparently the setpoint of the HPA axis is permanently above normal (Chapters 8 and 9).

Recognizability

Are individuals susceptible for stress-induced depression recognizable in terms of psychopathology? Some data seem to suggest this.

Recently a new subtype of depression has been hypothesized in which anxiety and signs of increased outward-directed aggression are the precursor and 'driving' symptoms (Chapter 9). Mood lowering is a later occurring phenomenon, if it occurs at all. Some episodes remains restricted to signs of anxiety and aggression dysregulation, in others mood disturbances also occur, and a full blown depression develops. In view of these findings this subtype of depression was named anxiety/aggression-driven depression. Character-neurotic traits were found to be common in this depression type, and so were 5-HT disturbances, relative to the rates found in other types of depression. The 5-HT disturbances are trait-related, causing, so the hypothesis reads, lability of anxiety and aggression regulation. Anxiety and (suppressed or manifest) anger are key elements of the group of stress-syndromes. Because of labile anxiety and aggression regulation in concert with neurotic personality traits sapping coping abilities, anxiety/aggression-driven depression qualifies as a stress-inducable depression par excellence.

The (still hypothetical) construct of anxiety/aggression-driven depression is the first stress-induced depression characterized in some detail both psychopathologically, psychologically and biologically. Of course no exclusivity is claimed. It is very well possible that other types of stress-induced (or inducable) depression may exist. Further research should clarify this matter.

Diagnostic strategies

The current way of diagnosing psychiatric disorders, in this case depression, is categorical in nature. A clinical construct is defined on several axes and all axial criteria have to be satisfied in order to qualify for a certain diagnosis. Moreover, refined syndromal differentiation has been shifted to the background. For a particular diagnosis x out of a series of y symptoms have to be present, no matter which ones. Each diagnostic construct, therefore, covers a variety of syndromes. Psychiatric research, however, demands diagnostic precision, foremost with regard to symptomatology. This is particularly true for biological research. It is unlikely that one will elucidate the biological underpinnings of vaguely defined, heterogeneous diagnostic constructs. Accordingly, the characterization of anxiety/aggression-driven depression was based on a different diagnostic approach (Chapters 1 and 9). A four-tier diagnostic procedure was followed: characterization of depression on a categorical, syndromal, symptomatological and functional level. Functional analysis means attempts to define and assess the psychic dysfunctions generating the phenomena the observer perceives and the patient experiences as psychopathological symptoms. This latter step is considered quintessential for refined diagnosing and should be further developed.

Applying this way of diagnosing, the following observations were made. Anxiety and aggression dysregulation are central to the development of anxiety/aggression-driven depression; 5-HTergic disturbances are linked to particular psychic dysfunctions underlying the depressive syndrome and, finally, certain neurotic liabilities of those patients interfere with coping abilities. Those features would have escaped attention or at least registration had the usual categorical way of diagnosing Axis I and II disorders been applied.

Functional analysis of the prevailing syndrome(s) will provide the diagnostician with a detailed 'map' of those functions of the 'psychic apparatus' that operate abnormally and those that function within normal limits. Psychic (dys-)functions, moreover, are much better measurable and quantifiable than entire syndromes or categorical entities. Applying and elaborating the functional approach, a psychiatric physiology will gradually develop, elevating psychiatric diagnosing on a true scientific footing.

For biological research, functional analysis of the psychiatric syndrome is essential. It is the most refined and reproducable way to define the phenomena of which one hopes to unravel the biological underpinnings. This will increase the chance of uncovering meaningful and valid data on the complex relationships between abnormal brain functions and abnormal behaviour.

The key questions raised at the end of the Introduction to this book, then, permit the following answers:

1 Stress may induce depression; the evidence in favour of this statement is quite strong and so far no contradictory findings have been reported.

2 Stress is no universal depressogenic condition; particular vulnerabilities increase the risk of stress-induced (or inducible) depression. One (for the time being still hypothetical) subtype of depression thought to be particularly stress-sensitive is anxiety/aggression-driven depression. Whether other vulnerable subtypes exist, awaits further studies.

3 Categorical diagnosing by itself is a crude method to define abnormal mental states; too crude a method for biological psychiatric research, including research into the effects of stress on brain functioning. The multi-tier approach, culminating in exploration and assessment of the psychic dysfunctions underlying manifest psychopathological phenomena, seems to be the optimal starting point to maximize the yield of human brain and behaviour research.

Name index

Subject index

CPSIA information can be obtained at www.ICGtesting.com
Printed in the USA
BVOW021434211012

303519BV00003B/1/P